SURGICAL TECHNIQUES IN OTOLARYNGOLOGY HEAD AND NECK SURGERY

Series Editor: **Robert T Sataloff** MD DMA FACS

FACIAL PLASTIC AND RECONSTRUCTIVE SURGERY

SURGICAL TECHNIQUES IN
OTOLARYNGOLOGY
HEAD AND NECK SURGERY

Series Editor: **Robert T Sataloff** MD DMA FACS

FACIAL PLASTIC AND RECONSTRUCTIVE SURGERY

Authors

Anthony P Sclafani MD FACS
The New York Eye and Ear Infirmary
Professor, Department of Otolaryngology
New York Medical College, Valhalla
Center for Facial Plastic Surgery
Chappaqua, New York, USA

Thomas C Spalla MD
Attending Surgeon, Department of Surgery
Cooper University Hospital
Assistant Professor
Cooper Medical School, Rowan University
Camden, New Jersey, USA
Adjunct Professor, Drexel University College of Medicine
Department of Otolaryngology—Head and Neck Surgery
Philadelphia, Pennsylvania, USA

JAYPEE

JAYPEE BROTHERS MEDICAL PUBLISHERS (P) LTD

New Delhi • London • Philadelphia • Panama

Jaypee Brothers Medical Publishers (P) Ltd

Headquarters

Jaypee Brothers Medical Publishers (P) Ltd
4838/24, Ansari Road, Daryaganj
New Delhi 110 002, India
Phone: +91-11-43574357
Fax: +91-11-43574314
Email: jaypee@jaypeebrothers.com

Overseas Offices

J.P. Medical Ltd
83, Victoria Street, London
SW1H 0HW (UK)
Phone: +44-2031708910
Fax: +02-03-0086180
Email: info@jpmedpub.com

Jaypee-Highlights.
Medical Publishers Inc
City of Knowledge, Bld. 237
Clayton, Panama City, Panama
Phone: +1 507-301-0496
Fax: +1 507-301-0499
Email: cservice@jphmedical.com

Jaypee Medical Inc.
The Bourse
111 South Independence Mall East
Suite 835, Philadelphia, PA 19106, USA
Phone: +1 267-519-9789
Email: jpmed.us@gmail.com

Jaypee Brothers
Medical Publishers (P) Ltd
17/1-B Babar Road, Block-B
Shaymali, Mohammadpur
Dhaka-1207, Bangladesh
Mobile: +08801912003485
Email: jaypeedhaka@gmail.com

Jaypee Brothers
Medical Publishers (P) Ltd
Shorakhute, Kathmandu
Nepal
Phone: +00977-9841528578
Email: jaypee.nepal@gmail.com

Website: www.jaypeebrothers.com
Website: www.jaypeedigital.com

Inquiries for bulk sales may be solicited at: jaypee@jaypeebrothers.com

Surgical Techniques in Otolaryngology–Head and Neck Surgery: Facial Plastic and Reconstructive Surgery

First Edition: **2014**

ISBN 978-93-5090-631-6

Printed at : Ajanta Offset & Packagings Ltd., New Delhi

Dedication

This book would not have been possible had it not been for decades of dedicated facial plastic and reconstructive surgeons with the forethought and vision to describe and share their technique. Surgeons who have particularly influenced and inspired me in this endeavor include J Regan Thomas, M Eugene Tardy, John Conley, Peter Adamson and Dean Toriumi, among others, and as they did, it is incumbent on each new generation to expand, refine and promote the care we provide to patients. On a personal level, I would not have been able to complete this work without the unfailing support, encouragement and constructive criticism of my dear Peggy, Anthony, James and Matthew; without their love and support, this book would not have been possible.

— Anthony P Sclafani

I could not have undertaken this endeavor without the guidance I have received over the years from countless individuals. My education has come not only from those who are more advanced in years or training, but it continues to come from contemporary colleagues, fellows, residents, medical students, nurses, and most importantly, patients. Specifically, I would like to thank: Werner Roennecke, Scott McLean, and E Gaylon McCollough for their roles in my facial plastic surgery education. On a personal note, I would like to thank Tracey Saunders and my parents, Tom and Francene Spalla, for all of their love, support, and understanding over the years.

— Thomas C Spalla

Contributors

Yuan Y Liu MD

Attending Surgeon
Assistant Director
Plastic Surgery Fellowship
Cooper University
Health Center
Camden, New Jersey, USA

Grigoriy Mashkevich MD

Assistant Professor
Department of Otolaryngology—
Head and Neck Surgery
Division of Facial Plastic and
Reconstructive Surgery
The New York Eye and Ear Infirmary
New York, New York, USA

Anthony P Sclafani MD FACS

The New York Eye and Ear Infirmary
Professor, Department of Otolaryngology
New York Medical College, Valhalla
Center for Facial Plastic Surgery
Chappaqua, New York, USA

Thomas C Spalla MD

Attending Surgeon, Department of Surgery
Cooper University Hospital
Assistant Professor
Cooper Medical School, Rowan University
Camden, New Jersey, USA
Adjunct Professor, Drexel University
College of Medicine, Department of
Otolaryngology Head and Neck Surgery
Philadelphia, Pennsylvania, USA

Foreword

Surgical Techniques in Otolaryngology—Head and Neck Surgery is a six-volume compendium. In addition to being an integral component of the compendium, each volume was written to stand alone, as well. The volumes in this work include Atlases of Otologic and Neurotological Surgery, Rhinologic and Sinus Surgery, Laryngeal Surgery, Facial Plastic and Reconstructive Surgery, Pediatric Otolaryngologic Surgery, and Head and Neck Surgery. The authors of each volume have included not only background information and step-by-step details of surgical technique, but also "pearls" gleaned through vast experience. Each volume contains extensive illustrations and intraoperative photographs that illustrate and simplify the techniques described.

Surgical Techniques in Otolaryngology—Head and Neck Surgery is intended to provide clinicians with thorough, accessible and clinically useful details of surgery for nearly all disorders cared for by otolaryngologists. The work also serves as a companion to Sataloff's six volume "Comprehensive Textbook of Otolaryngology—Head and Neck Surgery" that was written simultaneously with the compendium on surgical techniques. Hopefully, Surgical Techniques will prove useful for otolaryngologists by making it easier to provide (and teach) state-of-the-art otolaryngologic surgery.

Robert T Sataloff MD DMA FACS
Series Editor
Professor and Chairman
Department of Otolaryngology—Head and Neck Surgery
Senior Associate Dean for Clinical Academic Specialties
Drexel University College of Medicine
Philadelphia, Pennsylvania, USA

Preface

Modification of the human body and face has been practiced since prehistory. From adornment with tattoos and piercings by the Neolithic man, to the treatment of facial trauma described in the papyri of ancient Egypt and Vedic texts of India to medieval techniques of repair of facial deformities, man has sought to control and modify his appearance. While Tagliacozzi is considered the father of plastic surgery, the techniques he described rely on centuries of prior work.

Truly modern plastic surgery developed out of the necessity to repair the frankly horrific injuries encountered during the First World War. Sir Harold Delf Gillies, an otolaryngologist, vividly described the methods he used to help the trauma victims he treated, and along with Blair, Morestin and others ushered in the age of modern facial plastic surgery. While many of these techniques may seem antiquated by today's standards, the thoughtfulness and precision with which he performed them and the level of detail in which he described them provides us with a platform from which to seek better outcomes. Gillies also serves as an example as to our responsibility to help promote better patient care.

This Atlas is not intended to be comprehensive. It features the techniques favored by the authors; indeed, as every practicing facial plastic surgeon knows, each patient is unique, and all surgery must be carefully selected and tailored to the individual. It is impossible to cover every nuance and each modification of every procedure. What we have sought to provide is a broad reference for facial plastic surgical procedures which will assist the reader in his/her approach to facial plastic surgery. As importantly, this volume will provide the necessary foundation to understand and incorporate into practice the variations in physical findings and in technique described in the companion textbook for this Atlas. We hope this text is a useful resource for the reader in his/her journey through facial plastic and reconstructive surgery.

Anthony P Sclafani MD FACS
Thomas C Spalla MD

Acknowledgments

The authors would like to thank Joe Rusko, Marco Ulloa and the entire Jaypee Brothers Medical Publishers (P) Ltd, New Delhi, India production team for their assistance in assembling this Atlas. We would also like to thank Robert T Sataloff, MD DMA FACS for the opportunity to contribute to this series.

Contents

CHAPTER 1

Introduction to Aesthetic Facial Plastic Surgery

Thomas C Spalla

BACKGROUND

Aesthetic facial plastic surgery encompasses a host of procedures, interventions and surgeries which aim to improve or correct one's appearance. Inherent in this is that the issue to correct is purely one of aesthetics, meaning that the issue does not compromise function and is not significantly deforming to the point of causing true psychological damage. However, certain conditions, such as severely protruding ears, correctable through otoplasty, blur this line. Accordingly, a severely ptotic brow can cause the patient to appear fatigued, upset, or angry while causing a visual field defect. In the vast majority of aesthetic facial plastic surgery, the aim is to provide the patient a measurable improvement in his or her appearance. Each person comes with his or her own desires, as they have generally given considerable thought prior to the consultation. The field of facial plastic surgery allows the surgeon to have a considerable impact in helping the patients achieve their goals. Through thoughtful interaction, carefully planned and well-executed surgery, and close follow-up, the facial plastic surgeon can have a career with immense challenge and variety which will be remarkably rewarding.

CONSULTATION

The patient consultation is critical when it comes to any surgical procedure, but its emphasis cannot be overstated when discussing aesthetic surgery. The interaction between the patient and physician will determine whether or not the patient decides to pursue surgery with that surgeon or chose to find another. The majority of patients seeking aesthetic rejuvenation are women, and they are educated and savvy when it comes to beauty. Oftentimes, they have spent hours reading articles on the Internet, perusing magazines and books on the topics, and have asked their friend's/aesthetician's/hair stylist's opinions. This also implies that they have usually researched you, the surgeon, prior to coming into the office. Therefore, they are already empowered, not only with knowledge of what they desire to change and how they feel it should be changed, but they are already forming opinions about you, even before you have ever met. Your reputation truly does precede you.

The consultation is a two-way process by which the surgeon gains insight into the patient's goals, fears, understanding of the procedures, and motivation for undergoing surgery. The surgeon also must determine whether or not the patient is a good candidate for surgery. Not only are medical comorbidities taken into account, but psychological factors must also be considered. On the other side, the patient gains insight into: expectations, risks, alternatives, the surgeon (experience, personality), the facility, the staff, the recovery process and the aftercare.

The most important part of the consultation for the surgeon is to listen. This may seem logical, but it bears mentioning. Too often, we are preoccupied with what we perceive as "wrong" and the ways in which it can be "fixed". However, our role is to meet the patient's goals within reason. This can only be met once we step back and hear what she is telling us. Perhaps what she perceives as heavy eyes is really a ptotic brow, or a nose which is "too big" is really an appropriate nose overshadowing a weak chin. Thorough training in facial plastic surgery allows us to recognize and correct these issues, but the art is in communicating this to the patient during the consultation while setting realistic expectations.

Once the agreed upon changes are understood and the surgeon feels that the patient is an appropriate candidate, the proposed surgical/procedural interventions can then be discussed with the patient and his or her companions. At this point, as with surgery which is not aesthetic, informed consent can be obtained.

CONSENT

Obtaining consent prior to proceeding with any surgical procedure is mandatory, and aesthetic surgery cannot be treated differently. The quality and depth to which a patient is consented reflects directly on the surgeon and his or her abilities.

Aesthetic surgery is fairly unique in that the patient has generally done some research (of varying quality and resources), and simply by coming in for the consultation, many of them have already made up their mind to undergo a surgery or procedure. The surgeon must practice some degree of restraint and not rush to sign up every patient who walks in the door. Take a few moments before obtaining consent to gain insight into his or her understanding of the procedure and its risks. The Internet is rife with discussions of plastic surgery nightmares, and while these should not be common, it is the surgeon's duty to put the patient's understanding and fears into perspective and create realistic risks and expectations of the proposed procedures.

Consent must be informed; merely obtaining a signature does not qualify. Obtaining consent is a process by which the surgeon and patient (or patient's surrogate) discuss the procedure(s), the rationale for choosing the intervention(s), the risks, the benefits, the expectations, and the alternatives to the procedure. It is the surgeon's duty to answer all questions posed regarding the intervention in language that is clearly understood by the involved party. After any clarifications are made, the patient (or surrogate) should be able to relay this information back to the surgeon to demonstrate understanding of the procedure(s). It is not possible, nor expected, that the surgeon convey every possible risk involved with the surgery. An attempt by the surgeon to list and attempt to explain every little thing that could go wrong during and after surgery will overburden the patient (or surrogate) with information, and the overall, and most important, messages will be lost. Additionally, having the patient sign a form that attempts to list every possible complication does not protect the surgeon legally and should be avoided, and this most certainly does not serve as "informed" consent.

The surgeon must make himself or herself and the staff available for follow-up questions or concerns the patient may have prior to surgery. Creating a policy of open and honest dialog with the patient will foster a long and fruitful doctor-patient relationship.

BEFORE AND AFTERCARE

The care provided to patients prior to, and after, facial plastic surgery is just as important, if not more so, than the surgeon's skill in the operating room. Undergoing any surgery can be particularly trying for patients and their caregivers, and since the postoperative care is so crucial with facial plastic surgery, the instructions must be clearly stated.

Prior to the procedure, part of the patient selection and consent process should be to review the required postoperative care. If your patient is unable or unwilling to follow the directions, then they are not likely to be a good candidate for the proposed procedure(s). Once the patient is scheduled for surgery, providing him or her with clearly written instructions helps to relieve the patient's anxiety in trying to remember everything that was discussed during the consultation. Each encounter the physician and physician's staff has with the patient affords the opportunity for continued education, discussion, and reassurance.

Once the patient is out of the early postoperative healing phase and questions arise, the surgeon may consider allowing the patients to e-mail photographs of any areas of concern. While photographs cannot substitute for a face-to-face examination, it can allow for a rapid assessment of the patient's concern and may allow the patient to avoid taking time out of his or her schedule if the issue does not require immediate assessment. Patient privacy statutes must be upheld with electronic communication, just as in every other means of patient contact. No matter what the medium through which the patient's concerns are addressed, open communication with the patient will allow for the best possible outcomes and satisfaction throughout all aspects of surgery.

FOLLOW-UP

In aesthetic facial plastic surgery, ensuring long-term follow-up with patients is essential for several reasons. The results from facial plastic surgery change with time, whether it is through the healing nature of the initial surgery or by aging, both intrinsic as well as extrinsic factors. Through the observation and photographic documentation of these changes, the facial plastic surgeon becomes a lifelong student and hones his or her craft throughout the years. Additionally, by maintaining these connections with patients, the surgeon is not seen as simply a technician, or simply as a means as a quick fix. It allows the patient to create a strong, and hopefully permanent, doctor-patient relationship. This bond not only allows the patient to present himself or herself to the surgeon with additional areas of concern in the future, but this open dialog often creates additional referrals to the facial plastic surgeon via the patient's friends and family members.

CHAPTER

2

Aesthetic Facial Analysis

Thomas C Spalla

INTRODUCTION

Assessing beauty is an exceedingly complex process by which the observer makes a rapidly calculated decision on whether or not the perceived subject possess favorable aesthetic qualities. What defines these qualities is truly in the eye of the beholder. However, when dealing with aesthetic facial plastic surgery, there are some generally agreed upon standards, or ideals, which surgeons judge as desirable. While this chapter focuses on these standards, surgeons must carefully consider each individual as unique and separate from the last. Performing the same rhinoplasty steps on each patient demonstrates a lack of attention to the patient's morphology and may not be in accord with the patient's desires, such as to preserve ethnicity. During the consultation process, the facial plastic surgeon must carefully listen to the hopes and expectations of the patient and must also take the time to educate the patient about the generally accepted ideal proportions while creating realistic expectations.

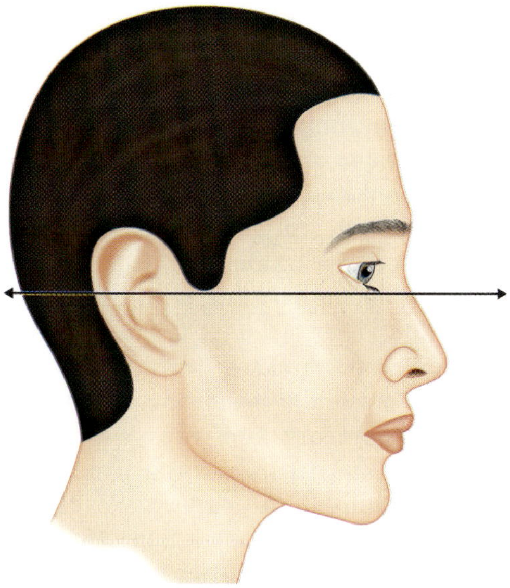

Fig. 2.1: The Frankfort horizontal

THE FACIAL PROPORTIONS

Frankfort Horizontal

Prior to discussing facial proportions, it is important to discuss the Frankfort horizontal (aka auriculo-orbital plane), which was developed for anthropologic measurements and is the standard reference plane for aesthetic measurements.[1] This allows for meaningful discussion between facial plastic surgeons and affords the opportunity for accurate assessment of results between patients and various surgeons. The imaginary line (Fig. 2.1) is drawn from the superior aspect of the external auditory canal through the inferior orbital rim.

Horizontal Proportions

The width of the face can be divided into five equal segments as demonstrated in Figure 2.2 going from helical rim to helical rim.

By examining the image, one can see:

Segment width = Eye width = Intercanthal width = Nasal base

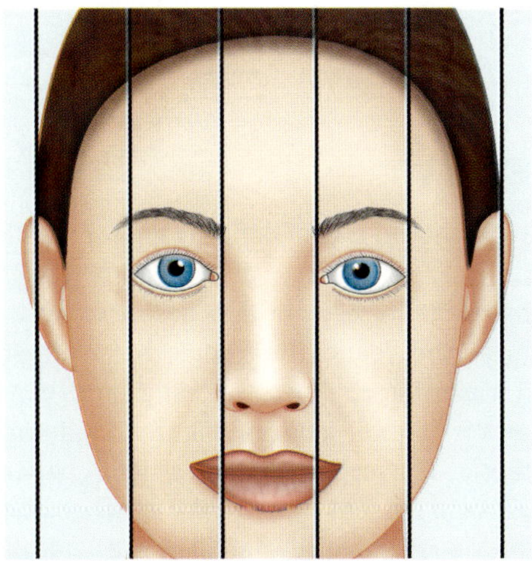

Fig. 2.2: The horizontal fifths of the face

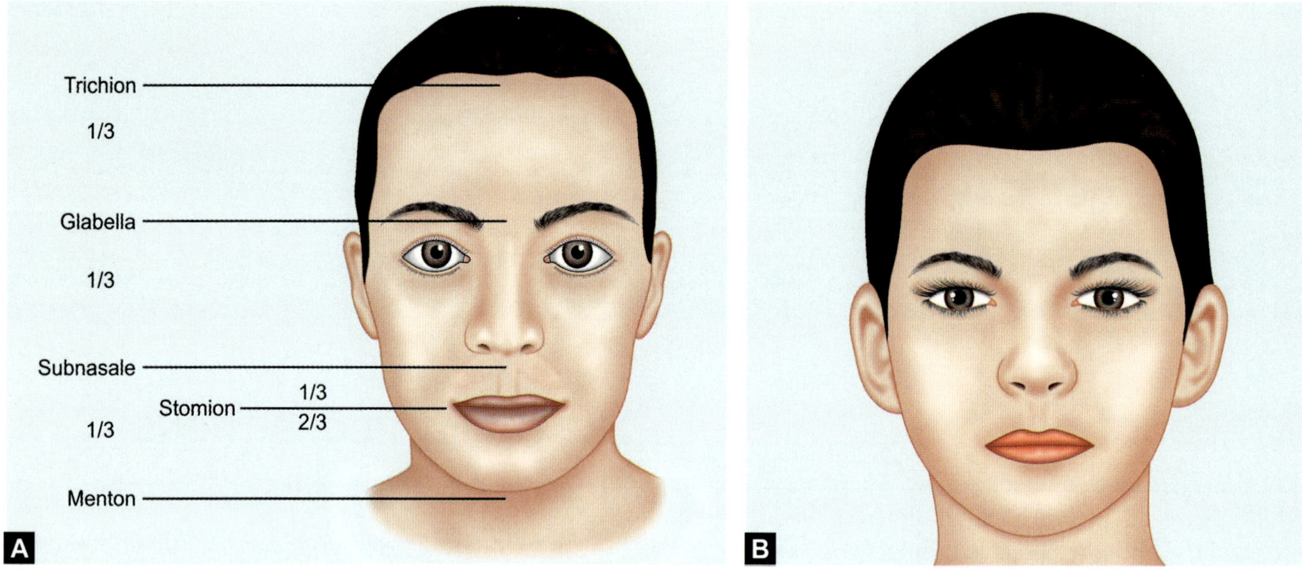

Figs 2.3A and B: (A) The vertical divisions of the face; (B) Subdividing the lower one-third of the face. From nasion to subnasale = 43% and from subnasale to menton = 57%

Vertical Proportions

The vertical dimensions of the face can be divided as demonstrated in Figure 2.3A. The distance from the trichion to the menton is the facial height. An alternative method for dividing the face is demonstrated in Figure 2.3B and the advantage of such a method is that the nasion (the deepest depression of the nose) is easier to define than the glabella and the forehead height is a relatively fixed structure.[2]

THE FOREHEAD

This region defines the upper one-third of the face. The hairline creates the defining point of the trichion and a gentle curvature towards the brow is desirable. The nasofrontal angle, as shown in Figure 2.4, should be between 115° and 135°.

THE BROW

The eyebrow should be the defining characteristics of the upper one-third of the face. Its appearance is extremely important in the female and the desirable aesthetic has evolved over the years. The female brow generally has a medial club-shape, tapers laterally, and arches with a peak at the lateral canthus. Figure 2.5 demonstrates this aesthetic. However, a recent article challenges the commonly held current ideal female brow aesthetics and notes that the height of the arch at the lateral canthus has slowly declined with time and the medial brow takeoff angle is more acute. The superior brow should be approximately 20–25 mm above the lateral canthus, and in older patients the apex of the arch can be more medial.[3]

The male brow is generally thicker and lies at the supraorbital rim. It is also less arched than the female brow. For this reason, a brow lift in a male must be given careful consideration to avoid feminizing the appearance.

THE NOSE

The nose is one of the defining characteristics of a person's face and alterations in its size and shape play a tremendous role in the way in which a person's face is perceived. A nose which is too large tends to mask features such as beautiful eyes or a nice smile. Similarly, a nose which is too small tends to make these facial features appear disproportionately large. The nasal plastic surgeon must have a firm grasp on nasal ideals, but he or she must also keep in mind the patient's wishes and desires while balancing a realistic aesthetic with the other facial proportions. Figures 2.6A to C illustrate some of the most common proportions.[1]

On anterior view, the nose should have a pleasing and gentle hourglass curvature, with a wider root sloping down and in to the narrower nasal bone region, and then gently widening to the nasal base. From a lateral perspective, the nasolabial angle (Fig. 2.6A) should be between 90–95° in a male and 95–105° in a female. Tip

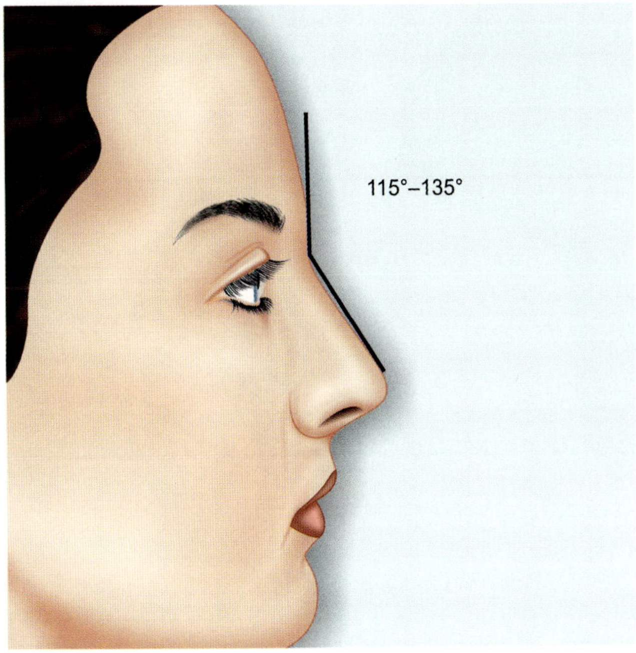

Fig. 2.4: The forehead and nasofrontal angle: The nasofrontal angle is created by a line from the nasion through the glabella and a second from the nasion along the nasal dorsum. This angle should be 115–135°

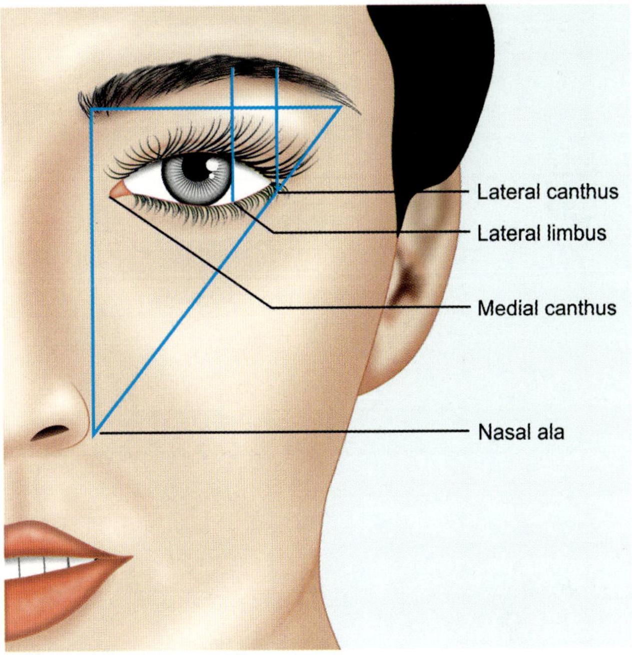

Fig. 2.5: The brow

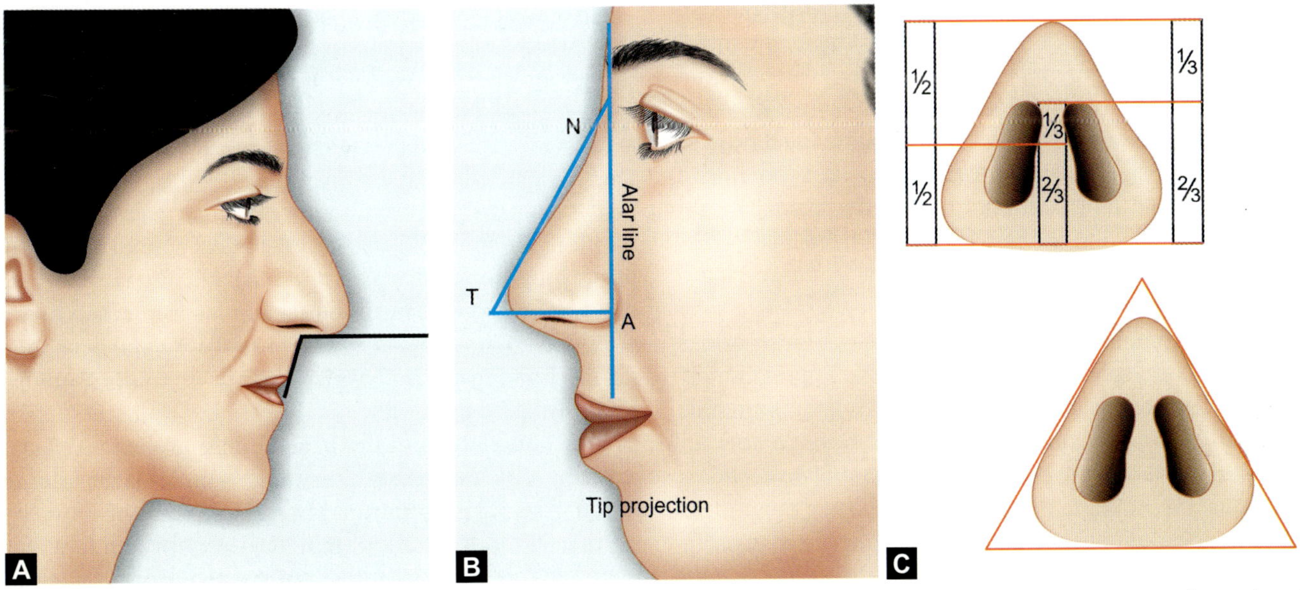

Figs 2.6A to C: (A) The nasolabial angle is created by an angle formed with a line from the subnasale through the most anterior portion of the columella and one from the subnasale through the vermillion border of the upper lip; (B) Goode method of determining nasal projection AT = 0.55 to 0.6 × NA; (C) Basal view and nasal proportions

projection is appreciated on the lateral profile. Several methods exist, but the Goode method (Fig. 2.6B) allows for a reproducible method for calculating the desired nasal projection.[1] A line is drawn from the nasion through the alar groove and a line perpendicular to this is taken through the tip. The ratio of the alar groove to tip length should equal 0.55:0.6 of the distance from the nasion to the alar groove.

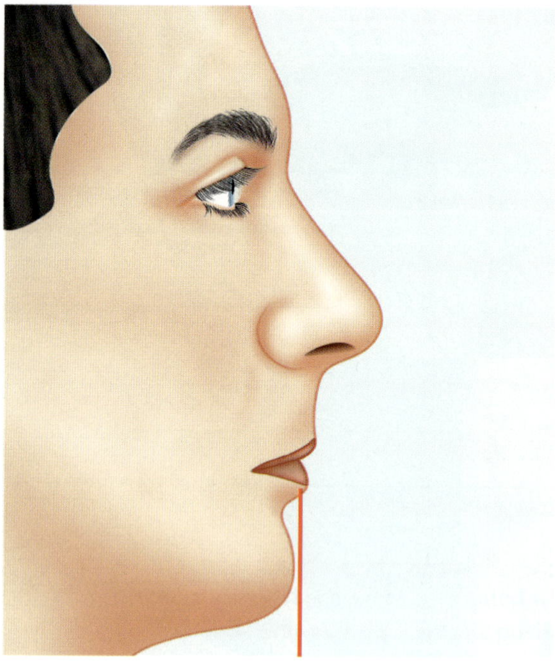

Fig. 2.7: Chin projection can be estimated by dropping a vertical line from the lower lip vermillion border

As illustrated in Figure 2.2, the nasal base width equals the intercanthal distance. However, in the non-Caucasian nose, the width may be up to 125% of the intercanthal distance. Nasal length is equal to 43% of the distance from the nasion to the menton as Figure 2.3B illustrates. The basal view of the nose (Fig. 2.6C) reveals the ideal nose to take the shape of an isosceles triangle. The tip to the nostril aperture should represent one third of the overall height of the nasal base and the nostrils should have a soft bean shape to them. Asymmetry in the nostrils is common and can be a difficult problem to correct.

Viewing the nose from the side (Fig. 2.6B) also brings attention to the columella which should lie approximately 2–3 mm below the level of the alae. Greater than this is referred to as a hanging columella and creates an undesirable view of the nose as seen on lateral projections. One must be careful to differentiate between a dependent or hanging columella and alar retraction which may occur with overaggressive cephalic trim of the lower lateral cartilages. The tip of the nose should have a gentle supra- and infra-tip break, or definitions between the tip and dorsum and the tip and columella, respectively.

THE CHIN

A strong chin is often associated with strength and masculinity and this feature is readily seen as a hyperbole in comic book characters. A retruded chin is often referred to as a "weak chin". A retruded chin from microgenia or micrognathia can cause the lower face to appear foreshortened while causing the nose to appear overprojected in the lateral view.

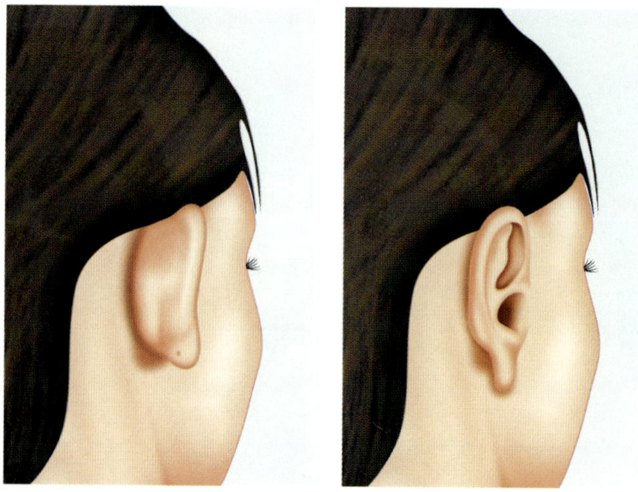

Fig. 2.8: The ear demonstrating the angle of protrusion as well as the distance from the mastoid skin

An easy way to estimate chin projection is to drop a vertical line from the lower lip vermillion border (Fig. 2.7). The male chin should lie at or beyond this by 2 mm, while the female chin should lie at or behind this by 2 mm.

THE EARS

The ears should not be overlooked in aesthetic facial analysis of the adult as adults are great candidates for otoplasty. In the child, the psychological consequences of protruding ears or of significant microtia often causes the child to be brought in to the facial plastic surgeon at an early age. An understanding of normal auricular accepted norms and proportions is necessary in understanding reconstructive methods.

The lateral edge of the helix should project 2–2.5 cm from the mastoid skin and the protrusion from the skull is 20–30° (Fig. 2.8). Alterations in cartilaginous development such as an underdevelopment of the antihelical fold can play a significant role in this projection. Width of the ear averages 32.5 mm in the female and 35.5 mm in the male, and length is 59 mm and 63.5 mm, respectively.[4,5]

CONCLUSION

This chapter provides an overview of some of the more common methods to determine ideal facial dimensions; numerous other methods exist. While beauty is subjective, the aesthetic facial plastic surgeon must understand the foundations of facial analysis to communicate results with other surgeons and patients, objectively assess his or her work, and use this foundation as a platform to build upon as definitions of physical perfection are sure to change.

REFERENCES

1. Powell N, Humphreys B. Proportions of the Aesthetic Face. New York: Thieme-Stratton; 1984.
2. Papel ID, Frodel JL, Holt GR, et al. Facial Plastic and Reconstructive Surgery, 3rd edition. New York: Thieme Medical Publishers, Inc.; 2009.
3. Griffin GR, Kim JC. Ideal female brow aesthetics. Clin Plast Surg. 2013;40(1):147-55.
4. Farkas LG. Anthropometry of normal and anomalous ears. Clin Plast Surg. 1978;5(3):401-12.
5. Weerda H. Embryology and structural anatomy of the external ear. Facial Plast Surg. 1985;2(2):85-91.

CHAPTER 3

Photography in Facial Plastic Surgery

Anthony P Sclafani

OVERVIEW

Quality, accurate and descriptive photographs of patients before and after treatment should always be taken. These serve as documentation and become part of the medical record, and can be used to assess the degree of change after treatment. They should also be used by the surgeon to critique his/her work in an effort to learn and improve results.

SPECIAL CONSIDERATIONS

Ideally, photographs should always be taken in the same lighting, pose, camera, focal distance and setting. However, even if not ideal, any opportunity for post-treatment photographs should be taken. Digital media have now supplanted film for photographs, and digital files are more durable, inexpensive and easier to store than film.

TECHNIQUES

A dedicated photography suite is helpful in maintaining consistency between photographs. A tripod-mounted single lens reflex (SLR) camera is positioned at head level. A camera mounted flash is supplemented by slave flashes placed at 45° angles to the seated patient, while an overhead flash eliminates back shadowing. While not always successful, effort should be made to photograph the patient in repose, without smiling. Standard photographs may be taken for each procedure, but should be supplemented as needed to demonstrate the specific areas of interest for each patient.

Face Lift/Midface Lift

- *Standard views*: Full face frontal, right and left lateral, right and left 45° oblique views. Views should include from the crown to the thyroid notch (Figs 3.1A to E).

Brow Lift

- *Standard views*: Full face frontal, right and left lateral, right and left 45° oblique views.
- *Supplemental views*: Close-up of forehead (hairline to lower lids) with eyes open, eyes closed, brows elevated and frowning (Figs 3.2A to I).

Blepharoplasty

- *Standard views*: Full face frontal, right and left lateral, right and left 45° oblique views.
- *Supplemental views*: Close-up of eyes (mid-forehead to mid-cheek) with eyes open in neutral gaze and in upgaze, and with eyes closed (Figs 3.3A to C).

Rhinoplasty

- *Standard views*: Full face frontal, right and left lateral, right and left 45° oblique, basal (worm's eye) views. Nasal tip should lie between brows in basal view (Figs 3.4A to F).

Botox

- *Standard views*: Full face frontal, right and left lateral, right and left 45° oblique views.
- *Supplemental views*: Close-up views of treatment area, both in repose and during animation (Figs 3.5A and B).

Dermabrasion/Chemical Peeling

- *Standard views*: Full face frontal, right and left lateral, right and left 45° oblique views.
- *Supplemental views*: Close-up views of specific scars, rhytids of interest.

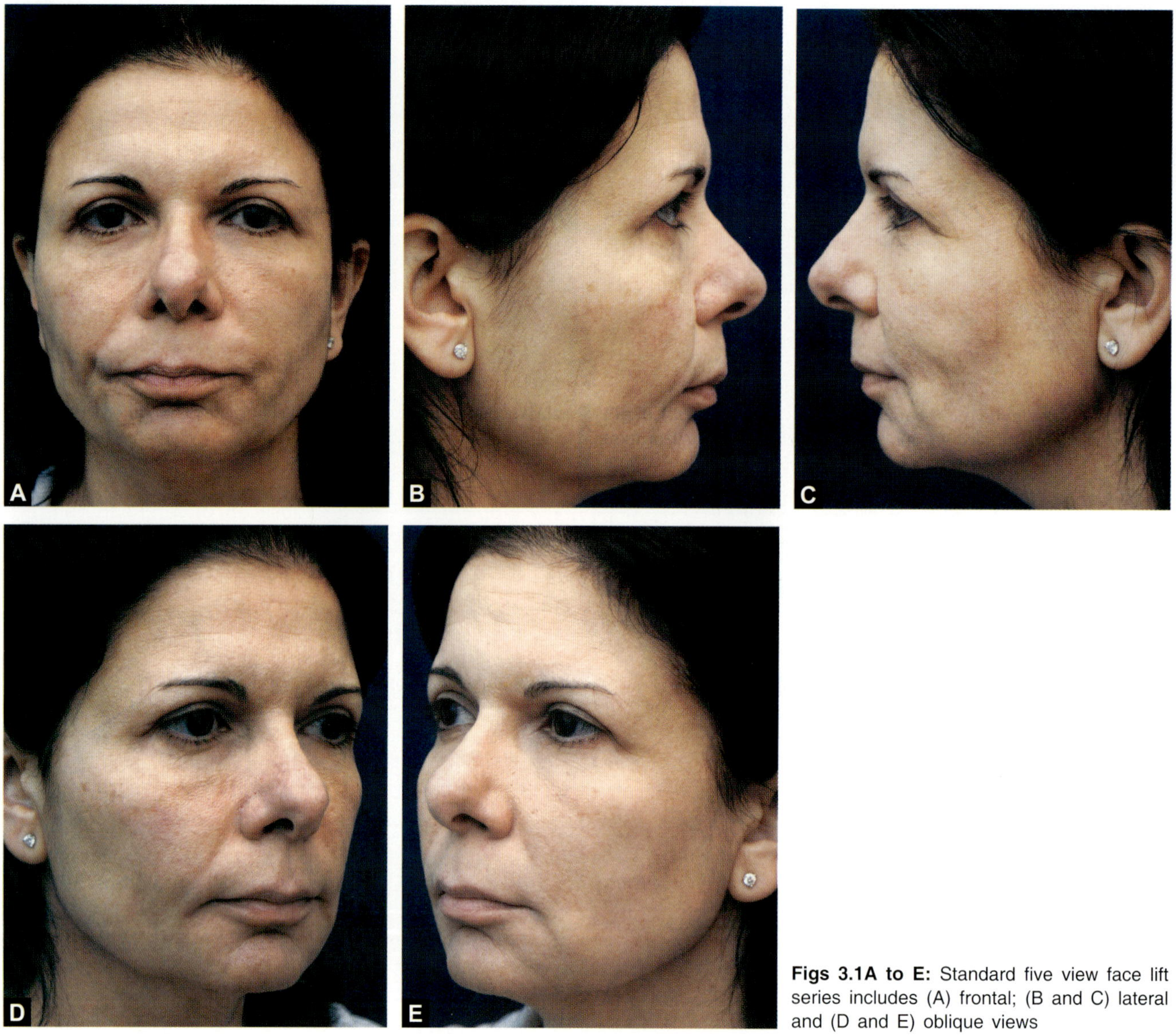

Figs 3.1A to E: Standard five view face lift series includes (A) frontal; (B and C) lateral and (D and E) oblique views

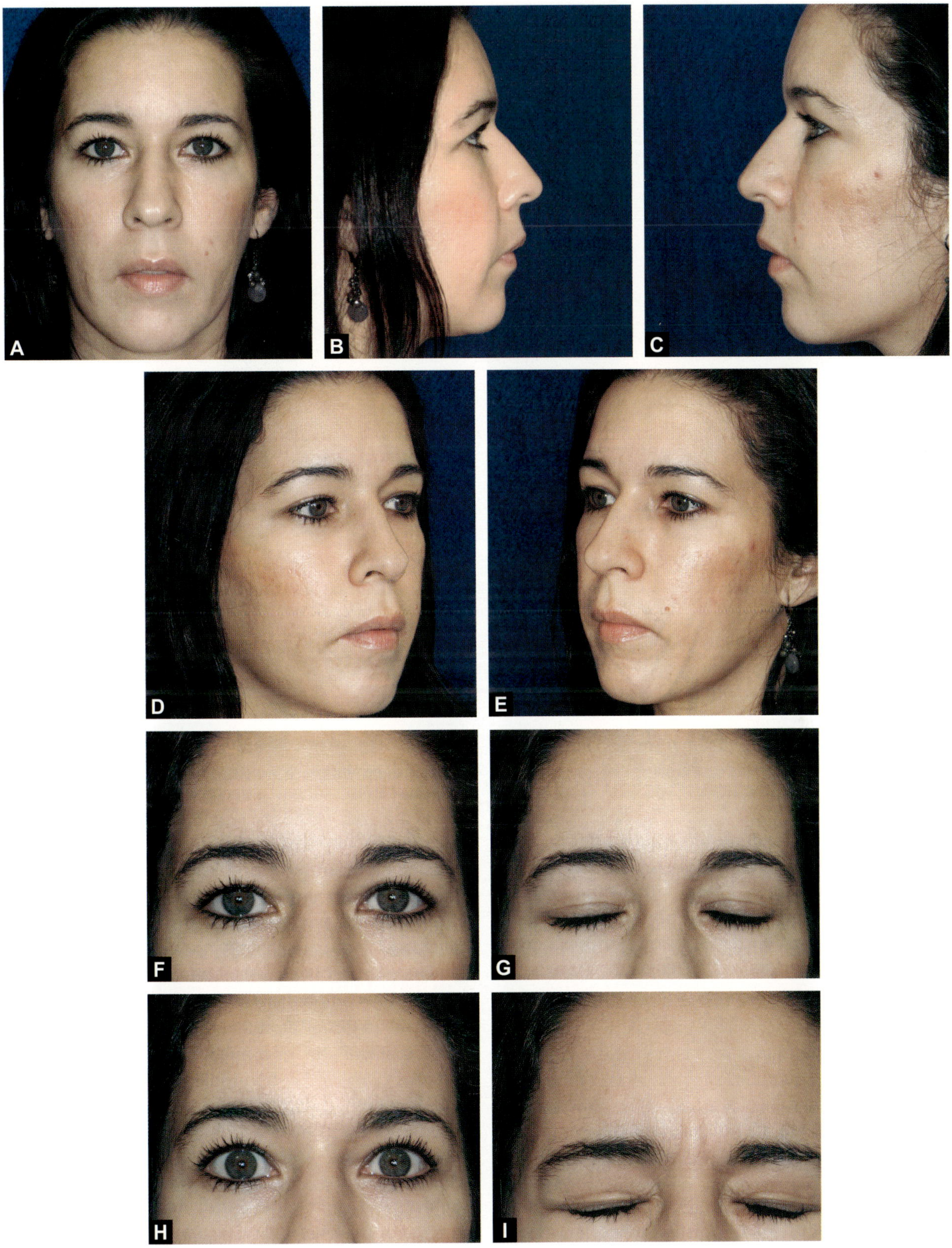

Figs 3.2A to I: Brow lift series of photographs includes (A to E) standard five view series, as well as (F) close-up of eyes open; (G) closed; (H) open with raised or (I) furrowed brows

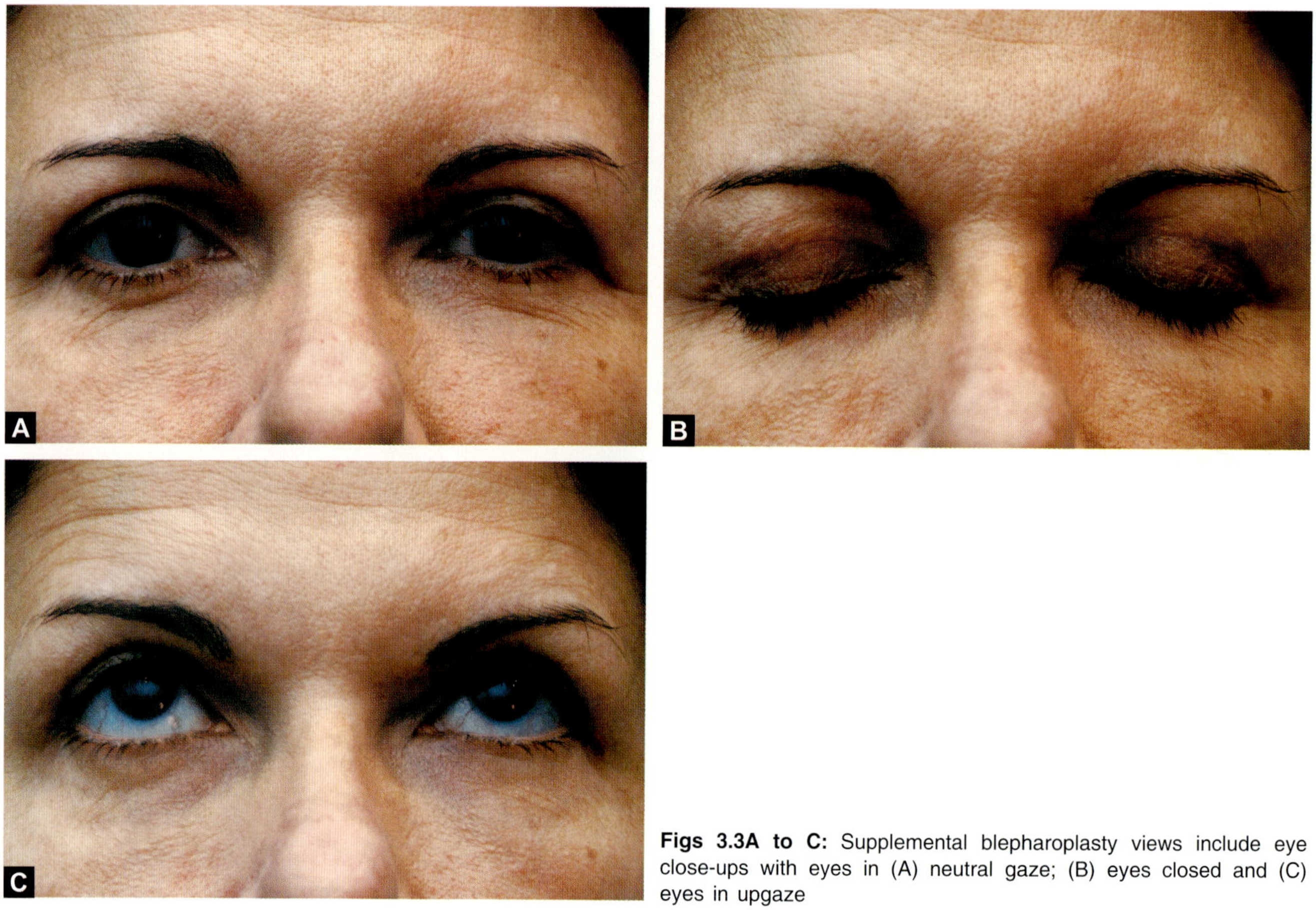

Figs 3.3A to C: Supplemental blepharoplasty views include eye close-ups with eyes in (A) neutral gaze; (B) eyes closed and (C) eyes in upgaze

Soft Tissue Fillers

- *Standard views*: Full face frontal, right and left lateral, right and left 45° oblique views.
- *Supplemental views*: Close-up frontal (± lateral and oblique) views of facial subunits being treated (Figs 3.6A to C).

Cheek Implants

- *Standard views*: Full face frontal, right and left lateral, right and left 45° oblique, basal (worm's eye) and bird's eye (Fig. 3.7).

Chin Implant

- *Standard views*: Full face frontal, right and left lateral, right and left 45° oblique views.

Auricular Surgery

- *Standard views*: Full face frontal, right and left lateral, right and left 45° oblique, posterior views. Hairband should be worn as needed to fully expose auricles.
- *Supplemental views*: Close-up lateral and oblique views of both ears (Figs 3.8A to E).

Facial Trauma

- *Standard views*: Full face frontal, right and left lateral, right and left 45° oblique, basal (worm's eye) and bird's eye views.

Hair Restoration

- *Standard views*: Full face frontal, right and left lateral, right and left 45° oblique, posterior views.

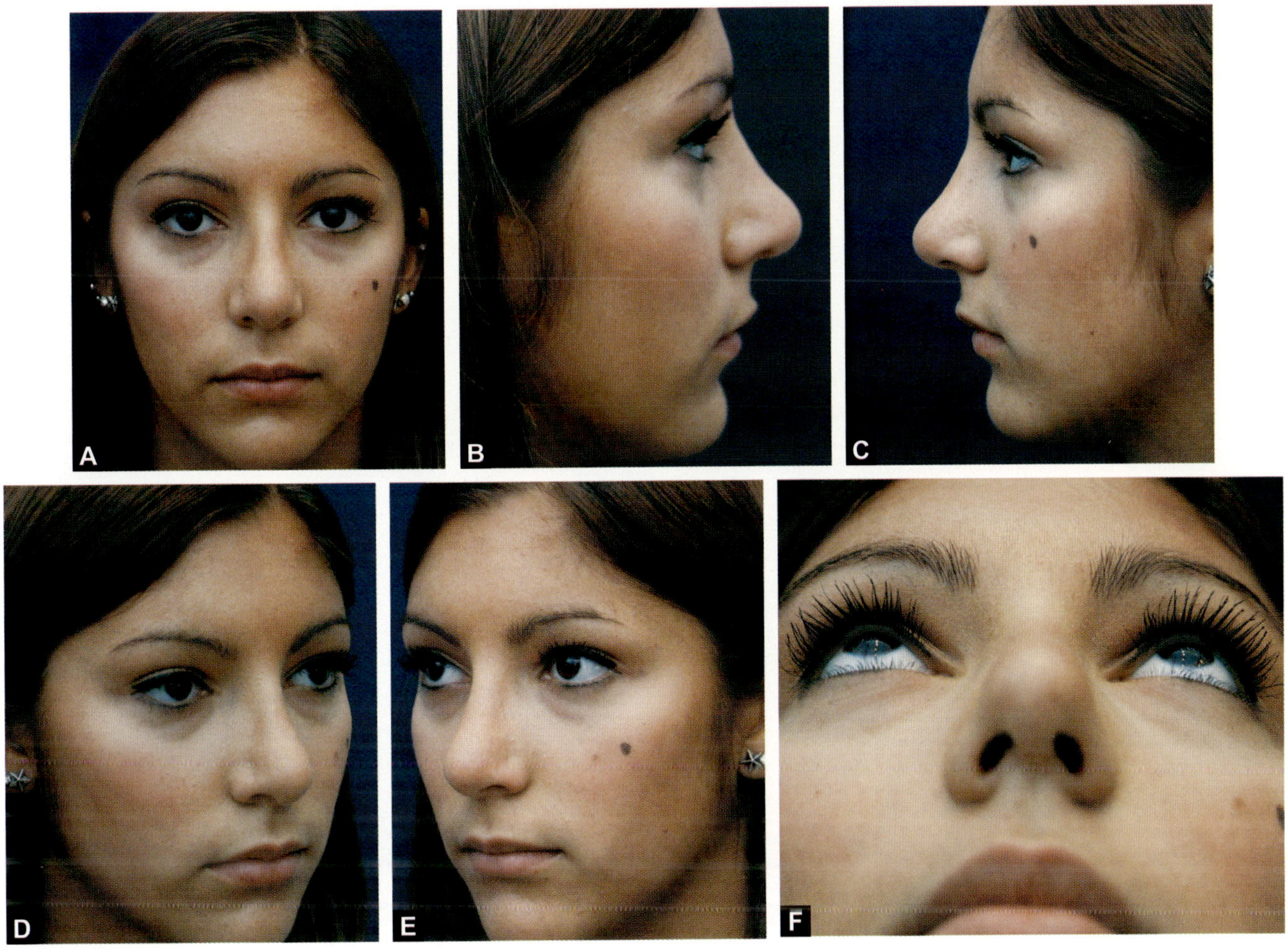

Figs 3.4A to F: Six view rhinoplasty series includes (A) frontal; (B and C) lateral; (D and E) oblique and (F) basal (worm's eye) views

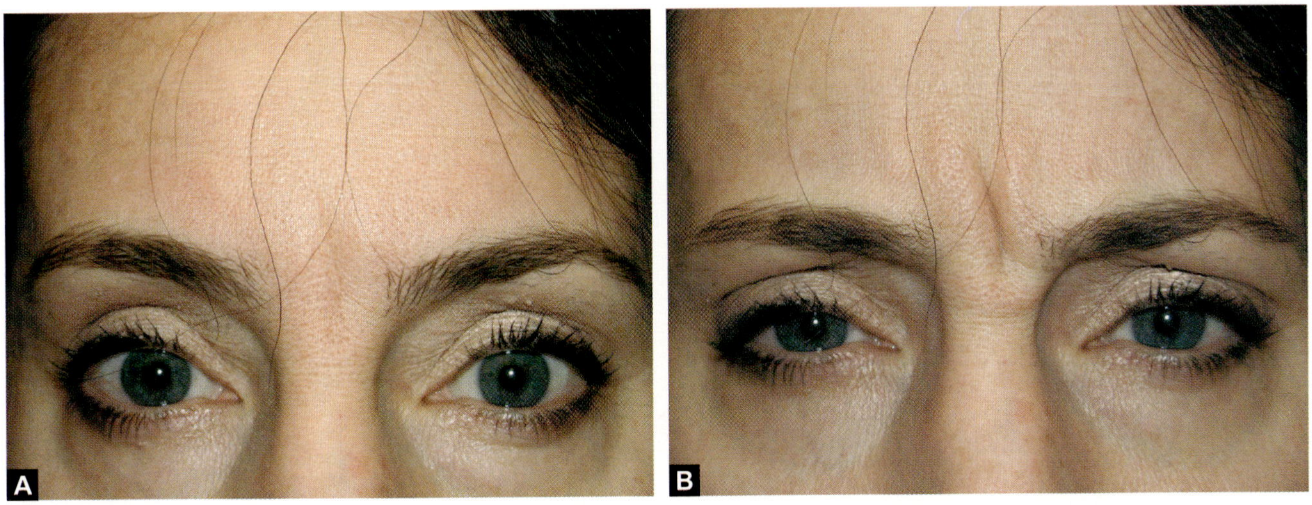

Figs 3.5A and B: Photographs to document the effect of botulinum toxin treatments should include close-up views of the treatment area in (A) repose and (B) animation

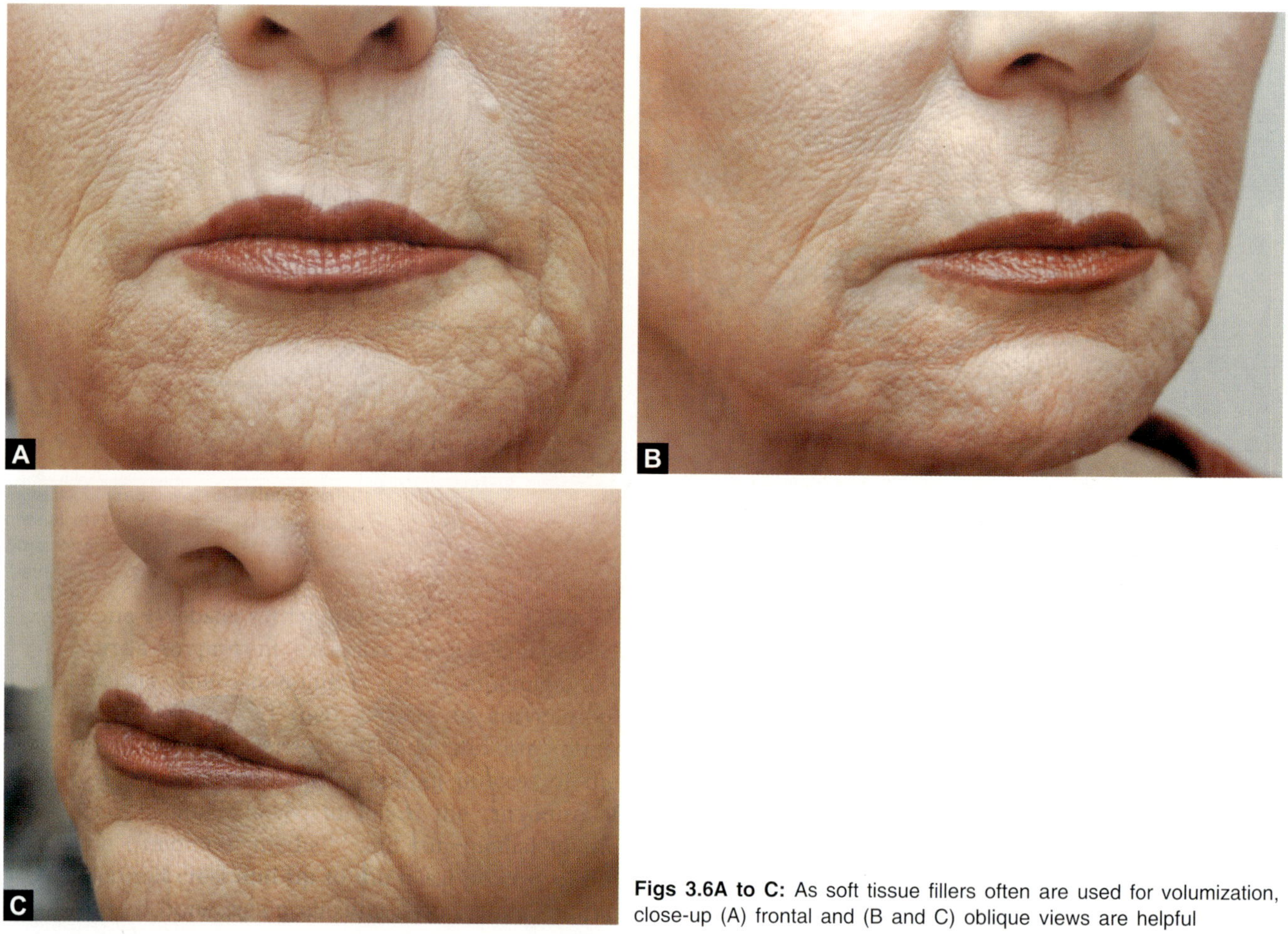

Figs 3.6A to C: As soft tissue fillers often are used for volumization, close-up (A) frontal and (B and C) oblique views are helpful

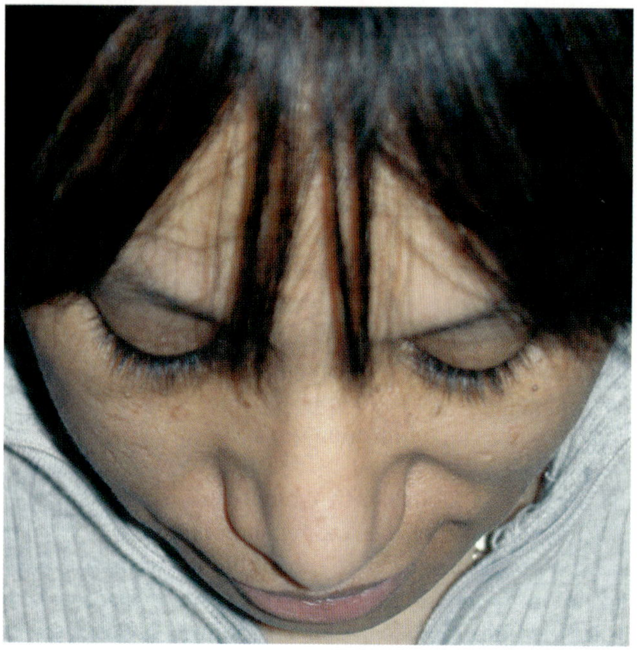

Fig. 3.7: Bird's eye view provides an excellent way to compare cheek contours

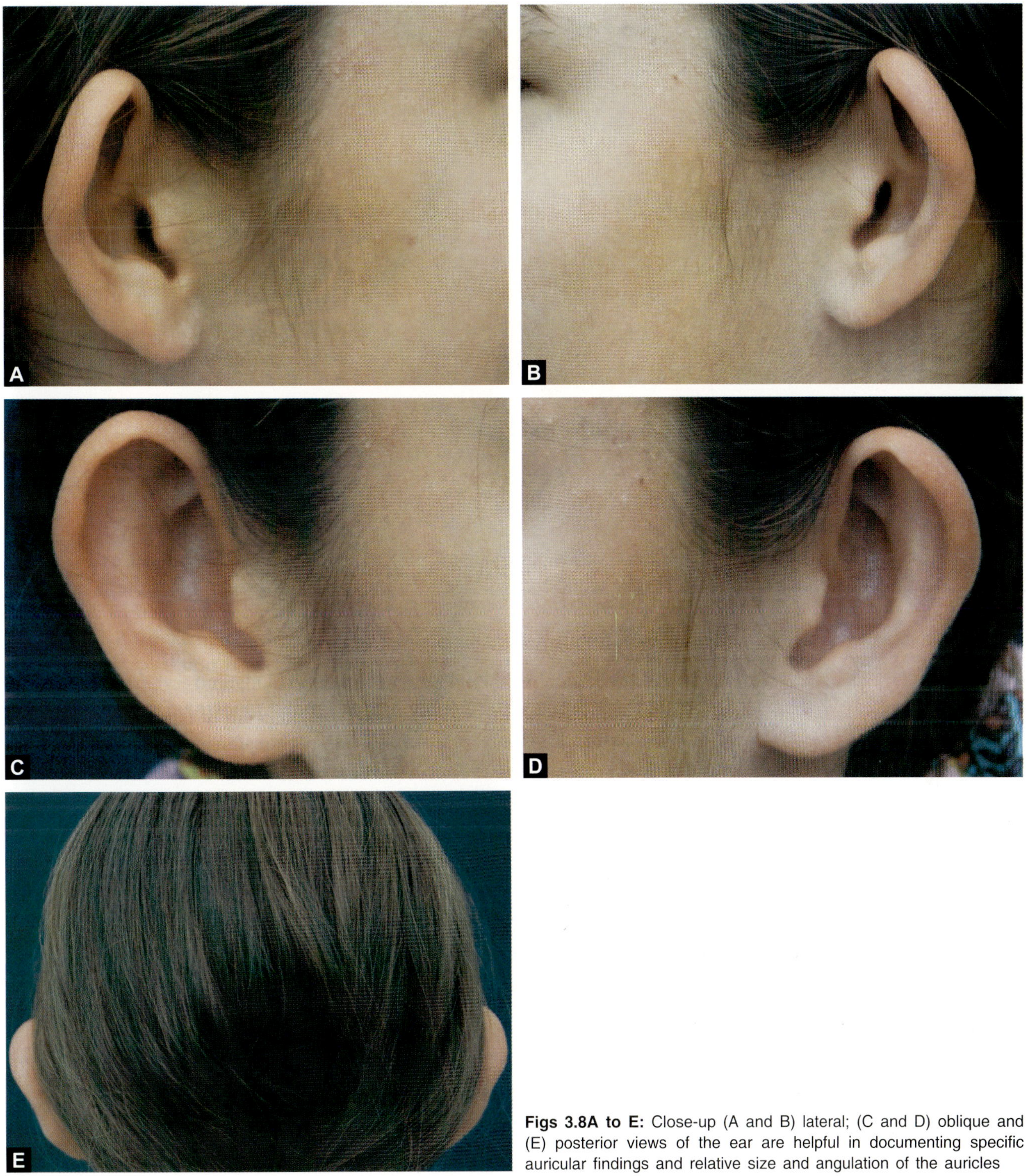

Figs 3.8A to E: Close-up (A and B) lateral; (C and D) oblique and (E) posterior views of the ear are helpful in documenting specific auricular findings and relative size and angulation of the auricles

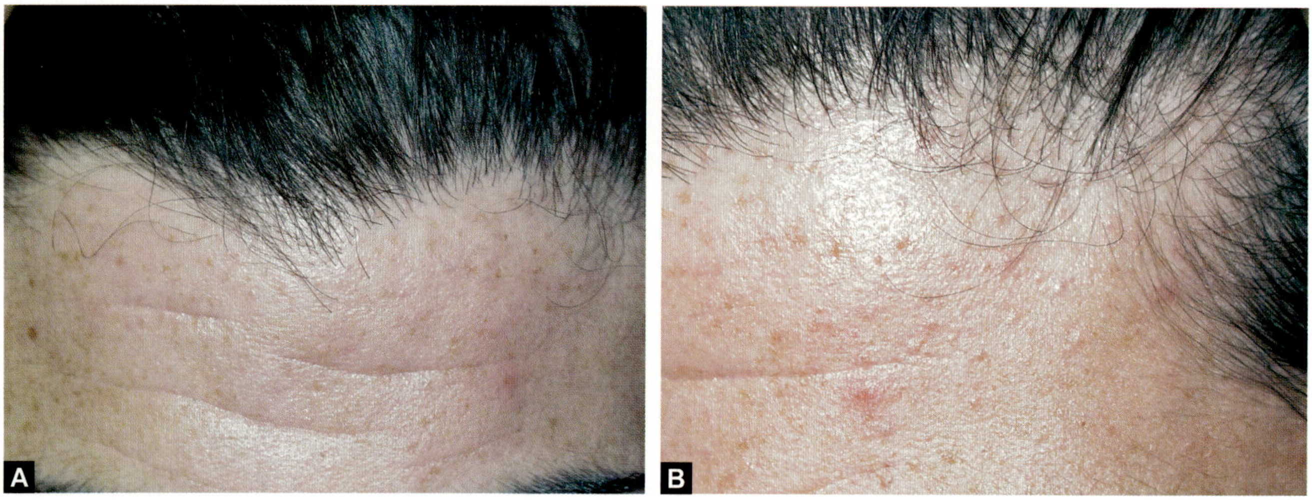

Figs 3.9A and B: Close-up views of the (A) frontal hairline and focal areas, such as (B) the temporal trough, reuseful in documenting the effects of treatment

- *Supplemental views*: Close-up views of the frontal hairline (Figs 3.9A and B) (include brows as reference point), crown (taken from the frontal position, with the patient leaning forward, head in hands and elbows on knees).

CHAPTER

4 Minimally Invasive Procedures in Facial Plastic Surgery

Anthony P Sclafani

OVERVIEW

Care of the skin has long been overlooked and relegated to over-the-counter cosmetics. However, a better understanding of skin physiology, the introduction of new topical medications and the rediscovery of the benefits of long-established topicals, along with patient emphasis on minimally invasive treatments has widened the options for skin care. The skin protects internal structures from environmental factors, is involved in internal heat regulation, serves as a water barrier and is the site of vitamin D production. Various proteins pigment the skin, most notably melanin, but hemoglobin also contributes to the color of skin.

The epidermis of the face is comprised of stratified squamous epithelial cells in four layers: (1) stratum corneum, (2) stratum granulosum, (3) stratum spinosum and (4) stratum basale (from outermost to deepest). Mitotic activity in the basal layer produces daughter cells which migrates upward, losing nuclei, accumulating keratin and ultimately sloughing off. Melanocytes are also present in the basal layer; these cells produce melanin-containing melanosomes and deposit this within the migrating epithelial cells. There are no blood vessels in the epidermis. The dermis is comprised of collagen, elastin and reticular fibers, as well as pain, mechanoreceptors, thermoreceptors, nerves, blood and lymphatic vessels, and adnexal structures such as hair follicles, sweat glands, apocrine glands and sebaceous glands. The dermis has a superficial papillary region (which has small papillae with which it interdigitates with the epidermal basal layer) and a deeper reticular portion. Epidermis lines the shafts of the adnexal units deep into the dermis.

Blood supply to the skin is provided by deep (running along the base of the dermis) and superficial (in the upper papillary dermis) dermal plexi. Loose areolar tissue and fat lies below the dermis, and fibrous septae from the dermis to the underlying muscles and bone compartmentalize the fat and stabilize the overlying skin.

SPECIAL CONSIDERATIONS

The external surface of the epidermis is covered by a thin acidic film formed by sebum and sweat known as the acid mantle. This serves to neutralize alkaline bacterial and viral products. The stratum corneum is composed of dead cells in which cytoplasm has been replaced by keratin.

Dermal thinning, flattening of the dermal papillae and disorganization of dermal collagen, accumulation of melanin and development of dyschromia can age the skin.

ALTERNATIVES TO PROCEDURE

Ablative skin resurfacing using erbium: yttrium aluminum-garnet (Er:YAG) laser (2,940 nm) or CO_2 (10,600 nm) can remove part or all of the epidermis and a portion of the dermis. In addition to thinning or ablating the epidermis (removing superficial rhytids and dyschromias), new collagen is produced in the dermis (tightening and smoothing the dermis). Other lasers with different wavelengths, such as the Q-switched ruby laser (694 nm) and the Q-switched neodymium: yttrium-aluminum-garnet (Nd:YAG) laser (1,064 nm) may also be used, and can more selectively target other chromophores, such as melanin and hemoglobin. Surgical lifting repositions skin but does not smooth it or change its quality.

TECHNIQUES

Topical Retinoids and Bleaching Agents

Topical retinoids are structurally related to vitamin A and can affect skin physiology. Topical retinol is modestly absorbed transdermally and is included in many over-the-counter cosmeceuticals. Tretinoin (Renova, Ortho Dermatologics, Valeant Pharmaceuticals International, Inc., Irvine, California, USA) has been shown to decrease sebaceous gland activity, thicken of dermal collagen and thin the epidermis. The cream should be used up to twice daily (if not limited by excessive drying of the skin), and results may take 8–10 weeks for gradual smoothing of fine lines and evening of complexion to appear. Patients are advised to use moisturizers, but at first, usage may need to be reduced in frequency and slowly increased as the skin "acclimates" to the tretinoin.

Dyspigmentation and dyschromias have traditionally been treated with hydroquinone (2–4%). This agent reversibly inhibits both deoxyribonucleic acid (DNA) and ribonucleic acid (RNA) synthesis, and is highly melanocyte specific in its cytotoxicity. Hydroquinone also competes with tyrosine for binding spots on tyrosinase and thus also competitively inhibits this enzyme necessary for the production of melanin. While generally quite safe, concerns have been raised as to the carcinogenic potential of hydroquinone, and ochronosis may develop, leading to a paradoxical blackened appearance with dermal thinning in treated areas.

Alternatively, 1–4% kojic acid, which also inhibits tyrosinase, may be used. Kojic acid has been shown to induce nondendritic melanocytes and lead to lower melanin content. It is, however, more irritating to the skin and is often combined with a corticosteroid.

Botulinum Toxin A

Clostridium botulinum was first isolated in the 1895, and botulinum toxin was isolated in the 1940s, after which its neurotoxic actions were delineated. There are seven subtypes of botulinum toxin, the most important of which is the botulinum toxin type A (BT×A). BT×A exists as a complex with hemagglutinins, which presumably protect it against the acid environment of the stomach, since these proteins dissociate at physiologic pH and leave the free toxin. The BT×A molecule has two chains, one which facilitates entry into the nerve and the active toxin. The toxin cleaves synaptosomal-associated protein 25 (SNAP-25), preventing fusion of presynaptic vesicles containing acetylcholine with the synaptic membrane. Over time, additional acetylcholine and vesicles are synthesized and additional nerve endings sprout and form new neuromuscular junctions. Currently, there are three preparations of BT×A approved for use in the US by the Food and Drug Administration (FDA): Botox Cosmetic (onabotulinumtoxin A, Allergan, Inc., Irvine, CA), Dysport (abobotulinumtoxin A, Medicis, Scottsdale, CA) and Xeomin (incobotulinumtoxin A, Merz Aesthetics, Inc. Franksville, WI). Since each commercial producer determines the "units" of each toxin with different methods, it is important to remember that units of these neurotoxins are not interchangeable.

Areas of Treatment

The three commercially available toxins are approved for treatment of glabellar rhytids, but off-label use has been described for treatment of forehead, lateral orbital, perinasal rhytids, contouring of the brows, fine radial lines of the lips, hyperkinetic activity of the mentalis muscle and treatment of platysmal bands, among other areas.

Technique of Botulinum Toxin Type A Treatment

All commercially available BT×A requires reconstitution prior to use with preservative free saline. The dilution volumes in the published literature range from 1–10 cc or higher, but most authors reconstitute BT×A with 2–5 cc. Smaller diluent volumes raise the concentration and hence the volume injected at any given point is smaller and less likely to spread to distant areas; however, higher concentrations produce a less "blended" effect.

The technique of BT×A injection depends on the anatomy of the area being treated. In general, the target muscles are thin and fairly superficial. Gentle palpation of the treatment area while the target muscle is actively contracted provides the injector with a more precise sense of muscle location, depth and strength. The required number of units is then deposited using a 30-gauge needle, avoiding widespread of toxin to prevent paralysis of nearby nontarget muscles. Figures 4.1 and 4.2 show common injection sites and dosages for specific effects.

Soft Tissue Fillers

Soft tissue fillers are materials that are injected into or just below the dermis which produce volume augmentation. When injected below a rhytid or skin fold, the skin above is smoothed, while if injected into an otherwise normal area, such as the lips or over the malar eminence, overt volume enhancement occurs. In general, the more superficially placed the filler, the more apparent the volume change. However, injections placed too superficially may lead to nodularity, skin discoloration and skin slough. Dermal fillers produce their effect through simple volume addition, stimulation of host tissue production, or both. Commercially available soft tissue fillers are generally approved for treatment of wrinkles and folds such as the nasolabial folds, but are commonly used in the face in an off-label fashion.

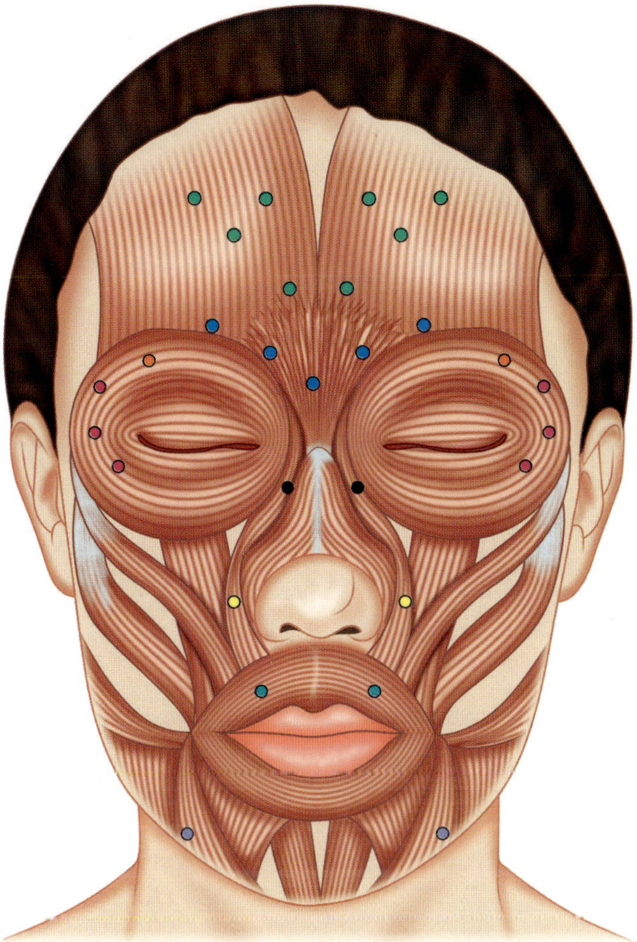

Fig. 4.1: Typical sites for BT×A injections. Green: Transverse forehead rhytids are generally treated with 20–30 units into the frontalis muscle, remaining at least 2 cm above the orbital rims to avoid brow ptosis; blue: oblique and transverse glabellar lines and furrows, as well as medial brow ptosis, are treated typically with 20–25 units into the corrugator and procerus muscles; orange: the lateral brow arch can be elevated 1–3 mm with 2–3 units injected into the lateral superior orbicularis oculi muscle just below the brow; red: crow's feet are effaced by injecting 7–15 units per side into the lateral orbicularis oculi muscle, remaining 1 cm lateral to the orbital rim; black: lateral nasal animation (bunny) lines are corrected with 1–3 units injected into the lateral nasalis muscle; yellow: an excessively "gummy" smile is corrected with 2–3 units per side injected into the levator labii superioris alaeque nasi muscle lateral to the lower pyriform aperture; aqua: fine, hyperkinetic radial lines of the upper lip can be treated with 1–2 units injected into the mid-paramedian lip; purple: down-turned mouth corners and folds (marionette folds) can be treated with 2–5 units per side injected along the lower mandibular border just lateral to the prejowl sulcus (units are given for botulinum toxin type A)

Injection Techniques

Soft tissue fillers should be injected using the smallest needle possible which allows passage of the material without clogging or altering the filler. The three basic techniques of injection are serial puncture, linear threading and fanning (Figs 4.3A to C). These techniques can be used together, and are chosen based upon the filler site being injected and plane to be filled. Serial puncture injections are best for placing filler into a more superficial layer like the mid-dermis, while linear threading works well when injecting deeper, looser planes like the subdermis, injecting as the needle is withdrawn to reduce the risk of vascular injection. Fanning injections are used when deeper, larger areas are injected and larger volumes are used so that fewer needle sticks are used and the filler is distributed more evenly.

For most soft tissue fillers, the correct plane of injection is essential for success. Mid-dermal injections are generally done with 30- or 32-gauge needles, with the needle inserted at a 30° angle to the skin; while the outline of the needle should be visible through the skin, if the gray of the steel is seen, the needle is too shallow and should be repositioned. Injections into the deep dermis or superficial subdermal plane are performed with a less acute angle and are generally done with larger bore needles (25–30 gauges).

Filler Materials

- *Hyaluronic acid derivatives*: Hyaluronic acid (HA) is a polysaccharide found in many parts of the body, but is especially found in the skin. HA injected intradermally is resorbed by the body within 48 hours, so HA-based fillers are chemically cross-linked to increased residence times. HA derivatives are hydrogels, sequestering water molecules within the quaternary structure of these polymers. Ultimately, HA derivatives are metabolized to CO_2 and water, while the risk of allergic reaction is quite low. HA derivatives vary in their macroparticle size, with larger sizes generally persisting for a longer period (9-12 months rather than 5-7 months) but requiring larger bore needles (27 rather than 30 gauge) and deeper (subdermal, rather than mid-dermal) placement. HA derivatives produce their effect predominantly through the volume they occupy, although there is some evidence that dermal placement leads to a thin capsule of collagen around the implant. Excessive or poorly placed HA can be enzymatically removed with hyaluronidase. HA derivatives are an excellent first option for most facial applications.
- *Calcium hydroxylapatite*: Calcium hydroxylapatite (CaHA) soft tissue filler is composed of CaHA beads suspended in a water, cellulose and glycerine carrier. After injection, the carrier molecules are resorbed, leaving behind the CaHA beads, which are

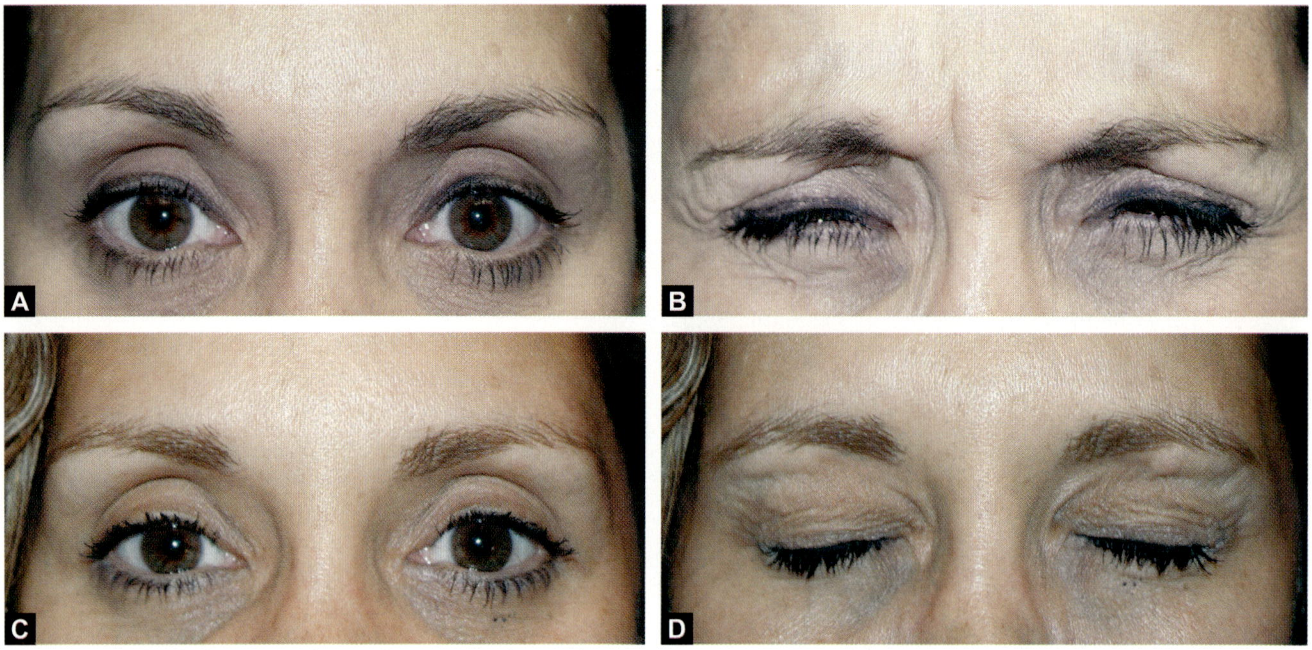

Figs 4.2A to D: Patient with mild medial brow ptosis and hyperkinetic lines of the glabella. (A) Repose, pretreatment; (B) Animation, pretreatment; (C) Repose, post-treatment; (D) Animation, post-treatment

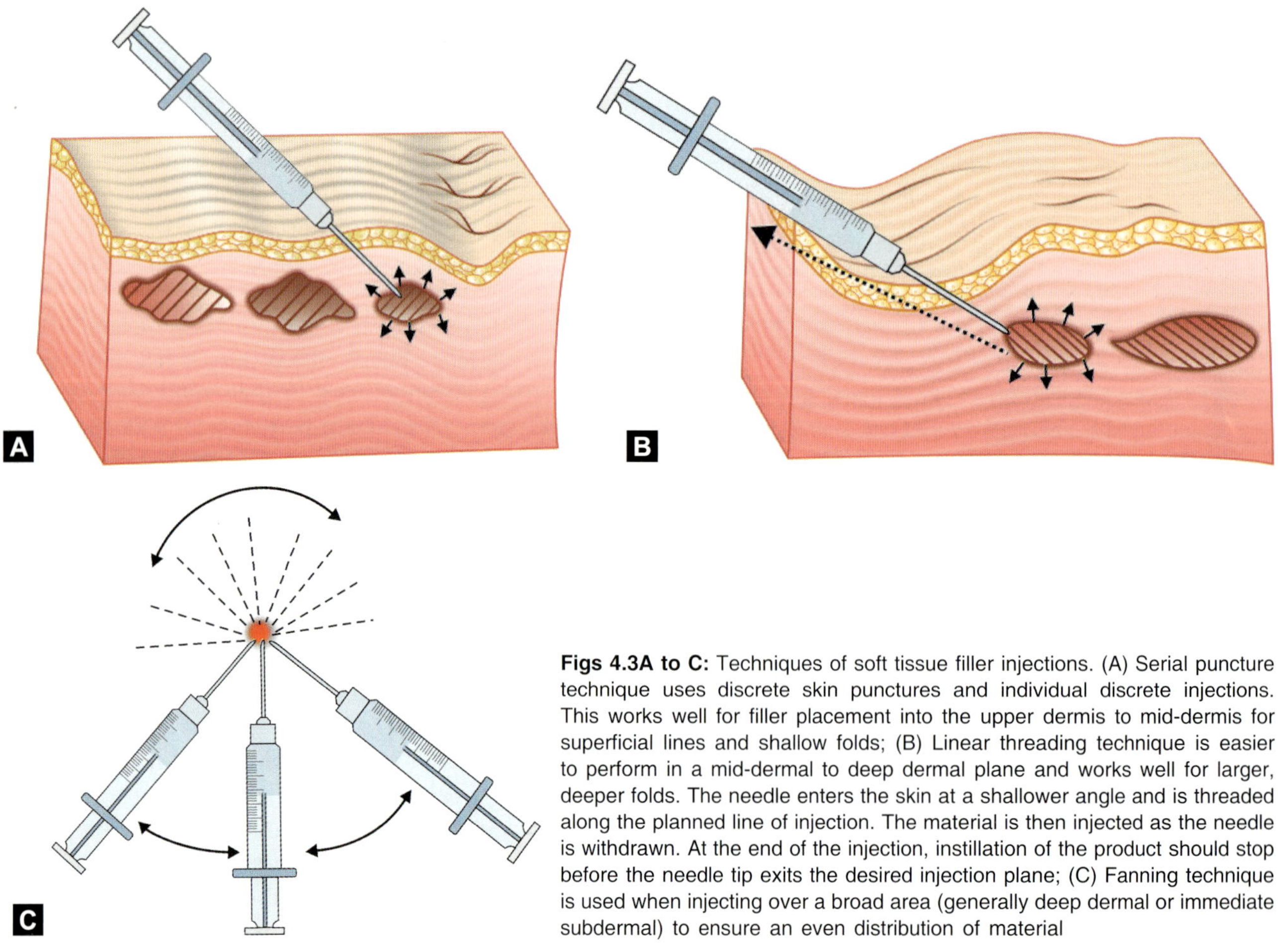

Figs 4.3A to C: Techniques of soft tissue filler injections. (A) Serial puncture technique uses discrete skin punctures and individual discrete injections. This works well for filler placement into the upper dermis to mid-dermis for superficial lines and shallow folds; (B) Linear threading technique is easier to perform in a mid-dermal to deep dermal plane and works well for larger, deeper folds. The needle enters the skin at a shallower angle and is threaded along the planned line of injection. The material is then injected as the needle is withdrawn. At the end of the injection, instillation of the product should stop before the needle tip exits the desired injection plane; (C) Fanning technique is used when injecting over a broad area (generally deep dermal or immediate subdermal) to ensure an even distribution of material

progressively surrounded by a fibrotic response. Since this collagenesis ultimately contributes to the overall volume, treated areas are generally not overcorrected, as the collagen replaces the carrier molecules in a nearly 1:1 ratio. Typical clinical efficacy of CaHA lasts for 12–15 months, although hydrolysis of the CaHA beads may take several years. Because of its dense nature, CaHA must be injected through a 25–27 gauge needle and must be placed deep to the dermis. In addition to the FDA-approved use for nasolabial folds, CaHA has been used for volume augmentation of the malar and mental areas, jawline and even the nasal dorsum. Injection in a superficial plane will produce a gritty and nodular appearance.

- *Poly-L-lactic acid*: Poly-L-lactic acid (PLLA) is sold as a dry powder of PLLA beads, which the physician reconstitutes with saline. These are then injected through a 25-gauge needle into the subdermis to a slight degree of overcorrection. The saline carrier is rapidly resorbed, and little to no effect of treatment is noted by the morning after treatment. Over the next several weeks, progressive fibrosis develops around the individual PLLA beads, producing a thickening of the dermis. Generally, several treatments spaced at least 4–6 weeks apart are required to produce a clinically significant result. Two years persistence of effect has been shown, and clinical effects may last longer. The PLLA beads slowly degrade to CO_2 and water. The most dramatic effects of PLLA use has been shown for large volume augmentation, including to treatment of human immunodeficiency virus (HIV)-associated antiretroviral therapy (HAART), as well as enhancement of mid and lower facial volume. To ensure even deposition in large areas, a grid pattern is injected and the treatment area is immediately massaged. It is essential that PLLA be rehydrated and mixed thoroughly prior to use, and large depot injections are discouraged to avoid subcutaneous nodule formation. Patients are also instructed to perform vigorous massage of the treated areas for 5 minutes five times a day for 5 days.
- *Polymethylmethacrylate*: Polymethylmethacrylate (PMMA) filler is a suspension of 20% PMMA beads in 80% (bovine) collagen gel. The partially denatured collagen is included to stimulate a controlled foreign body response. PMMA is injected into the subdermis through a 25-gauge needle, avoiding large depot injections and placement in the lips. Nodularity has been associated with PMMA, and has traditionally been treated with intralesional corticosteroid injections.

Dermabrasion

Dermabrasion involves the mechanical planning of the skin to a desired depth, removing the epidermis and a portion of the dermis. Epidermal cells lining the shafts of adnexal structures migrate to re-establish a complete epidermal layer over the treated area, while dermal collagen production aids in effacing rhytids.

Dermabrasion is powered by a mechanical driver and effected by a wire brush or diamond-coated fraise spinning at 1,200–1,500 rpm. Dermabrasion is contraindicated in patients with a history of cutis laxa, congenital ectodermal dysplasia and scleroderma, and the use of estrogens, oral contraceptives, or other photosensitizing medications should be discontinued prior to treatment. Active herpetic infection is a contraindication to dermabrasion. Patients with a history of herpetic infections should be pretreated with antiviral medications and continued on these until the skin is completely re-epithelialized.

Extent of Undermining/Dissection

Scars may be treated individually, but dermabrasion is generally performed over aesthetic facial units, such as cheeks, forehead or upper lip, when facial rhytids are treated. In either case, it is important to lightly "feather" the edges of the dermabraded areas to avoid an abrupt transition from treated to nontreated skin.

Tissue Modification

- *Layers*: Dermabrasion requires that the skin be fairly rigid, so that the depth of planning can be controlled. Traditionally, the skin was frozen by applying topical dry ice. A simpler solution is injection of a dilute anesthetic solution in the treatment area to distend and tighten the skin. The skin is then manually tensed and the dermabrader wheel is pulled towards the operator and perpendicular to the direction of the wheel movement in a steady, sweeping action over the treatment area, leaving untreated areas free of skin debris (Fig. 4.4A). It is important to maintain taut skin and ensure even pressure against the skin to produce a uniform plane of abrasion and avoid gauging the skin. Dermabrasion of the epidermis is bloodless, and punctuates bleeding signals penetration into the papillary dermis. The wheel is spun in the direction of any nearby mobile structures (such as lips or eyelids), so that the skin of these structures is not pulled into the dermabrader. Once the treatment area is abraded uniformly, additional dermabrasion can be performed

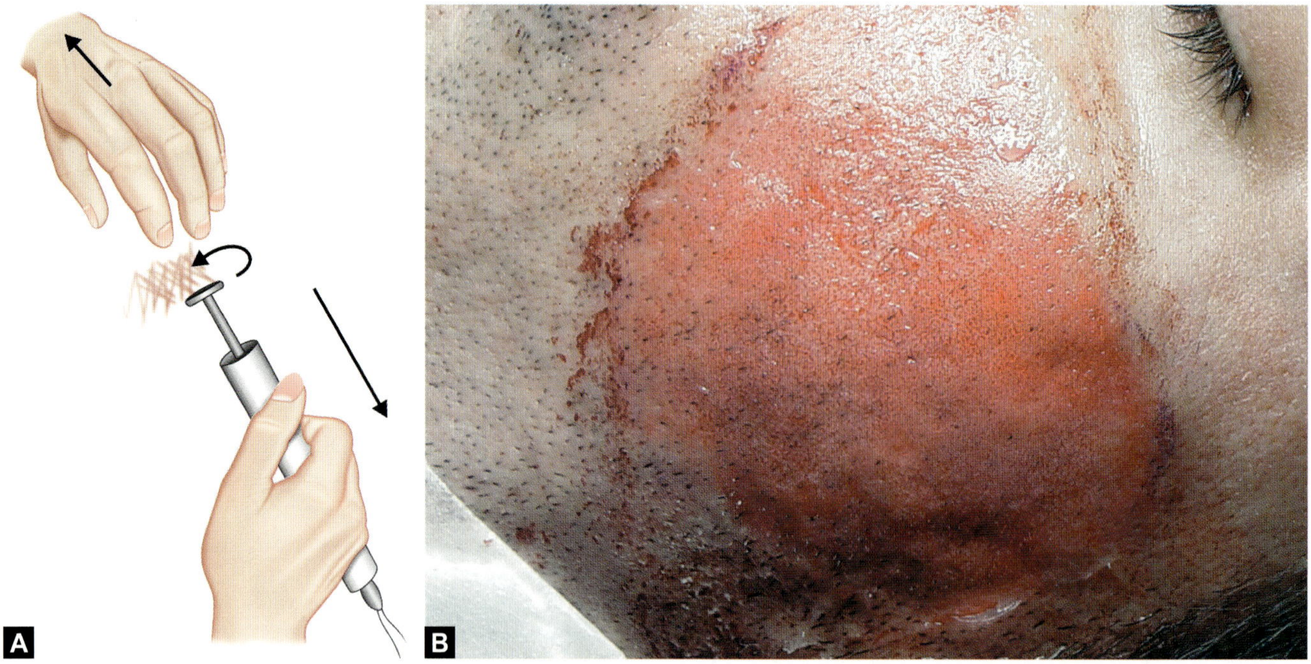

Figs 4.4A and B: Dermabrasion. (A) After the skin turgor is increased by instillation of a tumescent solution, the skin is placed on traction and the dermabrader wheel is stroked gently toward the surgeon. The dermabrader wheel should always rotate towards any nearby mobile structure, such as the lip; (B) After dermabrasion, petechial hemorrhage indicated papillary dermis exposure. The dermabrasion is blended with the surrounding skin by lightly dermabrading the edges

to plane further down into the dermis (Fig. 4.4B). A sterile gauze soaked in a dilute vasoconstrictor can be applied to the skin to control bleeding. Successive layers of abrasion should be done at a 45° angle to the prior level to avoid ridges. The reticular dermis should be avoided and its exposure is marked by more diffuse bleeding. Once the area of interest has been abraded, the edges of this area should be lightly abraded to blend the level in with the surrounding skin.

- *Dressings*: After dermabrasion is complete, another sterile gauze soaked in a dilute vasoconstrictor is applied to the treated area for 3–5 minutes to staunch any oozing, and the treated skin is then liberally coated with an antibacterial ointment such as mupirocin.

CHEMICAL PEELING

Chemical peeling involved application of a chemical solution to the skin which damages the skin in a controlled way so that portions of epidermis and dermis are removed and the skin is allowed to re-epithelialize in a smooth and even way. Superficial peels are defined as those which are limited in effect to the epidermis, medium depth peels penetrate to the superficial and mid-dermis, while deep peels remove skin down to the deep papillary and upper reticular dermis. Superficial peels, such as salicylic acid and glycolic acid peels, are easily applied by simply coating the skin for a defined period of time and then neutralized with water or saline. These "lunchtime peels" will not be discussed.

35% Trichloroacetic Acid Peel

Trichloroacetic acid (TCA) is a keratocoagulant agent which can be used in concentrations of 20–50%. A concentration of 30% or higher is generally required to penetrate into the papillary dermis, and pretreatment with a superficial peel, such as Jessner's solution, can facilitate deeper penetration by thinning the epidermis. Pretreatment with topical tretinoin for 4–6 weeks preoperatively will do the same. Stronger solutions are more effective in effacing fine rhytids and superficial skin blemishes, but are also associated with longer recovery times and a higher risk of hypopigmentation. Because a 50% TCA solution will penetrate into the reticular dermis, the risk of scarring is higher and it is not widely used. TCA peels are generally well-tolerated, requiring minimal analgesia. While oral benzodiazepines can be administered, they are not always required, as most patients experience a mild burning sensation for 2–3 minutes easily managed with a hand-held fan.

Treatment

A critical step in any chemical peel is a thorough degreasing of the skin. Failure to do so will lead to uneven application of the peeling agent and subsequently an uneven effect. A gauze pad soaked in rubbing alcohol or isopropyl alcohol is vigorously rubbed over the skin to remove any residual make-up, skin oils and other debris left on the skin after the patient has washed her face. A cotton tip applicator is dipped in a freshly mixed solution of TCA and excess solution is expressed against the side of the container. The cotton tip is then lightly swept across the treatment area is a broad, even stroke with uniform pressure. This process is then repeated and the treatment area uniformly covered. A light erythema develops initially and later develops into a white "frost" as the peel penetrates more deeply and proteins are coagulated. A solid frost on a base of erythema indicates penetration into the superficial to mid-dermis (Figs 4.5A to C). Some areas of skin require more layers of peeling agent than others to attain the same degree of frosting and depth of penetration. Deeper penetration in focal areas of deeper rhytids, dyschromias or scars can be achieved with more vigorous rubbing, while discrete areas of deeper penetration can be obtained by using a splintered applicator shaft dipped in the TCA solution to treat areas such as etched rhytids. A dry cotton tip applicator is available to dry any tears, which, if allowed to drip along the skin, would dilute the TCA and cause uneven peel depth.

Extent of Undermining/Dissection

The edges of the treated skin are feathered to better blend in with surrounding skin in terms of texture and color. The surrounding skin is lightly treated with the peeling solution to produce only a mild erythema, instead of the full frost in the center of the treated skin.

Baker-Gordon Peel

The Baker-Gordon peel was introduced in the 1960s and is a modified phenol peel. Pure phenol is a keratocoagulant, and the Baker-Gordon peel adds agents to increase the depth of penetration. The Baker-Gordon peel is a fresh mixture of 3 cc of 88% phenol, 2 cc distilled water, 8 drops Septisol and 3 drops croton oil (mnemonic for the ingredients, in order of volume used: "Pretty Damn Safe Concoction").

Transdermal phenol absorption can lead to cardiac arrhythmias. For maximal safety, patients with renal, hepatic or cardiac comorbidities are not considered candidates for any phenol-containing peel. Patients should be well-hydrated, and should receive a liter of crystalloid intravenously prior to the procedure and an additional liter during the procedure. Any phenol peel should be applied slowly over facial units (e.g. forehead, cheeks, perioral, etc.), with 10–15 minutes intervals between units. Since the Baker-Gordon peel can be painful, it should be done under intravenous sedation with cardiac monitoring.

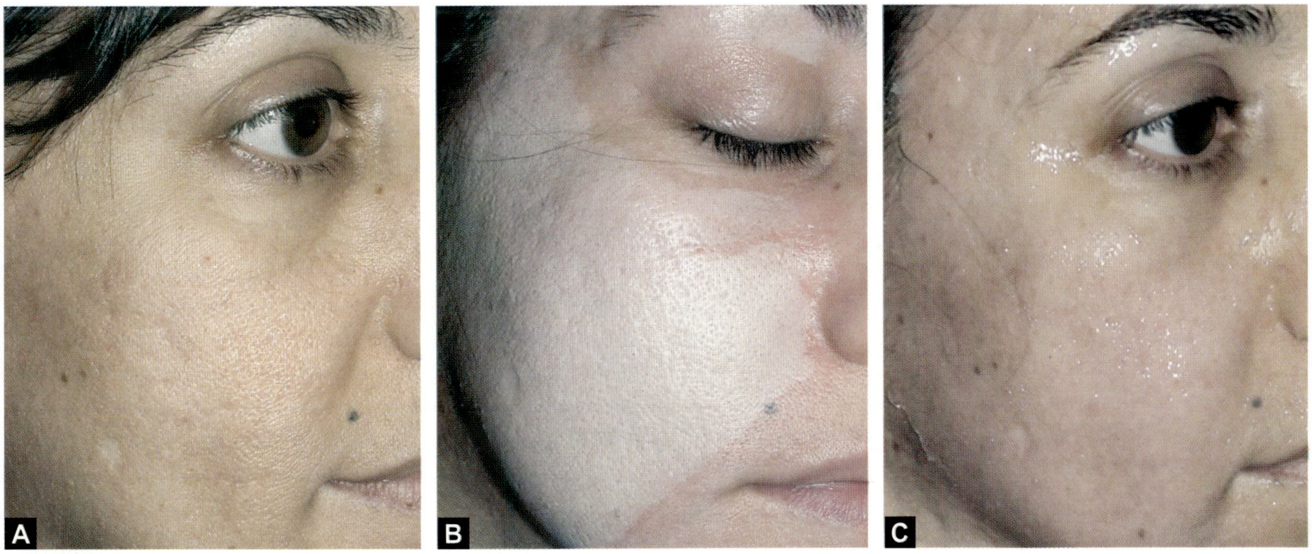

Figs 4.5A to C: 35% Trichloroacetic acid (TCA) peel. (A) Pretreatment; (B) Dense frosting indicated mid-dermal penetration; (C) One week after peel, with mild post-treatment erythema

Treatment

The Baker-Gordon peel mixture is a suspension, and should be mixed freshly in the operating room by the physician. Fresh 88% phenol must be used, as old solutions will absorb atmospheric moisture, diluting the phenol and causing an increase in its keratolytic capacity. The other components are added to the phenol and the mixture must be stirred immediately before each application. As with the TCA peel, a coating of peeling solution should be applied to produce an even depth of peeling, indicated by a dense white frost. The skin of the face is peeled in units, with an appropriate time period between units. A deeper level of penetration can be obtained by applying occlusive zinc oxide tape immediately after each unit is applied. Taped Baker-Gordon peels will penetrate to the mid-reticular dermis with an increased risk of postoperative scarring.

Extent of Undermining/Dissection

As with any chemical peel, the edges of the treated skin must be feathered to better blend in with surrounding skin in terms of texture and color. The surrounding skin is lightly treated with the peeling solution to produce only a mild erythema. Since application of a Baker-Gordon peel will lead to permanent dysfunction of melanocytes with decreased melanin production in the treated area, peeled skin will be lighter than untreated skin. It is essential to continue the peel into the hairline and below the jawline to avoid a visible transition. Patients are committed to lifelong sun avoidance and sun protection.

Dressings

After a medium or deep chemical peel, the skin is liberally coated with a topical emollient such as Eucerin, Crisco or petrolatum.

AUTOLOGOUS FAT TRANSFER

Autologous fat transfer offers the option of providing additional soft tissue volume using the patient's own tissue in a relatively noninvasive way. Harvested fat is isolated from a distant site, gently purified and then reintroduced into the facial soft tissues in areas that require additional volume. The transferred fat will survive only if it develops a vascular supply from the surrounding tissues quickly. After a brief period during which treatment related edema resolves and some fat is resorbed, the soft tissue volume augmentation is relatively stable as the remaining fat has become vascularized. Many techniques exist for autologous fat transfer, and the one described below is a modification of that popularized by Coleman (Figs 4.6A and B).

Incision Placement

Autologous fat transfer to the face rarely requires more than 20–30 cc of fat, and frequently less fat is used. Fat can be harvested from a number of areas, even in thin patients: the most common areas are the periumbilical area and the upper thighs. After a small amount of local anesthetic is injected, a small stab incision with a #15 blade is made, often in the inner lip of the umbilicus.

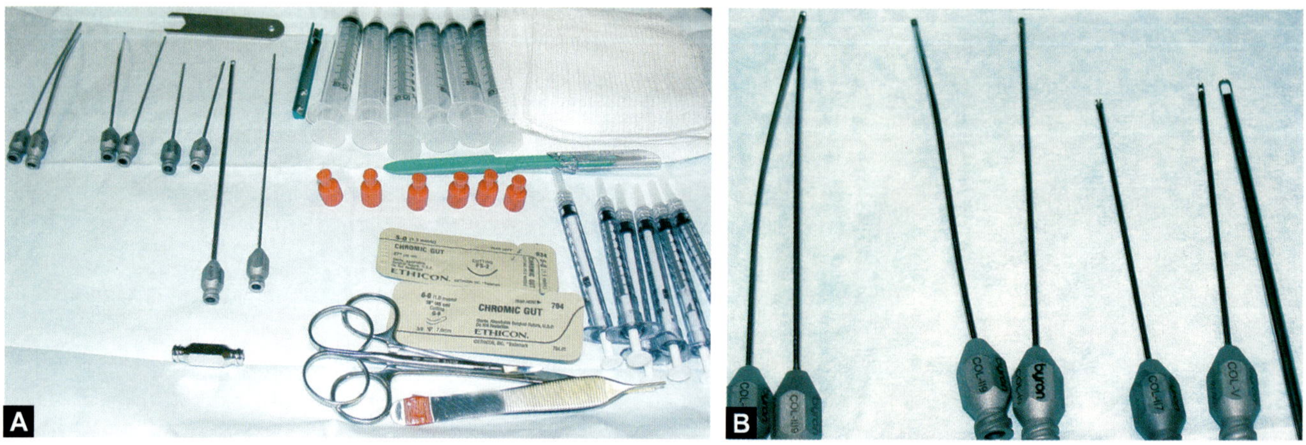

Figs 4.6A and B: Fat transfer instruments. (A) Instrumentation is relatively simple, requiring basic instruments and dedicated suction and injection cannulae; (B) Aspiration cannula (far right). Injection cannulae come in a variety of sizes, curved or straight, blunt or sharp-ended with an end or side port

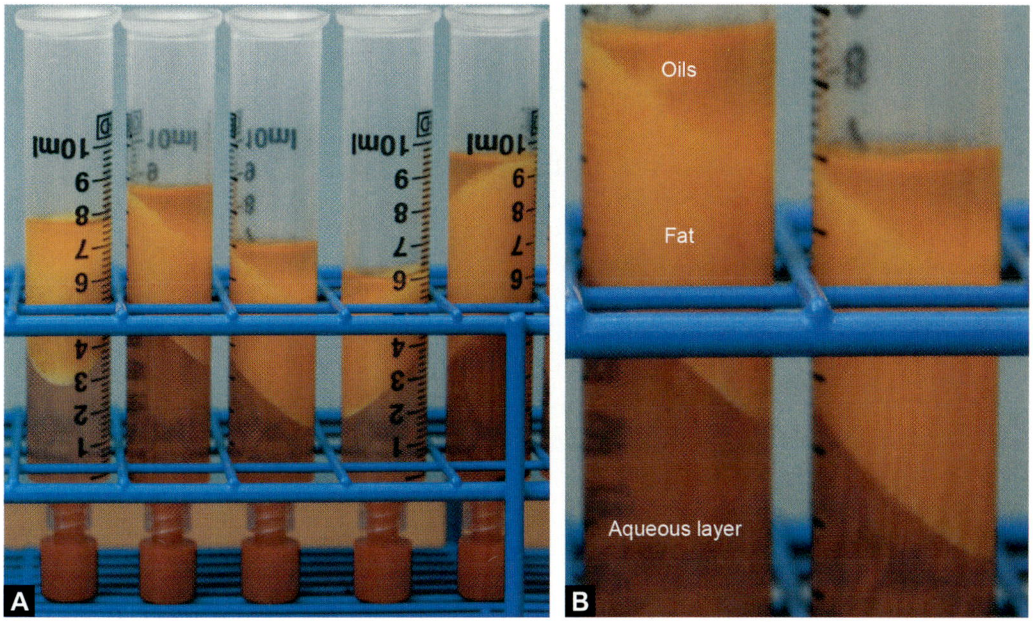

Figs 4.7A and B: (A) Harvested fat after centrifugation; (B) Supernatant oil is wicked away, while the infranatant aqueous layer is drained, leaving purified fat

Small stab incisions are made peripheral to the area of the face to be treated, and only large enough to accommodate the fat infiltration cannulae.

Extent of Undermining/Dissection

At the harvest site, a small caliber, blunt tip, multiport cannula is introduced through the incision and passed radially from the incision in the area of planned fat harvest though the subdermal fat. As the cannula is withdrawn, a tumescent solution (90 cc of lactated Ringer's solution with 10 cc of 1% lidocaine with 1:100,000 epinephrine, yielding a solution of 0.1% lidocaine with 1:1,000,000 epinephrine) is infiltrated gently. This anesthetizes the patient, distends the fat pockets and creates small "pretunnels" throughout the fat to be harvested.

A dual port Coleman fat harvest cannula is then attached to a 10 cc syringe and the plunger is pulled back 5–7 cc after the cannula tip is placed in the subcutaneous tunnel. Holding the plunger in the retracted position to generate a gentle vacuum, the cannula is then passed in a fan-like pattern with the dominant hand, while the nondominant hand manually compresses the skin and subcutaneous fat around the tip of the cannula. The to-fro motion of the cannula tip shears small parcels of fat that are aspirated into the syringe. Once 4–6 cc of fat is aspirated, the cannula is removed from the syringe, a sterile cap is placed on the syringe hub and the plunger is removed. Syringes of collected fat are then placed sterilely into a centrifuge and then spun for 3 minutes at 1,000 rpm (Fig. 4.7A). At this point, three layers are easily visible in the syringe: (1) a supranatant layer of oil released from fragmented adipocytes, (2) a fat layer and (3) an infranatant layer of blood and tumescent solution (Fig. 4.7B). The oil layer is first decanted and then further removed with a wick of half-inch sterile gauze. The cap on the syringe hub is released and the infranatant removed. If desired, platelet rich plasma or platelet rich fibrin matrix can be mixed with the fat at this point. The syringe plunger is replaced and the syringe connected via a female-to-female connector and loaded into individual 1 cc syringes.

Tissue Modifications

Fat Placement

Using one of a number of blunt tipped cannulae, sequential passes are made in the sites to be augmented, and small parcels of fat are deposited in multiple planes in the desired areas. Ideally, multiple passes are made and small amounts (0.1 cc) are infiltrated per pass. A criss-cross pattern is used to avoid ridges and lumpiness, using two or more entry sites located at least 1 cm from the edge of the treatment area. Overcorrection is recommended, and as with fat harvesting, edges should be "feathered" to avoid obvious transition zones. If properly placed, entry

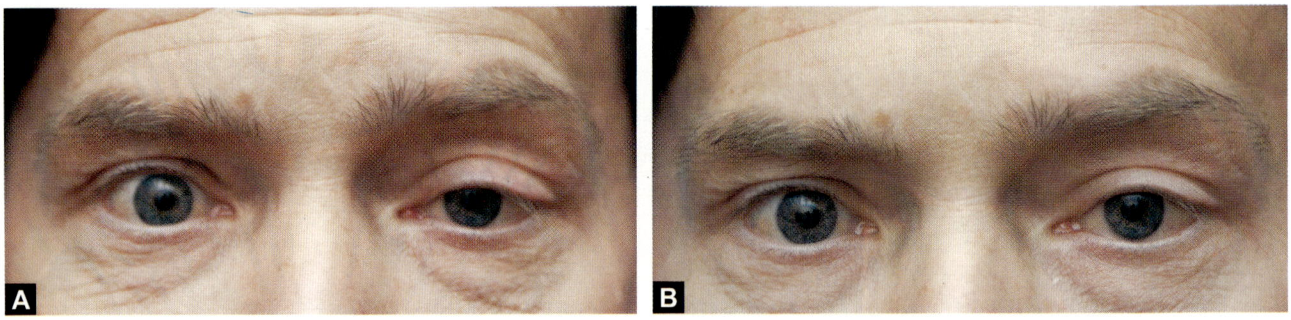

Figs 4.8A and B: (A) Left upper lid ptosis after aggressive treatment of blepharospasm; (B) Improvement 5 minutes after instillation of apraclonidine drops

incisions are sufficiently distant from the target area that the first 1 cm of tunnel collapses onto itself and prevents extrusion of fat from the treatment area.

Closure

Facial stab incisions are closed with a 5-0 fast absorbing gut suture and coated with a triple antibiotic ointment. A 4-0 or 5-0 chromic suture may be used to closure the umbilical incision, but some surgeon prefer to leave this incision alone, as residual tumescent solution will drain for a few hours after the procedure.

Dressings

A small sterile gauze dressing is placed over the umbilical incision and is changed several times over the first 12 hours as needed. No dressings are placed over the face.

POTENTIAL COMPLICATIONS

Botulinum Toxin A

Complications of BT×A are related to unwanted effects on nontarget muscles, the most significant being eyelid ptosis after treatment for the glabella. While the exact mechanism of ptosis after glabellar treatment is still under debate, the most commonly discussed theory is that diffusion of the toxin solution below the orbital rim affects the levator palpebrae superioris muscle, allowing the upper lid to descend. Injection at least 2 cm above the orbital rim is recommended to avoid ptosis. However, if ptosis does occur, it is generally self-limited, recovering in 2–6 weeks spontaneously. Patients without contraindications may treat the ptosis symptomatically with topical alpha-adrenergic eye drops (over-the-counter phenylephrine or naphazoline, or 0.5% apraclonidine (Iopidine) until the ptosis resolves (Figs 4.8A and B). Other cosmetic concerns may result from failure to account for the subsequent actions of antagonist muscles; treatment is directed towards restoring the balance of tonic muscular contraction. For example, a "Mephistopheles" or "quizzical" appearance may result after treating the central frontalis muscle, while the temporal edge of the frontalis is still functional and able to elevate the brow tail and arch excessively. A small amount of additional toxin can be placed in the superior portion of the lateral frontalis muscle to allow the brow tail to drop slightly and correct the brow shape.

Topical Retinoids and Bleaching Agents

Topical bleaching agents and retinoids are generally well-tolerated, especially since the epidermis remains intact. These topical agents may initially be drying or irritating to the skin, and topical moisturizers may be indicated or the frequency of use may need to be reduced.

Soft Tissue Fillers

Vascular Compromise/Skin Slough

The most feared complication of soft tissue fillers is vascular compromise. The most classical location for this is the glabella, but can occur anywhere. Occasionally, significant amounts of filler placed in a small area may lead to venous compromise. This is typically associated with late, throbbing pain and discomfort and venous congestion. Intra-arterial injection in the glabella produces immediate blanching of the skin, and is more likely with smaller gauge needles and when the needle is being advanced, rather than withdrawn, during injection. If blanching is noted, injection should stop immediately, the skin gently massaged and warm compresses and nitroglycerine paste applied in order to limit the area of vascular compromise. If a HA product has been injected, hyaluronidase [ovine hyaluronidase (Vitrase, Bausch and Lomb, Rochester, NY)] can be injected to spur the resorption of the injected HA. Patients should be followed closely and local wounds treated with topical or oral antibiotics; debridement may be necessary, but should be very conservative.

Infection, Early versus Late

Infections, although uncommon, may occur soon after treatment or several months later. Early infections generally are easier to diagnose, and should be treated with 2–3 weeks of an appropriate antibiotic. Late infections may present as minimally erythematous nodules weeks to months after treatment, and may represent activation of a low grade infection associated with bacterial biofilm. These infections should be treated with a prolonged course of oral antibiotics; combination therapy with a macrolide and a tetracycline is recommended.

Nodules/Granulomas

Some soft tissue fillers are prone to forming nodules by virtue of their composition. Particulate fillers, such as CaHA and PLLA, can be forced into accumulations by the action of muscle contraction; these fillers should not be used in highly mobile areas such as lips. PLLA may form nodules if the powder is insufficiently rehydrated. Local injection with sterile saline may help disperse these accumulations of product if treated early.

Visibility

Visibility of fillers is a result of improper placement. HA products injected above the mid-deep dermis will be evident as a gray discoloration, and if not improved sufficiently by massage can be treated with hyaluronidase. CaHA will impart a nodulogranular appearance if injected into the dermis. When injecting CaHA, it is important to remove pressure from the syringe plunger as the needle-tip, nears the skin entry site to avoid depositing filler in the dermis. Dermabrasion can be considered to remove filler from the superficial dermis.

Chemical Peels

Dyspigmentation

Uneven peel depth, as well as prolonged inflammation, can lead to uneven pigmentation. Uncomplicated, rapid re-epithelialization is essential to prevent hyperpigmentation. Lines of demarcation between treated and untreated skin result from inadequate feathering at the peel borders.

Infection

Excessive crusting may predispose to bacterial, fungal or viral infection. Patients should be medicated with an oral antiviral for 2 days prior to peeling and until the skin re-epithelialization is complete. Postoperative compresses with a dilute acetic acid (vinegar) solution are antibacterial and will also facilitate healing. *Staphylococcus aureus, Pseudomonas aeruginosa, Escherichia coli and Candida albicans* are common pathogens which should be considered if an infection is suspected.

Scarring and Persistent Erythema

Any delay of wound healing, whether because of infection, excessive and untreated crusting or excessive depth of peeling predisposes to scarring, and may necessitate treatment with corticosteroid injections or tape, pulse dye laser or silicone sheeting. Post-treatment erythema is expected after medium or deep chemical peels. Infection or other inflammatory conditions will prolong erythema. Erythema lasting longer than 30 (medium peels) or 90 (deep peels) days, especially if accompanied by pruritus, may be associated with the development of skin thickening or scarring.

Autologous Fat Transfer

- *Resorption and lipid cyst*: The key biological process involved in successful fat transfer is the rapid revascularization of the transplanted adipocytes. Over the first several days, adipocytes are dependent upon local tissues for oxygen and nutrient delivery. Ultimately, neovascularization occurs to support the transferred fat cells, but in the interim a portion for these cells will undergo necrosis. While this cellular debris is generally resorbed, not infrequently the lipid releasate may become encapsulated and form a lipid cyst, which infrequently requires aspiration; untreated lipid cysts may lead to postoperative nodules or excessive fibrosis. More importantly, the inevitable loss of some viable adipocytes requires overcorrection at the time of treatment. However, it is important to transfer small parcels of fat cells in discrete, separate tunnels, raising the surface area (contacting the local tissue): transferred fat volume to maximize the revascularization of fat. Transfer of large boluses of fat increases the likelihood of lipid cysts as well as fat resorption.
- Seroma or hematoma can develop if adequate vasoconstriction is not achieved in the treatment area or if the technique is overly rough. Small cannulae

are most effective in limiting tissue trauma. Seromas or hematomas may require aspiration, and less commonly, open evacuation.

- Generally, noticeable asymmetry is not observed in patients treated with matching volumes of fat bilaterally. However, small areas if treated with dissimilar volumes of fat will lead to asymmetry. Additional fat correction may be required to address this problem.
- *Ridges*: Ridges or rippling may be noticed postoperatively at the donor site if the harvesting passes are not fanned evenly or feathered peripherally. In facial areas treated with autologous fat, patients will often complain of firmness of treated areas and a sharp edge at the junction with untreated tissues. This is especially true in the early postoperative period, and generally resolves along with edema. However, irregularities and ridges, especially in areas of thin skin, may occur. Small amounts of additional fat may be required to smooth the transition between treated and untreated tissue.

AFTERCARE

Botulinum Toxin A

After BT×A treatment, patients are instructed to avoid recumbent position, head-hanging, vigorous activity or manipulation of the treated area for 4–6 hours after treatment.

Fillers

Cool compresses are applied for the first 2–4 hours after treatment. After most soft tissue fillers, patients are instructed to avoid manipulation of the treated area for 2–3 days; however, PLLA is prone to development of subcutaneous nodules, and patients are advised to perform vigorous massage for 5 minutes five times a day for 5 days.

Dermabrasion

Treated areas are covered in a topical emollient (such as bacitracin, mupirocin, Vaseline or Eucerin) and patients are advised to wash with warm soapy water several times a day, reapplying the ointment afterward until the skin has completely re-epithelialized.

Chemical Peel

Dilute acetic acid compresses are applied several times a day, followed by application of an emollient such as Vaseline, Eucerin, petrolatum or Aquaphor.

Fat Transfer

Care after fat transfer is generally limited. Patients should avoid mechanical manipulation of the treated areas for several days. Cold compresses are discouraged, as the vasoconstriction induced may delay revascularization.

COMBINATION THERAPY

Dramatic results can be obtained from combining multiple minimally invasive treatments (Figs 4.9A to H). Sufficient time should be allowed to elapse after each treatment such that the full effect is realized (e.g. 1–2 weeks after BTxA, 2–4 weeks after a TCA peel) and the skin has fully healed, including resolution of edema.

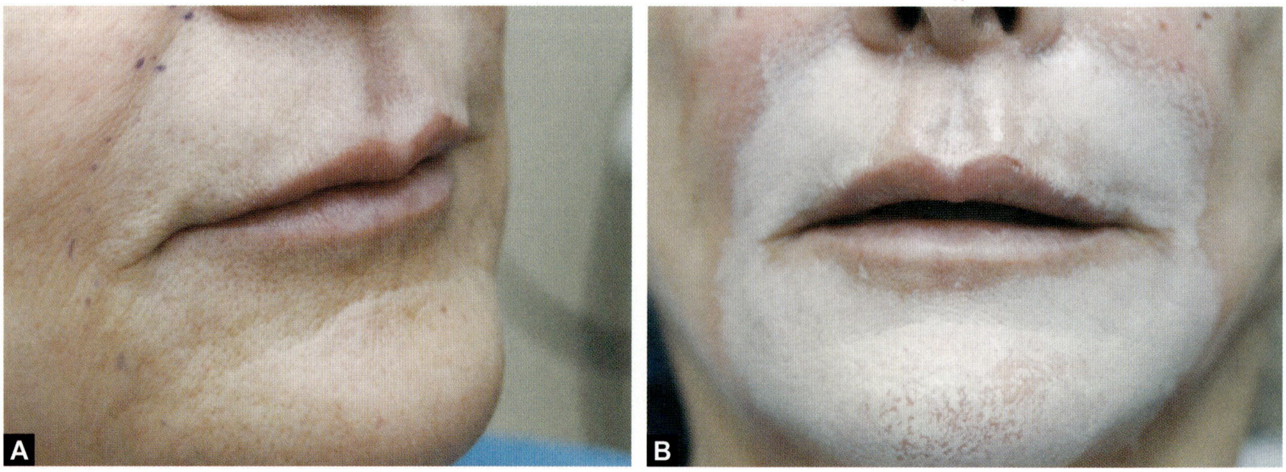

Figs 4.9A and B

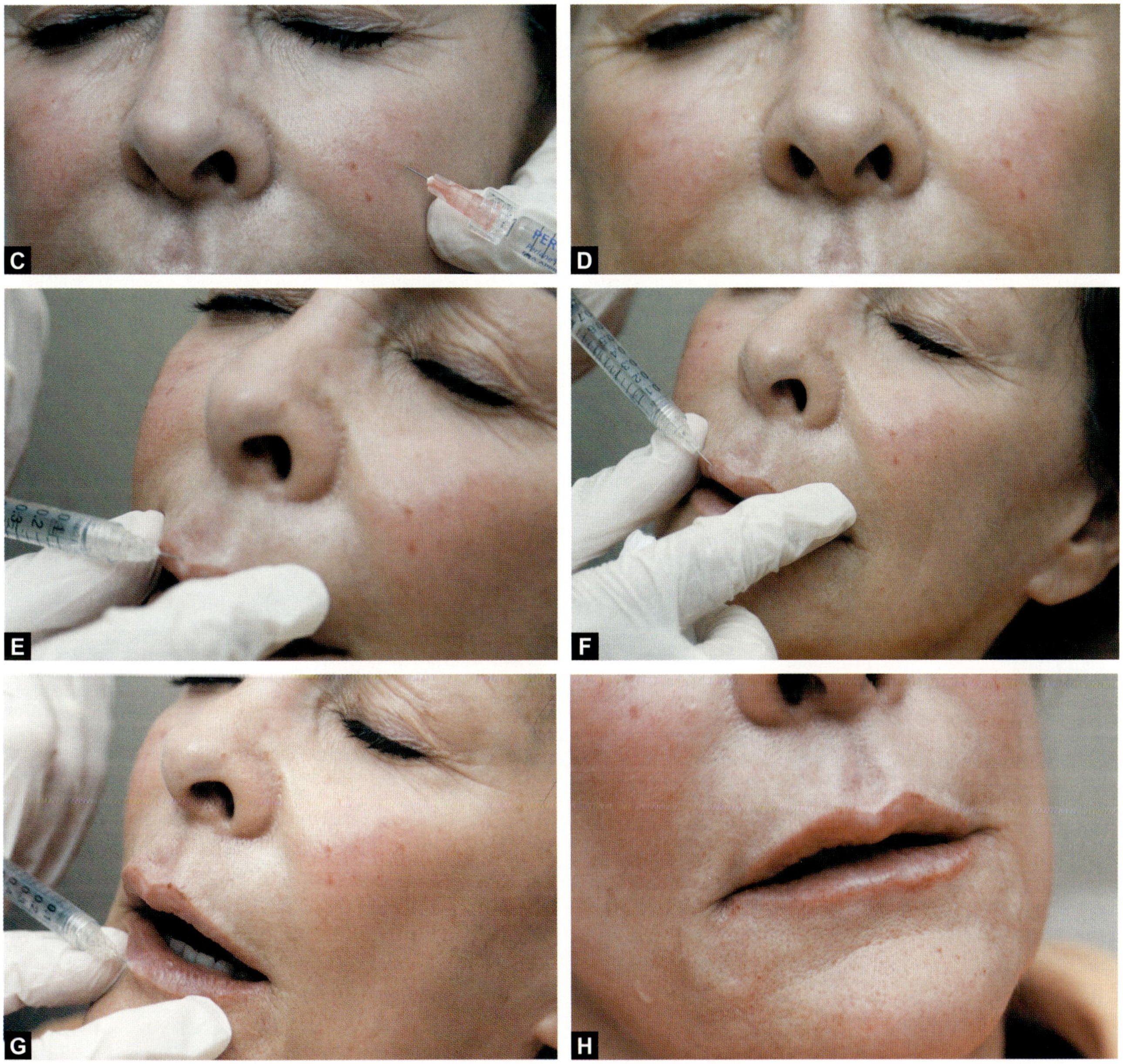

Figs 4.9A to H: Combining minimally invasive treatments can effectively improve trouble areas. (A) Mild perioral and midfacial findings 4 years after a superficial muscular aponeurotic system (SMAS) rhytidectomy were treated first with (B) 35% trichloroacetic acid (TCA) perioral peel followed 4 weeks later by soft tissue filler therapy; (C) Midfacial volume was augmented with deep injections of Perlane (infraorbital hollows were also filled with suborbicularis injections of Restylane); (D) Difference can be seen after treatment of right side; (E) Lip contours were revived with Juvederm injection at the vermilion border; (F) While upper lip volume and projection was enhanced with Juvederm injection into the central vermillion; (G) The lower lip required only vermillion border injections; (H) Appearance immediately after treatment

BIBLIOGRAPHY

1. Bray D, Hopkins C, Roberts DN. A review of dermal fillers in facial plastic surgery. Curr Opin Otolaryngol Head Neck Surg. 2010;18(4):295-302.
2. Kim EK, Hovsepian RV, Mathew P, et al. Dermabrasion. Clin Plast Surg. 2011;38(3):391-5.
3. Langsdon PR, Rodwell DW, Velargo PA, et al. Latest chemical peel innovations. Facial Plast Surg Clin North Am. 2012;20(2):119-23.
4. Pu LL, Coleman SR, Cui X, et al. Autologous fat grafts harvested and refined by the Coleman technique: a comparative study. Plast Reconstr Surg. 2008;122(3):932-7
5. Sclafani AP, Fagien S. Treatment of injectable soft tissue filler complications. Dermatol Surg. 2009;35:1672-80.

CHAPTER 5

Face Lift and Neck Lift

Anthony P Sclafani

OVERVIEW

Rhytidectomy refers to a set of procedures designed primarily to rejuvenate the mid and lower face and neck. A misnomer, rhytidectomy does not cut out wrinkles but primarily is a surgery of tissue repositioning, so the term is used here primarily because of its common use. Rhytidectomy may involve the midfacial tissues, the lower face or the neck, and is more usefully described by the specific techniques, planes and maneuvers used to rejuvenate the face. This chapter will discuss the midface lift, face lifts such as the lateral SMASectomy, superficial musculoaponeurotic system (SMAS) lift, deep plane face lift and platysmaplasty. The incisions employed, the planes dissected, the tissues removed, the vectors of tissue suspension and the tissue fixation employed will determine the aesthetic effects and the longevity of these procedures.

A number of processes occur simultaneously and to varying degrees in the face which contribute to facial aging. Superficial skin rhytids develop, associated with dermal thinning and beginning with fine, etched lines in the skin, gradually deepening to more significant wrinkles. Areas of hyperkinetic muscle contraction, such as the crow's feet and glabella, will furrow the overlying skin, and failure of the muscle to fully relax will led to standing rhytids. Soft tissues, such as the jowls, may descend, as retaining ligaments and skin lose elasticity and stretch. Finally, bony resorption may occur, changing the underlying foundation of facial appearance.

SPECIAL CONSIDERATIONS

As with any aesthetic procedure, a careful facial analysis should be performed, and true tissue malposition should be verified. Other processes of facial aging, such as hyperkinetic or static rhytids, soft tissue volume deficiencies, or bony resorption are not well treated by rhytidectomy. In particular, patients with significantly volume deficiency will look "pulled" or "surgical" after rhytidectomy. A proper aesthetic diagnosis is essential to the success of any cosmetic procedure, but especially rhytidectomy.

As many of these procedures entail wide dissection and large skin-soft tissue flaps, patients taking anticoagulants have especially high risk of developing hematoma. Appropriate management of anticoagulant therapy is essential and should be ensured, in cooperation with the patient's primary care physician. Casual use of low dose aspirin by the patient should be discontinued at least 7 days prior to surgery. Tobacco use can lead to tissue ischemia and skin loss, and patients should be instructed to discontinue use for at least 6 weeks before surgery; alternatively, some authors argue that the more robust blood supply associated with the deep plane face lift makes this technique more appropriate for active smokers. Perioperative hypertension is also associated with higher incidence of hematomas, and should be aggressively managed preoperatively and postoperatively.

ALTERNATIVES TO PROCEDURE

Proper diagnosis of the patient's needs will dictate the appropriate surgical rhytidectomy procedure. Non-surgical alternatives to rhytidectomy are primarily those which attempt to redrape the skin by augmenting facial volume: soft tissue fillers and fat transfer, primarily. Customized malar implants can also be used to fill submalar deficiency. Alloplastic chin augmentation will secondarily improve the appearance of the cervicomental angle, as will submental liposuction alone. Energy-based skin rejuvenation may provide some tightening of the facial skin, but this is rarely sufficient to correct significant skin laxity and ptosis.

TECHNIQUES

Superficial Musculoaponeurotic System Face Lift

Incision Placement

The SMAS face lift is typically conducted after addressing submental and subjowl fat deposits with liposuction (discussed elsewhere). Standard postauricular, peritragal, and temporal incisions are made, and may incorporate the previously made liposuction incisions (Fig. 5.1). The postauricular incision in males is made in the postauricular sulcus, as opposed to on the conchal bowl in females. The incision runs up to the level of the external meatus, where it crosses the mastoid skin until reaching the hairline. A broken line "Z" incision is incorporated just behind the postauricular crease to prevent webbing. If significant posterior elevation is anticipated, the incision turns and runs inferiorly along the hairline; otherwise, the incision courses back into the occipital hair-bearing scalp and gently curves inferiorly. A curvilinear temporal incision can be made extending in hair-bearing skin and curving gently anteriorly, but if significant superior elevation of the skin flap is anticipated, this should be avoided to prevent unnatural elevation of the temporal hair tuft. Instead, the incision is made across the base of the sideburn and up along the anterior edge of the lower temporal hairline.

Traditionally, a retrotragal incision (Fig. 5.2A) is used only in females, and a pretragal incision (Fig. 5.2B) is made in males to avoid advancing the beard onto the tragus.

Extent of Undermining/Dissection

A subcutaneous dissection is then performed, advancing 4 cm (short flap) to 10 cm (long flap) from the tragus and preauricular incision, to a point as far anterior as a line drawn from the lateral canthus to oral commissure (Fig. 5.3). Using scissors, a skin flap can be elevated in the occipital region while taking care to avoid injury to the great auricular nerve (Fig. 5.4). After freeing up the earlobe, the scissors can be directed toward the lower neck through the superficial subcutaneous plane. The tips of the scissors are advanced medially with a spreading action (Fig. 5.5A), creating a series of subcutaneous tunnels which can then be connected by pressing the partially opened blades of the scissors against the intervening tissue bridges (Fig. 5.5B). In the cheek, dissection remains below the malar arch to avoid disruption of the temporal branches of the facial nerve.

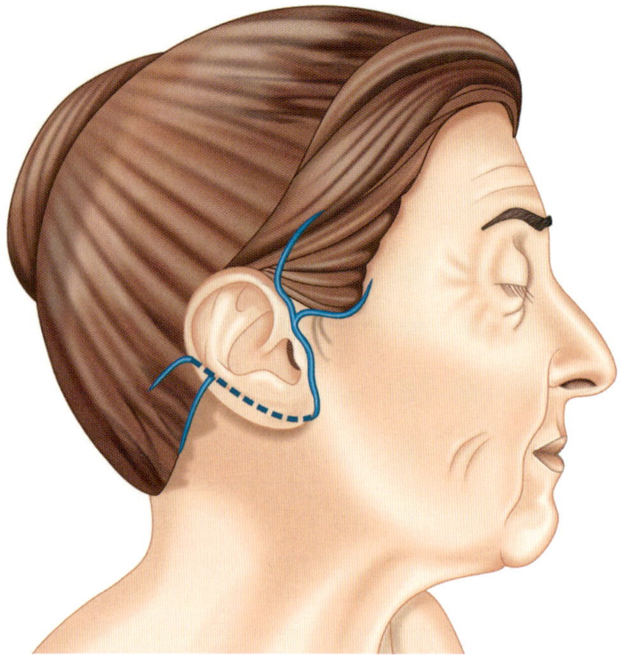

Fig. 5.1: Standard face lift incisions run around the ear and into or along the temporal and occipital hairlines

Tissue Modifications

- *Incision*: A vertically oriented strip of SMAS is incised approximately 2 cm anterior to the skin incision, exposing the parotidomasseteric fascia, and may curve around the earlobe. Using blunt dissection, the SMAS is elevated (Fig. 5.6) from below the zygoma inferiorly to its junction with the platysma. Anterior to the parotid, dissection may continue superficial to the masseter to avoid facial nerve branches. Inferiorly, the lateral aspect of the platysma is then identified and a minimal subplatysmal elevation is conducted. Facial nerve branches can be protected by spreading the scissors in a vertical direction toward the skin flap.
- *Tissue advancement*: Kocher clamps are then applied to the edges of the SMAS flap medial to the tragus and below the mandible (Fig. 5.7A), and the optimal vectors of SMAS advancement which smooth the jawline and rejuvenate the neck are assessed. If necessary, the SMAS can be split and two distinct vectors developed (Fig. 5.7B).
- *Suturing*: The SMAS-platysma flap is then secured with a superoposterior vector of traction to the thickened, relatively immobile SMAS in the pretragal area [Loré's fascia (LF)] at the level of the helical root with a 3-0 polydioxanone suture (Fig. 5.8). If there was significant superior mobilization, the SMAS can be incised, resected and sutured below and parallel to

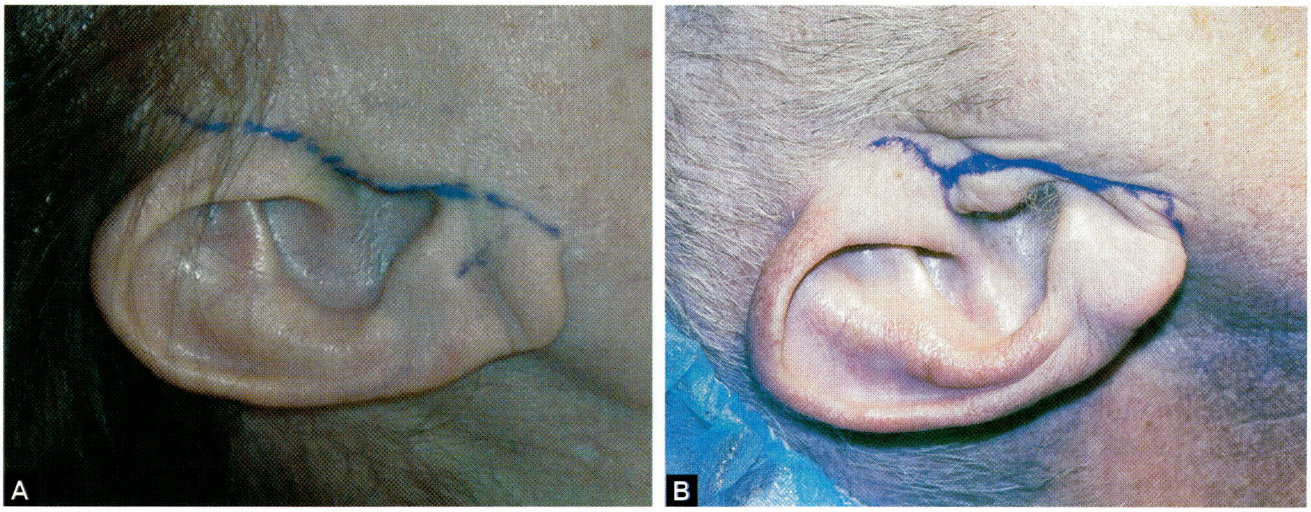

Figs 5.2A and B: (A) The preauricular incision can run on the inner surface of the tragus to camouflage part of the incision and (B) In men, because of beard hair, the incision should run in a pre-existing preauricular crease

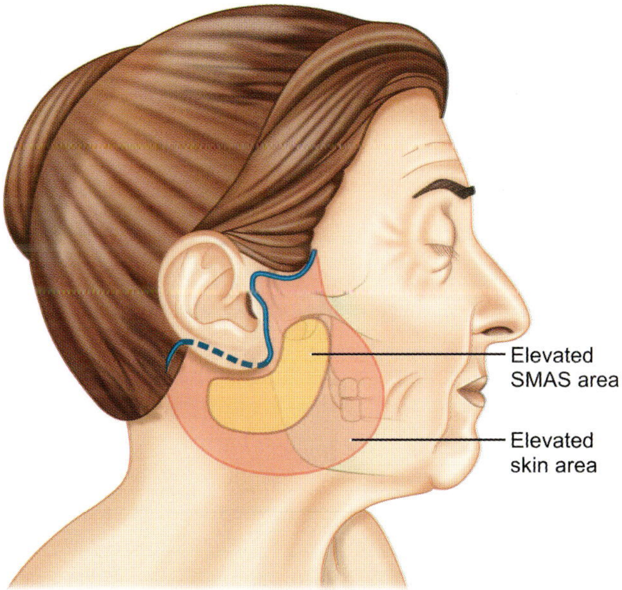

Fig. 5.3: A superficial muscular aponeurotic system (SMAS) face lift elevates a skin flap followed in addition to a SMAS flap

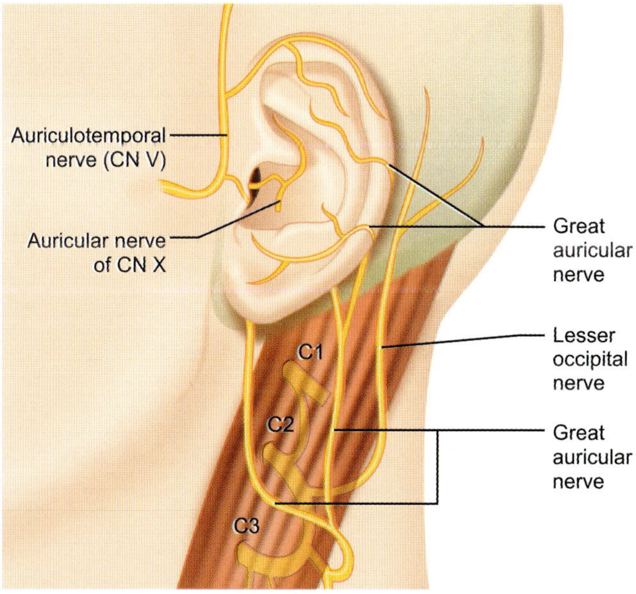

Fig. 5.4: Care should be taken to preserve the great auricular nerve during dissection

the malar arch. The SMAS flap below the mandibular angle, where the platysma interdigitates with the SMAS, is sutured posterosuperiorly to the mastoid periosteum and conchal bowl periosteum. After realigning and placing key sutures to align the SMAS-platysma flap, excess SMAS is trimmed, and the SMAS closed along the incision's length with interrupted 3-0 polydioxanone sutures.

Closure

- *Skin excision*: Prior to wound closure, the skin is redraped and excess skin is excised. It is essential that the continuity of the occipital (and if cut, the temporal) hairline be restored. "Pilot" cuts (Fig. 5.9) through obviously excess skin can be made at critical areas (such as the points at which the occipital incision

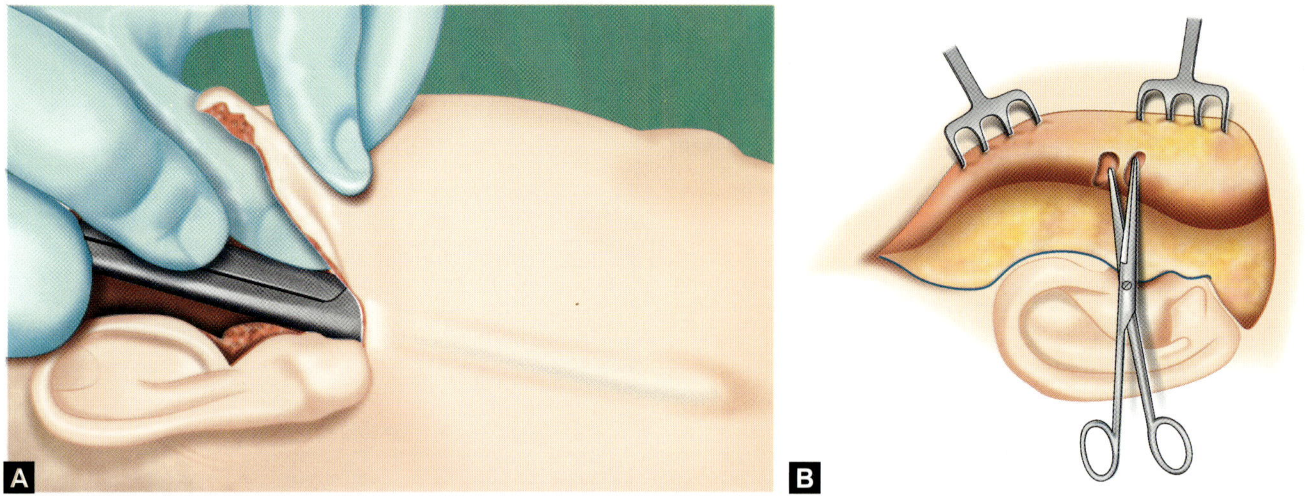

Figs 5.5A and B: (A) Skin flaps should be raised in the subcutaneous plane. During dissection, the impression of the scissor tips are seen; (B) Separate subcutaneous tunnels are developed, which are connected by straddling the intervening tissue bridges with partially opened scissors and gently pushing

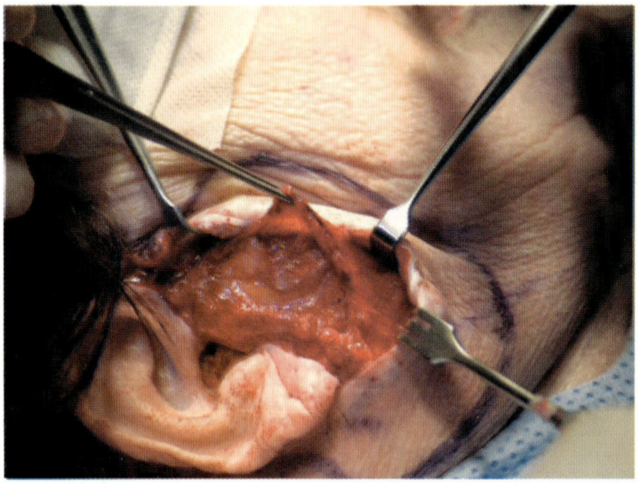

Fig. 5.6: Superficial musculoaponeurotic system flap is elevated and held in the forceps. Loré's fascia (LF) is seen closer to the ear

meets the hairline and the postauricular crease) and temporary 3-0 nylon sutures placed. With the flap temporarily suspended, more exact excision of skin can be performed. It is essential to avoid excessive skin excision and skin closure tension. Skin excision should not be relied upon to elevate the facial soft tissues. If a retrotragal incision was used, the portion of skin which will overlie the tragus should be defatted carefully prior to wound closure.

- *Layers/sutures*: Once the SMAS has been advanced and sutured, the elevated skin can be easily redraped so as to produce the desired aesthetic effect while minimizing standing cone deformities. Skin is resected differentially based on the vectors of traction and elevation and the degree of skin redundancy; care is taken to avoid undue tension on the skin flap. The incisions are then closed in a two layer fashion, using 3-0 Vicryl for dermal closure. The temporal and occipital portions of the wound are closed with skin staples; the postauricular portion of the skin closure is accomplished with 4-0 chromic sutures. A deep suture should be placed from the deep tissues of the earlobe up to the perichondrium of the conchal bowl to stabilize the earlobe position and reduce the risk of a "pixie ear" deformity. Retrotragal closure is performed with a running 6-0 chromic suture, while the preauricular skin is closed with running or interrupted 6-0 polypropylene sutures.
- *Drains*: Active or passive drains may be placed to evacuate the sub-flap space but these should not be considered alternatives to ensuring hemostasis prior to wound closure. While monopolar cautery can generally be used over the sternocleidomastoid muscle (SCM), it is important to avoid injury to the great auricular nerve, which crosses the mid-point of the SCM and runs superiorly, with branches supplying the earlobe and lower conchal bowl. In this area and the anterior face and neck, bipolar cautery may be used carefully to control bleeding and limit potential injury to neural structures. Drains are generally placed in dependent areas and brought out of the skin (preferably through separate incisions) posteriorly. Multi-hole Jackson-Pratt or fluted Blake drains can provide active drainage, or Penrose drains can be used for passive drainage (Fig. 5.10). Generally, drains are removed within

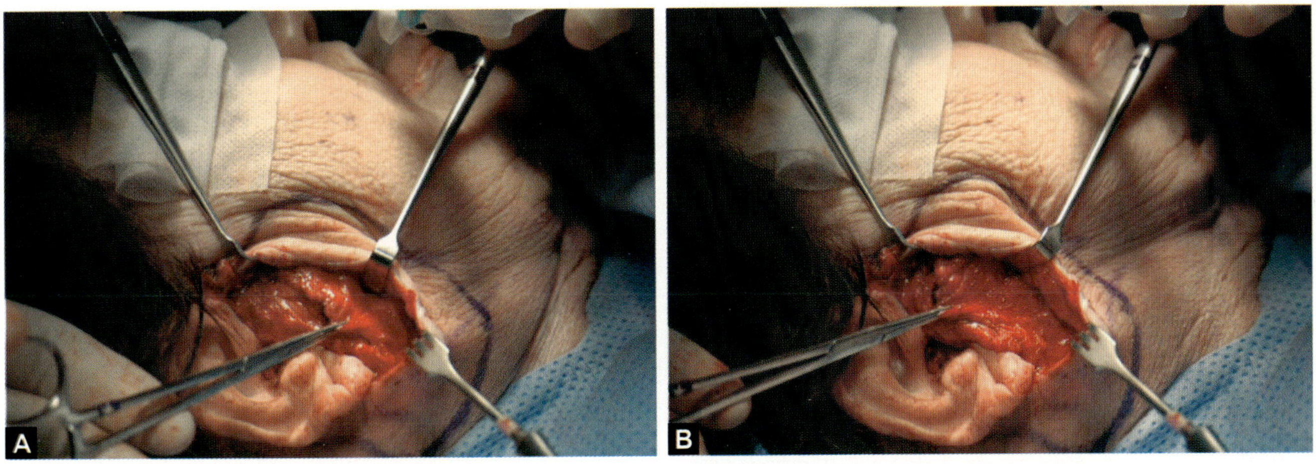

Figs 5.7A and B: (A) Kocher clamps are placed on the superficial musculoaponeurotic system (SMAS) flap and (B) retracted superolaterally until the optimal vector of pull is determined

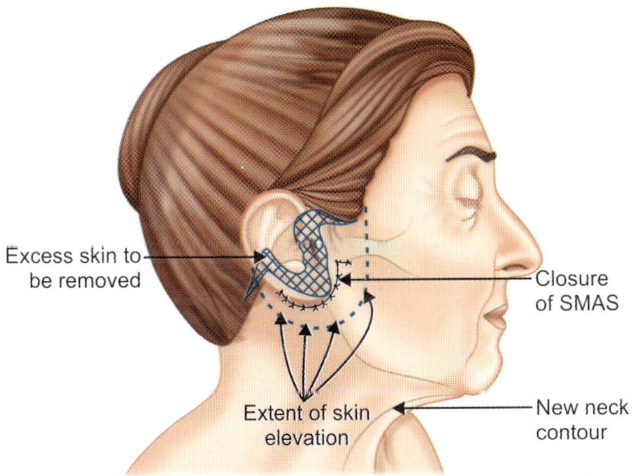

Fig. 5.8: After the superficial muscular aponeurotic system (SMAS) flap is retracted, excess resected and the SMAS repaired, the skin is retracted and redundancy is noted and excised

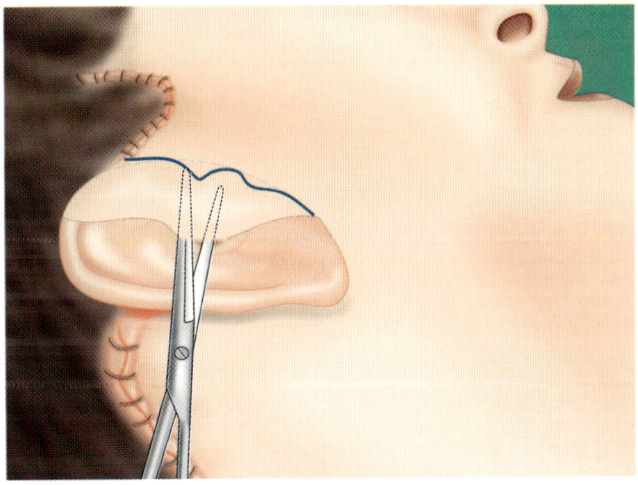

Fig. 5.9: The skin is sequentially resected and closed

24–36 hours of surgery. Alternatively, some surgeons now eschew drains in favor of platelet rich plasma or platelet rich fibrin matrix to avoid hematoma or seroma formation without drains.

- *Dressings*: A moderately compressive dressing is placed around both sides of the face and neck for 24–36 hours, following which it is replaced with a self-applied elastic strap dressing which the patient wears continuously for the first week and at night-time for the next 3 weeks.

Rhytidectomy with Lateral SMASectomy

Rhytidectomy with lateral SMASectomy was described as an alternative to the SMAS flap rhytidectomy, which required discrete elevation of the SMAS. Prior to its adoption, extensive SMAS dissection anterior to the parotid gland was thought necessary to invoke significant change in overall facial contour. However, this dissection was known to put facial nerve branches at higher risk. Advocates of the lateral SMASectomy approach argued that extensive SMAS dissection was not necessary in many patients, and that its risks outweighed the long-term benefits. Additional advantages of the lateral SMASectomy technique include decreased likelihood of tearing the superficial fascia and decreased postoperative dehiscence because SMAS flaps were not elevated. This rapid and relatively safe technique produces contouring of not only the nasolabial fold, but also the jowl and jawline. The lateral SMASectomy also generates a more superiorly oriented vector of lift.

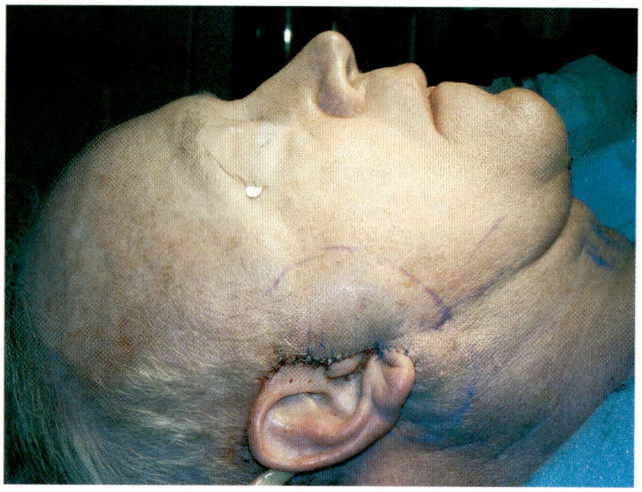

Fig. 5.10: Immediately after Penrose drain placement and skin closure

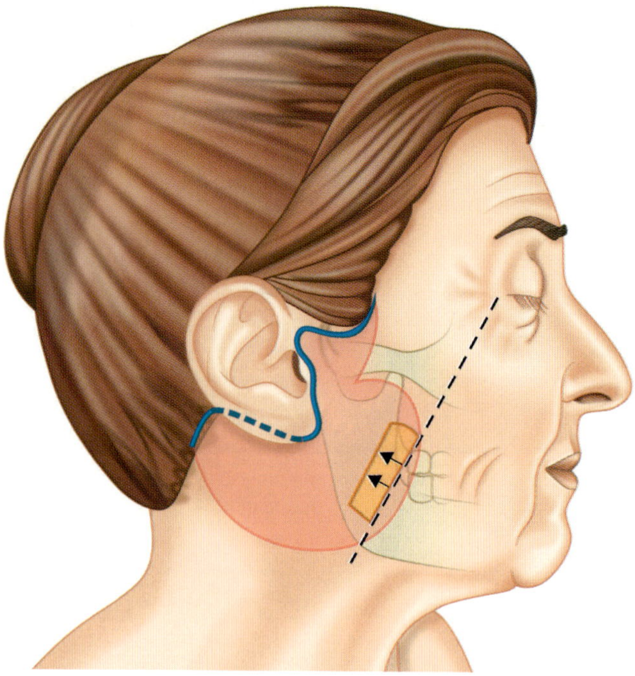

Fig. 5.11: Lateral SMASectomy requires a more modest skin flap elevation and superficial musculoaponeurotic system (SMAS) elevation

Incision Placement

Generally, the lateral SMASectomy is performed when a more vertical pull is desired and in cases of less skin redundancy. As such, the occipital extension of the standard SMAS face lift is usually omitted, with the incision typically ending in the postauricular crease at the level of the external auditory meatus or just slightly higher. The anterior portion of the incision is also quite similar to that in a SMAS face lift, although again typically shorter and with substantially less extension into the temporal hairline.

Extent of Undermining/Dissection

Typically, the lateral SMASectomy face lift uses a shorter skin flap than the SMAS face lift, with flaps extending 4–8 cm from the incision (Fig. 5.11). It is important that the flap is undermined sufficiently to expose the lateral SMAS.

Tissue Modifications

- *Incision*: A line is drawn from the lateral canthus to the mandibular angle, and the SMAS along the portion of this line between the lower aspect of the malar eminence and the angle of the mandible is incised. This effectively places the incision at the medial edge of Loré's Fascia (LF), a relatively fixed structure, and parallel to the nasolabial fold (Fig. 5.12). If additional neck contouring is desired, the inferior aspect of this incision can be extended inferior to run along the posterior border of the platysma.
- *Excision*: A rectangular window of SMAS 1–2 cm in width anterior to this incision is then undermined and excised. It is important to remain above the parotidomasseteric fascia for enhanced protection of the facial nerve branches as well as to reduce the risk of sialocele.
- *Tissue advancement*: As with the SMAS face lift, the edge of the SMAS is grasped with forceps and the optimal vector of elevation is determined; typically this more superolateral than in a standard SMAS lift.
- *Suturing*: The edge of the SMAS is then sutured to LF with multiple 3-0 polydioxanone suture. As the medial SMAS is typically more mobile than the lateral SMAS, the medial cheek tissues are elevated and securely resuspended.

Closure

- *Skin excision/burrows triangles*: As with the SMAS face lift, once the SMAS is suspended, the skin can easily be redraped and excess skin noted, marked and excised. Again, pilot cuts and temporary stay sutures at the superior aspects of the preauricular and postauricular incisions can be placed, allowing for more accurate determination of redundant skin. Also, defatting of the skin to overlie the tragus should be performed as well.
- *Layers/sutures*: As with the SMAS face lift, the lateral SMASectomy incision is closed in layers, with 3-0 Vicryl sutures dermally and 4-0 chromic sutures

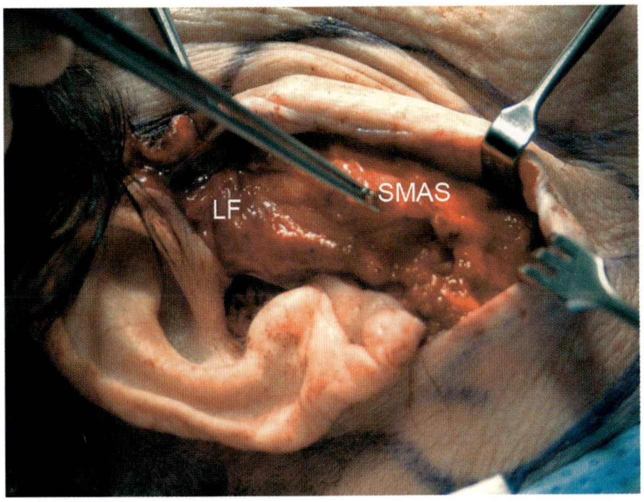

Fig. 5.12: Superficial musculoaponeurotic system (SMAS) flap and Loré's fascia (LF) noted

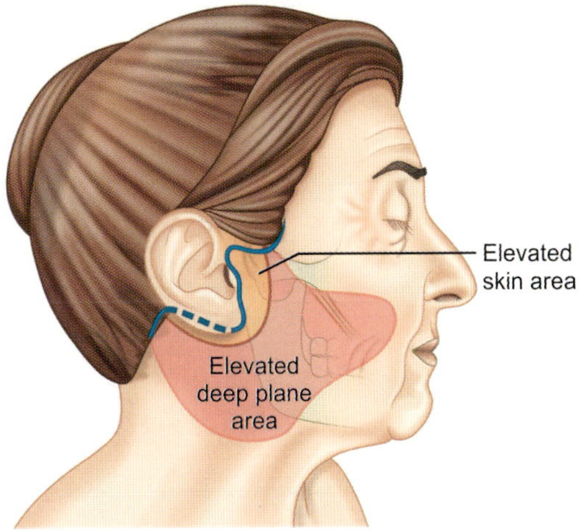

Fig. 5.13: Deep plane rhytidectomy dissection planes

in the postauricular crease. Again, post-tragal closure is accomplished with 6-0 chromic suture and the preauricular skin is closed with running or interrupted 6-0 polypropylene sutures.

- *Drains*: Active or passive drains can be used, although the undermined flap is smaller than with a SMAS face lift. Some surgeons opt to use fibrin glue or platelet rich plasma in lieu of drains.
- *Dressings*: The same dressing as after SMAS face lift is used to provide mild compression of the elevated flap against the underlying vascular bed.

Deep Plane Face Lift

The deep plane face lift addresses both the neck and lower face, and can be combined with other procedures such as submental liposuction, platysmaplasty and augmentation mentoplasty. Redundant skin may then be excised at this point without creating tension in the flaps.

Incision Placement

Standard temporal, preauricular and postauricular incisions similar to those used in the SMAS face lift are made extending from the temporal hairline, around the ear and into the occiput.

Extent of Undermining/Dissection

A short subcutaneous flap is then elevated that extends approximately 3 cm anterior to the tragus, staying posterior to a line drawn from the angle of the mandible to the lateral canthus, thereby exposing only LF.

Tissue Modifications

- *Incision*: A J-shaped vertical strip of SMAS is then incised, taking care to stay posterior to the course of the temporal branch of the facial nerve. The sub-SMAS plane is then entered and elevated inferiorly, dividing the zygomaticocutaneous and mandubulocutaneous ligaments. The plane is developed down into the subplatysmal plane, approximately 3–5 cm below the margin of the mandible (Fig. 5.13). The division of these ligaments allows for complete mobilization of the deep plane flap. More superiorly, the zygomaticus major muscle is identified below the malar eminence. The flap is then elevated over the muscle, in a superior to inferior fashion, avoiding injury to the zygomatic branch of cranial nerve VII (CN VII). Face lift scissors are spread in a vertical fashion to dissect the sub-SMAS plane parallel to the branches of the facial nerve (Fig. 5.14). The subplatysmal plane can be elevated far medially, but does not have to be carried across midline.
- *Tissue advancement*: Traction is then applied to the composite skin-SMAS-platysma flap in a superolateral direction, to create an initial vector parallel to and just below the axis of the mandibular ramus. The vector of elevation in the cheek is usually along a line running from the oral commissure to helical root. The short skin flap is similarly advanced.
- *Suturing*: The mobilized free edge of the SMAS-platysma flap is secured to the mastoid periosteum with interrupted 3-0 polydioxanone sutures posteriorly, and with the same sutures to LF in the preauricular area.

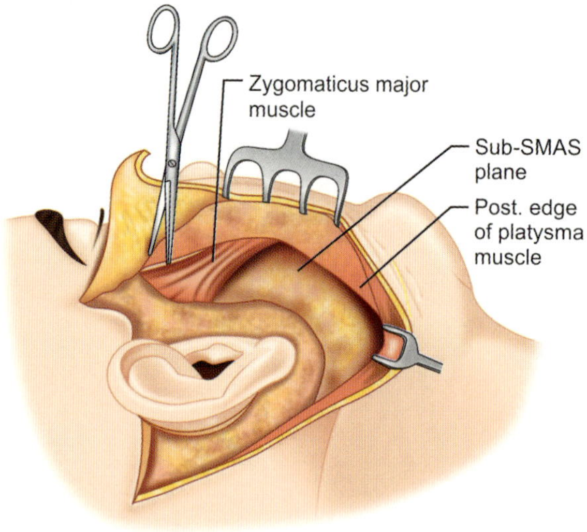

Fig. 5.14: After a short skin flap is developed, the superficial muscular aponeurotic system (SMAS) is incised and a sub-SMAS dissection performed. Dissection progresses over the zygomaticus major muscle

Closure

- *Skin excision*: After the flap is advanced, redundant skin can be assessed and the amount of skin resection determined. Contrary to the face lift procedures with separate skin and SMAS flaps, the deep plane face lift flap can tolerate a modest amount of tension on the skin closure due to its robust vascularity. As with the SMAS face lift, temporary tension sutures can be placed at strategic locations, allowing a more accurate assessment of skin to be made. Skin is excised and the flap thinned appropriately as necessary, such as the tragal skin coverage.
- *Layers/sutures*: The wound is closed in layers, with 3-0 Vicryl sutures dermally and 4-0 chromic sutures postauricularly. The tragus is closed with 6-0 chromic sutures and the preauricular skin is closed with running or interrupted 6-0 polypropylene sutures.
- *Drains*: Active or passive drains can be used for the first 24 hours.
- *Dressings*: A mildly compressive dressing is applied for the first 24 hours and followed by an elastic support garment.

Corset Platysmaplasty

Platysmaplasty is useful in patients with platysmal banding to create a more defined cervicomental angle and jawline. Ideal candidates are those with good skin elasticity, mild to moderate neck ptosis and thin skin. The procedure can be conducted under local anesthesia in qualified patients, removing the associated morbidity with general anesthesia. As with many techniques, platysmaplasty is often employed in conjunction with submental liposuction. Not only does this union allow for improved defatting of the neck, liposuction also aids in undermining the cervical skin in a relatively atraumatic fashion. Corset platysmaplasty can be used in concert with laterally-based face lift techniques.

Incision Placement

In the upright position, the anterior borders of the SCM muscles, the jawline, jowls, left and right bands of platysma muscle, and thyroid cartilage are identified and marked out on the skin. A 4 cm submental incision is made after infiltration with local anesthetic.

Extent of Undermining/Dissection

A subcutaneous plane is developed through a process of blunt and sharp dissection. Scissors are advanced just below the dermis, the blades spread open and the scissor withdrawn. The soft tissue bridges are then divided sharply, creating a dissection pocket ranging from the submental incision down to the thyroid notch and between the anterior edges of the SCM muscles.

Tissue Modifications

- *Incision*: The medial edges of the platysma are identified. Each side of the muscle can then be horizontally transected at the level of the hyoid (Fig. 5.15).
- *Excision*: In patients with particularly heavy platysmal bands, a strip of muscle from each medial edge can be excised and the subsequent raw edges cauterized.
- *Suturing*: A running suture of 3-0 polydioxanone is then used to bring the two edges of platysma together in the midline from the submental zone down to the thyroid notch. The running suture is then returned superiorly with wider tissue bites, and tied in the submental region. This is the corset portion of the procedure, which creates a double layer plication producing a smooth midline surface and superior tightening of the cervicomental angle. This anterior approach not only contours the submental region, but it also may correct submandibular ptosis. Oblique plication of the platysma in bilateral submandibular regions tightens the lateral platysma muscle, thus elevating ptotic submandibular glands. One technique employs a running locking suture from proximal to distal and a running "baseball-type" stitch from distal to proximal. This can be augmented with the

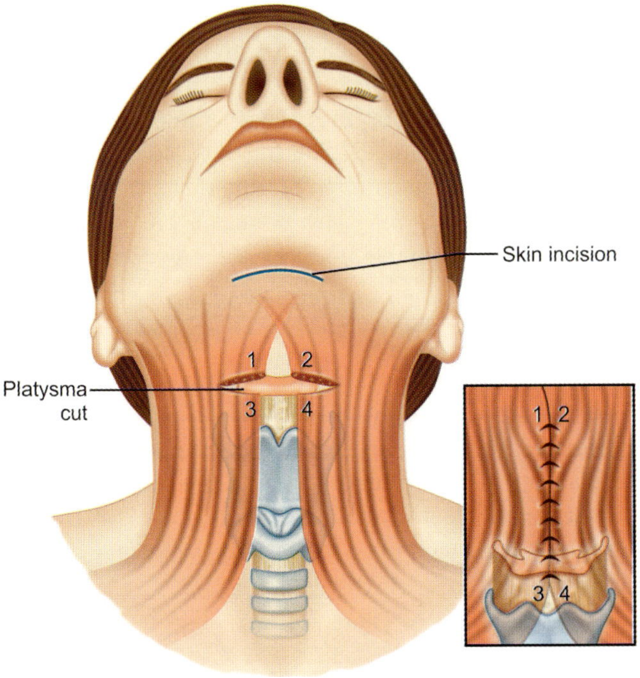

Fig. 5.15: Platysmaplasty included partial transverse transection of the medial edge of the platysma at the level of the hyoid and closure with a running suture

use of interlocking sling sutures from the right and left submental crease to the opposite mastoid process.

Closure

- *Layers/sutures*: The incision is then closed with 5-0 Vicryl dermal sutures and superficial 6-0 polypropylene sutures.
- *Dressings*: A postoperative compressive garment is then worn with frequent surveillance to ensure proper skin redraping.

POTENTIAL COMPLICATIONS

Risks of face lift surgery include hematoma, skin necrosis, scar widening, hypertrophy or keloid formation, hairline irregularities, alopecia, sensory nerve injuries, motor nerve injuries, infections, earlobe deformity and parotid gland injury. It is essential to obtain an informed consent for the procedure and to discuss with the patient preoperatively the risk of complications.

Hematoma

Hematoma is the most common complication of face lift surgery, occurring in 2–15% of patients. Risk factors include anticoagulant (including aspirin and nonsteroidal anti-inflammatory drug) use, hypertension and male sex. Patients should be taken off anticoagulants 2 weeks prior to surgery, if possible, and special care should be taken to avoid perioperative hypertension. Smooth emergence from anesthesia, avoiding coughing, gagging and straining, is also important to reduce the incidence of hematoma. An expanding hematoma generally is managed in the operation room (OR), removing clots, irrigating the wound and searching for a bleeding vessel, but often only diffuse oozing is found. Suspicious vessels should be cauterized or ligated, and suction drains and a pressure dressing should be applied. Major, nonexpanding hematomas can often be expressed through the postauricular incision line; a suture is removed and the wound opened. Minor hematomas can often be aspirated sterilely with an 18 gauge needle after the clot has liquefied (typically between 7 days and 10 days). All patients with a hematoma should be placed on 10–14 days course of oral antibiotics. Untreated hematomas, even minor ones, can lead to persistent skin discoloration, puckering and fibrosis.

Skin Necrosis

Skin necrosis occurs because of impaired circulation to the skin flap. Smoking greatly increases the risk of skin necrosis by a factor of 10, and the patient should refrain from smoking for 2–6 weeks prior to surgery and for an additional 2–4 weeks after surgery. If there is any concern that the patient is still smoking on the day of surgery, urine cotinine (a nicotine metabolite) can be rapidly measured. Other risk factors include long skin flap, peripheral vascular disease, connective tissue disorders and tension on the skin closure all raise the risk of skin necrosis. If an area of venous congestion develops, the area should be gently massaged frequently and the patient kept on antibiotics. If an eschar develops, the wound should be managed conservatively and followed closely until the wound achieves a satisfactory appearance.

Scar Issues

Issues related to the scar, such as scar widening, hypertrophy or keloid formation, hairline irregularities can ruin the outcome of an otherwise successful procedure. Excessive tension on the skin closure can lead to widening of the scar, scar hypertrophy and has been associated with keloid formation. Tension on the mobilized tissues should be borne by the deeper tissues, such as the SMAS, to reduce the risk of these complications. It is essential that when closing the temporal and occipital portions of the wound that attention is given to re-establishing a regular hairline and avoiding a step-off of the hairline. Temporary hair loss postoperatively, telogen effluvium, may occur but generally resolves in a few months; more permanent hair loss can occur, but this is generally due to transection of hair follicles or excessive wound tension.

Pixie Ear Deformity

An unstabilized earlobe will be pulled inferiorly by scar contraction postoperatively and lead to a "pixie ear" or "satyr ear" deformity. Suturing the deep tissues up to the inferior conchal bowl can secure the position of the earlobe, but if this deformity occurs a V-Y advancement is often necessary.

Nerve Injuries

The most commonly injured nerve during face lift surgery is the great auricular nerve, generally as it courses superiorly along the anterior SCM muscle, estimated to occur in 5-7% of patients. Motor (facial) nerve injuries are less common, occurring in 1-3% of patients. The two most common nerves injured are the temporal branch and the marginal mandibular branch of the facial nerve. Injury to the former causes an ipsilateral brow ptosis and paralysis, while injury to the latter will lead to an inability to properly evert the lateral lower lip and alter the smile. Paralysis noted once the patient awakens should be observed for a period of time sufficient for resolution of the effect of local anesthetic; if paralysis is still noted, surgical exploration and neurorrhaphy is generally not successful, but many of these injuries may be neuropraxic rather than from neurolysis and approximately 85% resolve over time. The temporal branches generally are at risk as they cross the midportion of the zygomatic arch with multiple rami, while the marginal mandibular nerve is at greatest risk once it crosses the mandibular border at the posterior edge of the prejowl sulcus. During a deep plane face lift, the sub-SMAS dissection follows the inferior border of the malar eminence over the zygomaticus major muscle. During this dissection, buccal branches may be encountered superficially anterior to the parotid gland; generally, sequelae are uncommon due to the interconnections of the upper and lower buccal branches.

Parotid Gland Injury

The proper dissection place over the parotid gland is below the SMAS and over the parotidomasseteric fascia. Injury or dissection deep to the fascia can lead to salivary leak and sialocele. These can be treated with aspiration and pressure dressings but may require open surgery.

AFTERCARE

After face lift surgery, patients should refrain from tobacco use for 2–4 weeks. An elastic face support typically works for the first week, and then nightly for an additional 3 weeks. Patients should expect moderate swelling for several weeks and should be told that they will be "presentable" some time between 3 weeks and 6 weeks after surgery.

BIBLIOGRAPHY

1. Baker DC. Complications of cervicofacial rhytidectomy. Clin Plast Surg. 1983;10(3):543-62.
2. Mitz V, Peyronnie M. The superficial musculo-aponeurotic system (SMAS) in the parotid and cheek area. Plast Reconstr Surg. 1976;58(1):80-8.
3. Pepper JP, Baker SR. SMAS flap rhytidectomy. Arch Facial Plast Surg. 2011;13(2):108.
4. Sykes JM, Liang J, Kim JE. Contemporary deep plane rhytidectomy. Facial Plast Surg. 2011;27(1):124-32.

CHAPTER 6

Blepharoplasty

Anthony P Sclafani

OVERVIEW

The eyes are a central focus of one's appearance, and distortion or disruption of the normal position, shapes, convexities and concavities of the eyelids may age a person's appearance (Fig. 6.1). A well-performed blepharoplasty will restore these contours to a youthful appearance (Fig. 6.2)

SPECIAL CONSIDERATIONS

The eyelids are delicate, three-dimensional structures with specific functions that, if disrupted, may lead to chronic dry eye, pain, vision disturbance. As upper lid movement accounts for 90% of eye closure, proper functioning and sufficient skin of the upper eyelid is necessary to prevent corneal exposure. Excessive upper lid skin should be distinguished preoperatively from eyelid ptosis or pseudoptosis caused by eyebrow ptosis (Fig. 6.3). Similarly, in the lower eyelid, "bags" under the eyes must be properly diagnosed as either skin redundancy or orbital fat pads or distinguished from lower lid laxity, suborbital hollowing and skeletonization of the infraorbital rim and malar bags. The "negative vector" eye, in which the cornea projects further anteriorly than the maxilla, is particularly at risk for postoperative lower eyelid retraction (Fig. 6.4). Lower lid support should be assessed with a "pinch" or "snap" test; lower lid laxity should be addressed with either a lateral canthoplasty or lateral retinacular suspension, depending on its severity.

ALTERNATIVES TO PROCEDURE

When evaluating a patient for upper lid blepharoplasty, the surgeon should consider whether the patient's issues are better addressed by ptosis repair. If there is coincident

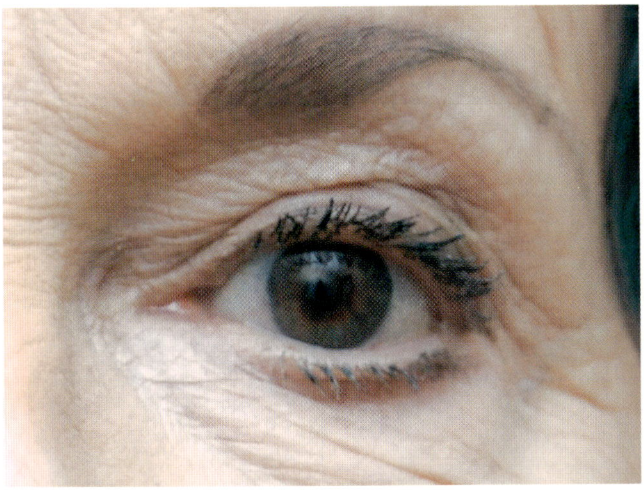

Fig. 6.1: The aging upper eyelid shows fine, loose, redundant skin, as well as pseudoherniated fat, seen here in the above the medial canthus. The aging lower lid is characterized by fine redundant skin and pseudoherniated fat pads. The lower lid, while not showing frank malposition, is rounded laterally

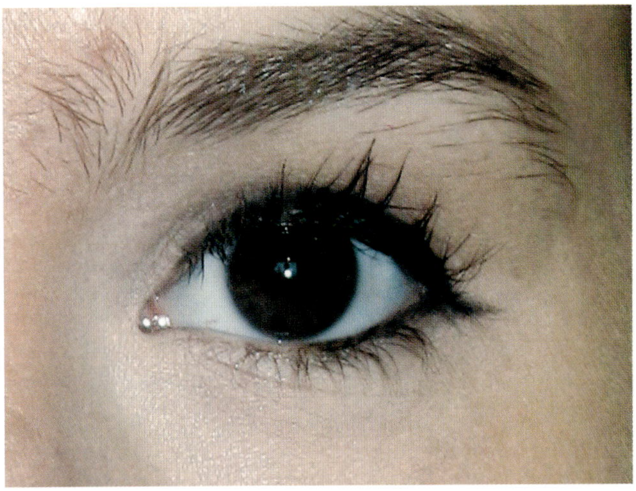

Fig. 6.2: The youthful upper lid is full without redundancy, with a subtle supratarsal crease. The lower lid is smooth and short, forming a smooth junction with the cheek

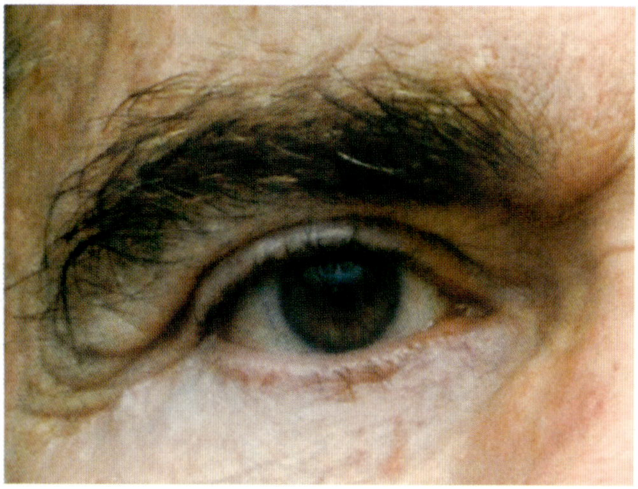

Fig. 6.3: Brow ptosis will force thicker, infrabrow skin to slide down over the upper lid

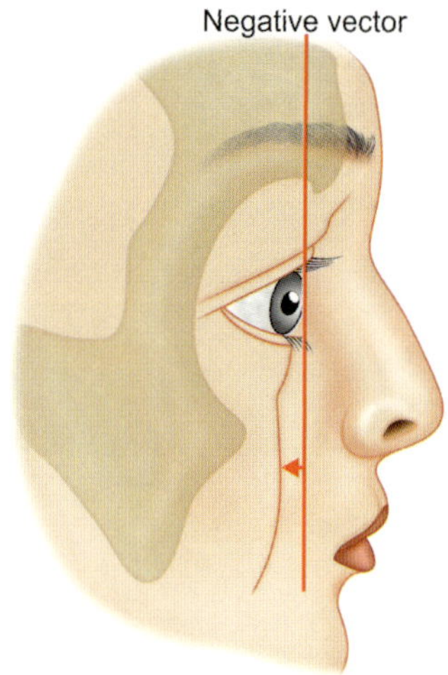

Fig. 6.4: The anterior extent of the cornea in the negative vector eye extends beyond the cheek

brow ptosis present, the eyelid should be evaluated when brow has been manually elevated to an aesthetic position; a brow lift can be performed in addition to or instead of an upper blepharoplasty as indicated. In the lower lid, fine lines can be treated with botulinum toxin A or skin resurfacing techniques such as chemical peels or laser skin resurfacing. Mild convexities caused by pseudoherniated orbital fat pads can be treated by tightening the lower eyelid skin with skin resurfacing techniques or soft tissue fillers; more significant deformities require removal or repositioning of the pseudoherniated fat. These convexities may be accentuated by associated infraorbital hollowing, which can be treated with a midface lift. Lower lid rounding and laxity can impart significant aging on a patient's appearance, and can be treated with a lateral canthopexy or canthoplasty.

TECHNIQUES

Upper Eyelid Blepharoplasty

Incision Placement

The upper lid skin incision is placed so that the lower limb of the ellipse (and thus the ultimate scar) rests along the supratarsal crease. The incision limb on the supratarsal crease is marked first; if there is an ill-defined crease, it should be found between 8 mm and 12 mm from the lashes in women and 6–10 mm in men. With the eyes closed and the brow manually elevated by the surgeon to the appropriate height, smooth forceps are used to grasp clearly redundant skin, and the superior edge of the planned skin excision is marked sequentially across the eyelid. While it is preferable to avoid extending the incision across the lateral orbital rim, skin redundancy generally requires it. Lateral to the canthus, the inferior limb of the incision sweeps superolaterally and rests within a crow's feet rhytid, if present, with the superior limb following appropriately (Figs 6.5A and B). Local anesthetic is injected subcutaneously, using 1–2 cc per upper lid. The skin is then incised with a #15 scalpel, and sharp Iris scissors are used to dissect the skin from the underlying orbicularis oculi muscle. In patients with relatively thin skin, hyaluronidase (5–7.5 units/cc) can be mixed with the local anesthetic prior to injection. This will allow the skin to be grasped with a fine forceps and "crimped" along the planned incisions with a von Graefe forceps, creating a "roll" of skin pedicled on the eyelid; the crimping apposes the upper and lower incision lines (Figs 6.6A and B). A sharp Iris scissor is used to directly excise this roll of skin at its junction with the remainder of the upper lid, and if done gently, the skin edges of the incision remain apposed and bleeding is minimal (Figs 6.7A to D). The skin edges are then gently and sequentially separated with sterile cotton applicators in a nasal to temporal direction, and all bleeding is controlled with a bipolar forceps cautery.

Extent of Undermining/Dissection

The tissues of the upper lid are easily retracted and significant undermining is not required.

Tissue Modifications

- *Excision*: If not already removed with the skin, a strip of orbicularis muscle is removed below the inferior limb

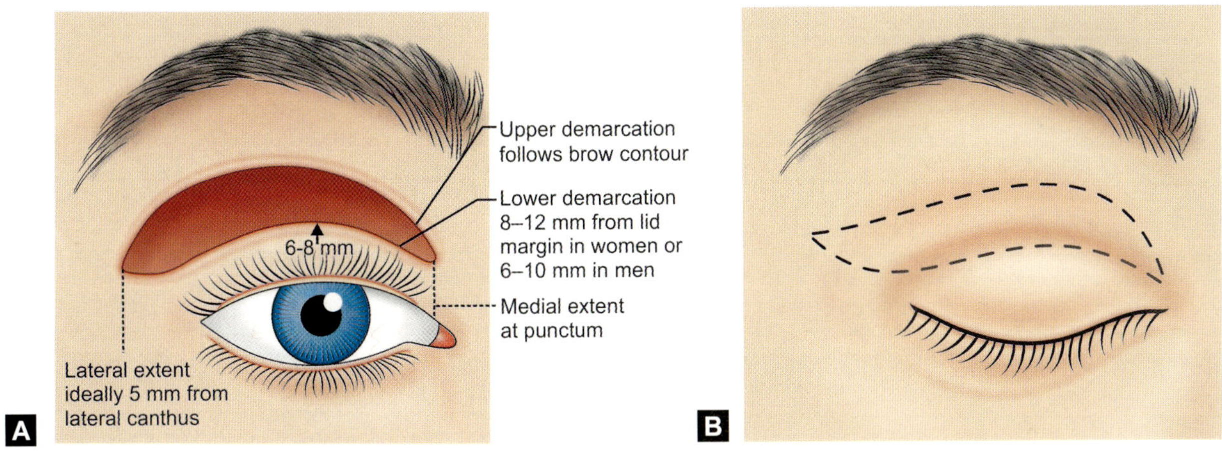

Figs 6.5A and B: Typical skin resection in upper lid blepharoplasty

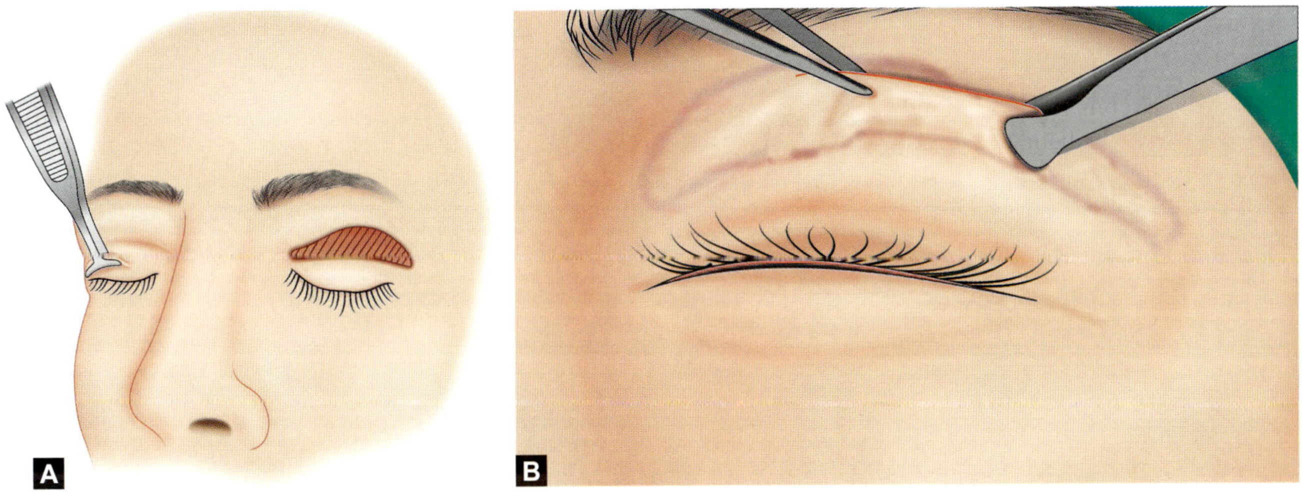

Figs 6.6A and B: The upper lid skin marked for excision is crimped with a von Graefe forceps, forming a discrete roll of skin

of the incision for added definition of the supratarsal crease and to expose the orbital septum (Fig. 6.8). Once the septum has been exposed, soft tissues can be gently swept superiorly for better visualization. With the upper eyelid held closed, gentle pressure is applied to the globe with a finger just above the lashes (this pressure is intermittently released and held only when necessary) and the supratarsal area observed for bulging of orbital fat pads. The nasal fat pad is distinguishable from the other orbital fat pads by its lighter, whitish-yellow color. The nasal fat pad is identified and the soft tissue over it is grasped with a forceps and lightly cauterized with the bipolar cautery (Fig. 6.9). The cauterized tissue is incised with Iris scissors, and the process is repeated until gentle pressure causes fat to herniate through the incision. This fat is then grasped and associated soft tissue swept back into the orbit gently with a cotton applicator (Fig. 6.10). Vessels associated with the fat are cauterized and divided while the fat is gently teased out further. Once the fat can be advanced no further with gentle traction, a mosquito hemostat can be applied at its base at the orbital septum. This clamp should be held gently by an assistant to avoid traction on more posterior structures while a #15 scalpel is used to excise the fat and the stump cauterized prior to releasing the hemostat. Alternatively, the author prefers to simply cauterize the stump with a bipolar cautery (Fig. 6.11) and cut with a sharp iris scissor sequentially instead of applying the clamp, as this makes it easier to identify and cauterize small vessels that may retract behind the orbital septum when

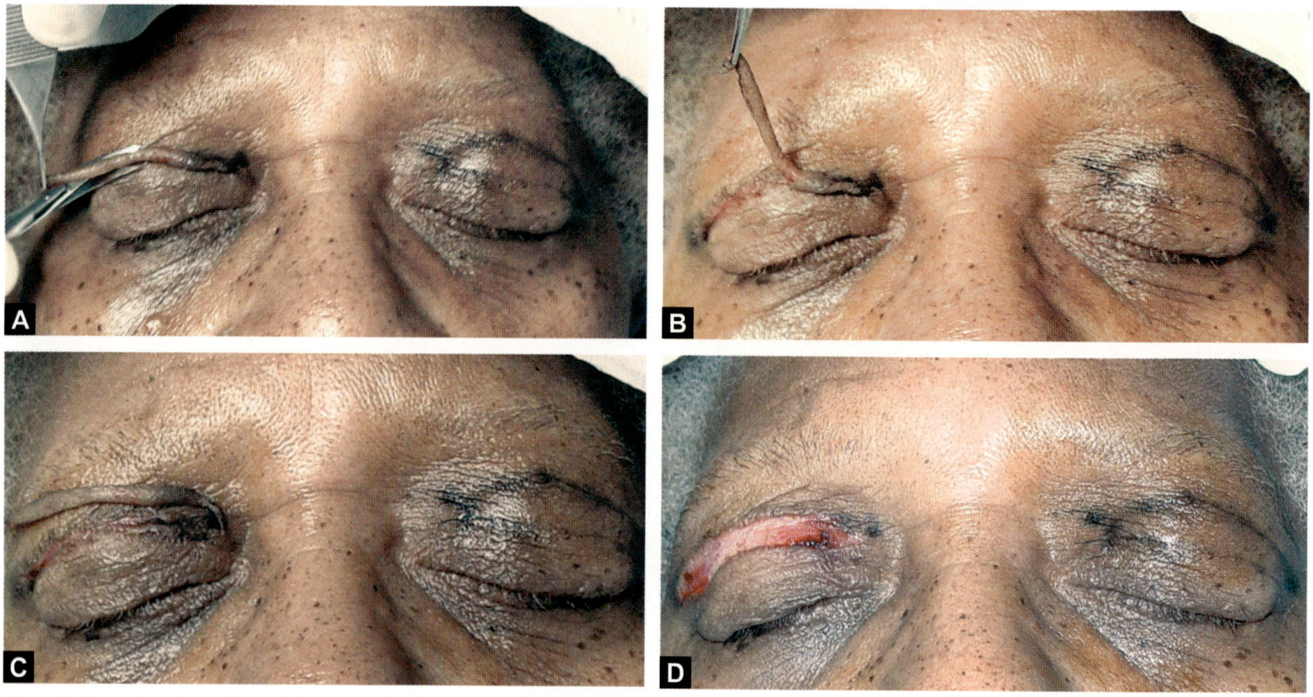

Figs 6.7A to D: Once the roll is formed, (A) curved iris scissors are used to excise the redundant skin; (B) If care is taken, redundant skin is precisely excised, skin edges stay opposed and bleeding is minimal, even when; (C) the skin is fully excised. (D) The wound edges can then gently be separated and any bleeding vessels cauterized

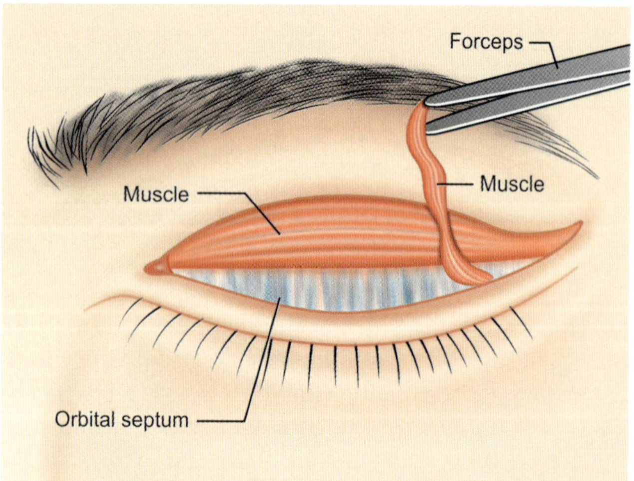

Fig. 6.8: After skin excision, a strip of orbicularis oculi muscle just above the tarsus is resected, and the orbital septum is exposed

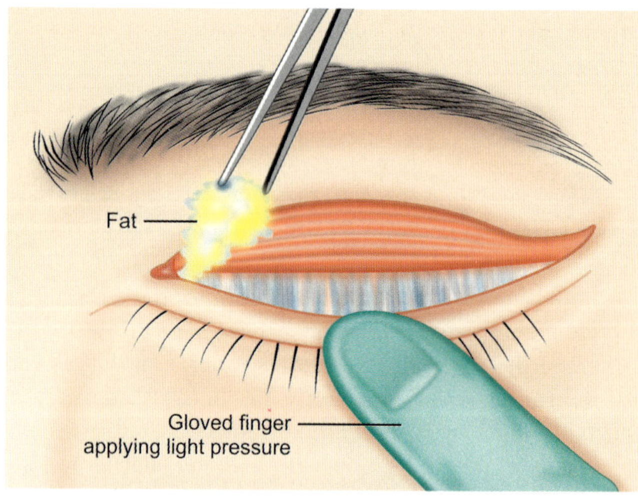

Fig. 6.9: With gentle palpation over the closed eyelid, bulges corresponding to the orbital fat pads are identified. The septum is grasped, cauterized and incised to expose the fat

pressure on the globe is released. It is important that the assistant maintain light pressure on the globe after the fat has been divided in order that the stump remains visible so hemostasis is ensured prior to allowing it to retract behind the septum. Attention is then directed towards the central fat pad, where the same steps are repeated.

- *Suturing*: Fullness of the lateral upper lid may be caused by a ptotic lacrimal gland. The orbital septum is opened and the caudal portion of the gland is exposed. A 4-0 polypropylene suture is passed through the gland capsule and then sutured to orbital periosteum on the inner aspect of the superior orbital rim.

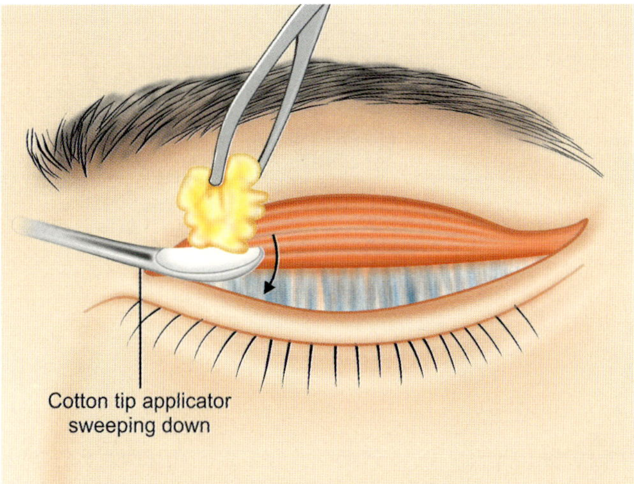

Fig. 6.10: The fat is grasped and dissected away from surrounding soft tissue with a cotton-tipped applicator, cauterizing any blood vessels during dissection

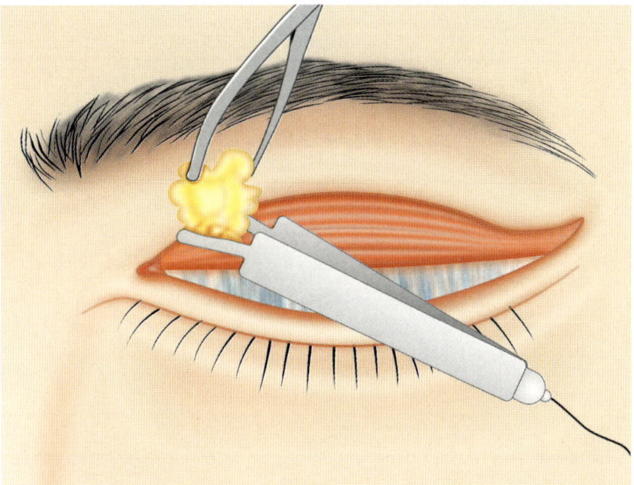

Fig. 6.11: Once the fat has been fully dissected, the base is cauterized and divided at the level of the orbital septum

- Closure
- *Layers*: Upper lid closure is performed in a single layer. Simple 6-0 fast absorbing gut sutures are first placed to approximate and align the skin edges at the medial and lateral limbuses and above the lateral canthus. A 6-0 polypropylene suture is then passed through the skin adjacent to the medial end of the incision; this suture then closes the wound in a subcuticular fashion until exiting through the skin adjacent to the lateral end of the incision (Fig. 6.12). After gentle traction is applied to the suture ends, these are taped down rather than tied, facilitating suture removal. The thicker skin lateral to the lateral orbital rim may require supplemental simple 6-0 polypropylene sutures.

Lower Eyelid Blepharoplasty

Incision Placement

- *Subciliary*: In cases where sufficient excess lower lid skin exists to warrant skin excision, a subciliary incision is used. A small volume of local anesthetic (2% lidocaine with 1:200,000 epinephrine) is injected subcutaneously along the planned incision. Beginning medially below the medial punctum, an incision 2–3 mm below the lashes is made and extended laterally along the lid and into a lateral orbital rhytid, extending up to 1 cm lateral to the canthus (Fig. 6.13). Further handling of the lid skin is done based on the degree of anticipated skin resection.
  - *Skin flap*: In cases with significant excess skin, a skin flap can be raised, carefully elevating the lower lid skin from the orbicularis oculi muscle. Bleeding is generally more significant than with a skin-muscle flap, and should be carefully controlled with an electrocautery. The skin flap is elevated down to the level of the inferior orbital rim.
  - *Skin-muscle flap*: Most subciliary cases are amenable to a skin-muscle flap. This technique provides access to the orbital fat pads and allows for skin resection, but also preserves the lower lid sling support provided by preserving orbicularis oculi muscle along the lid margin. The subciliary skin incision is made from medial to lateral, incising only skin with a #15 scalpel. At the lateral orbital rim, blunt spreading with a Stevens scissors in a vertical direction splits the fibers of the orbicularis oculi muscle until the orbital rim periosteum is exposed. The scissor tips are then turned medially and a submuscular plane is developed below the skin incision. Finally, with one blade of the scissors external and one blade in the deep pocket, the incision is completed to fully divide the tissues at the skin incision (Figs 6.14A to D). By angling the scissors such that the deep blade of the scissors is caudal to the incision, the muscle is split to leave a strip along the upper border of the incision (Fig. 6.15). This plane is followed inferiorly to the orbital rim.
- *Transconjunctival*: In cases where little to no skin excess exists, a transconjunctival approach is used.

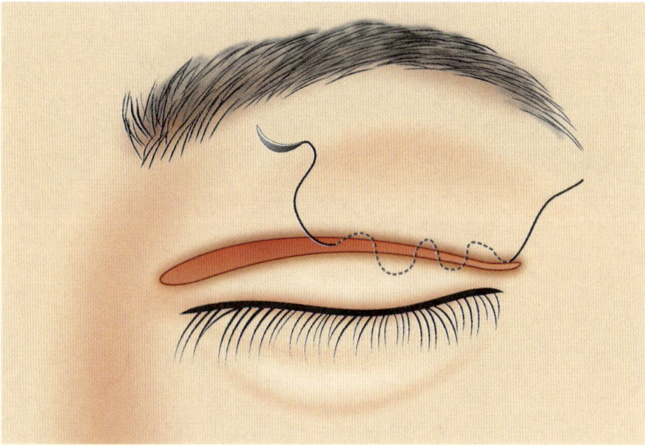

Fig. 6.12: The upper lid incision is closed with a running subcuticular suture taped externally

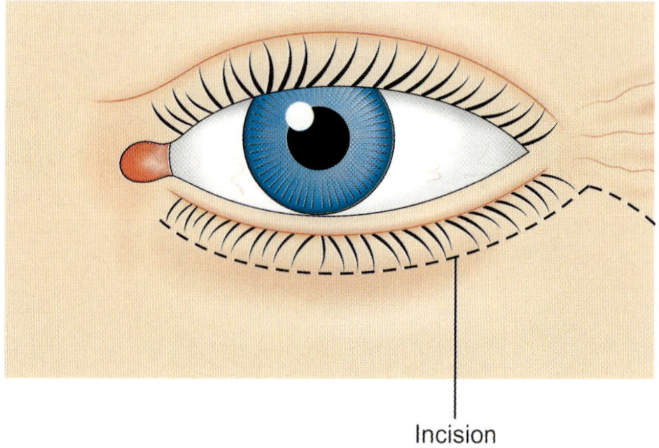

Fig. 6.13: The subciliary incision is made 2–3 mm below the lashes, from just below the inferior punctum medially to run in an inferior crow's feet rhytid laterally

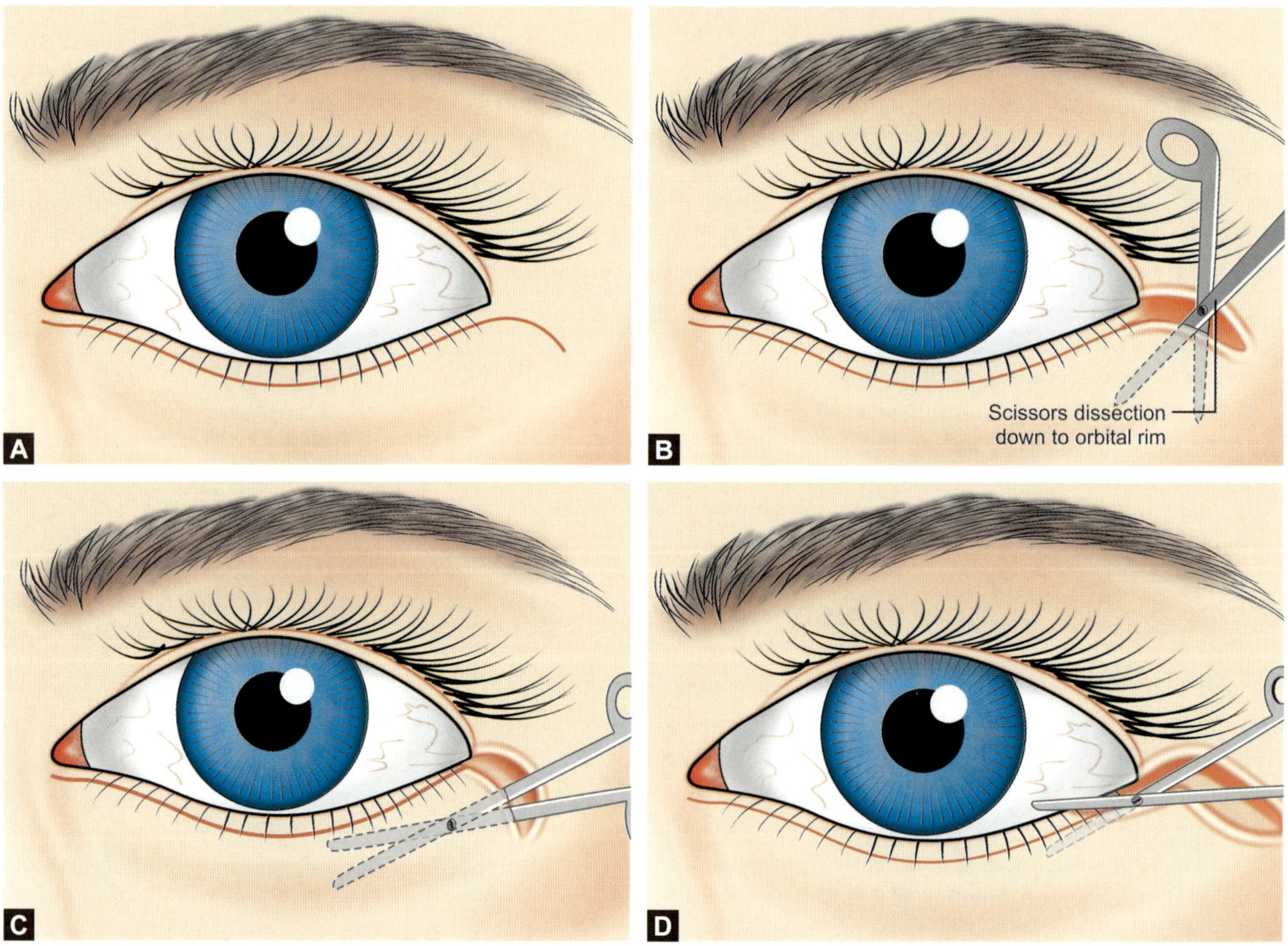

Figs 6.14A to D: (A) A skin-muscle flap lower blepharoplasty begins with a subciliary skin incision usually extending into a lateral orbital rhytid; (B) Scissors are used to bluntly divide the orbicularis muscle and define the lateral orbital rim; (C) The scissors are turned medially while remaining in a preseptal, submuscular plane, and blunt dissection progresses to the medial extent of the incision; (D) The scissors are used to divide the soft tissue below the incision. The scissor is angled so that the external blade is closer to the lid margin than the lower blade, ensuring that a strip of muscle is left along the upper margin of the incision for lid support

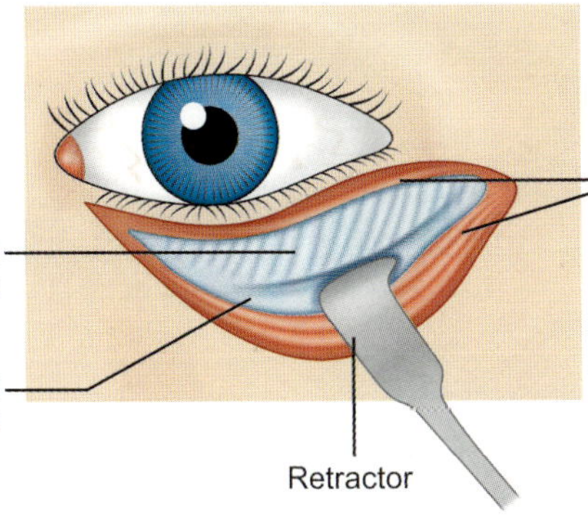

Fig. 6.15: After completing the skin-muscle flap dissection, the lower eyelid flap can be retracted inferiorly to expose the orbital septum down to the level of the inferior orbital rim

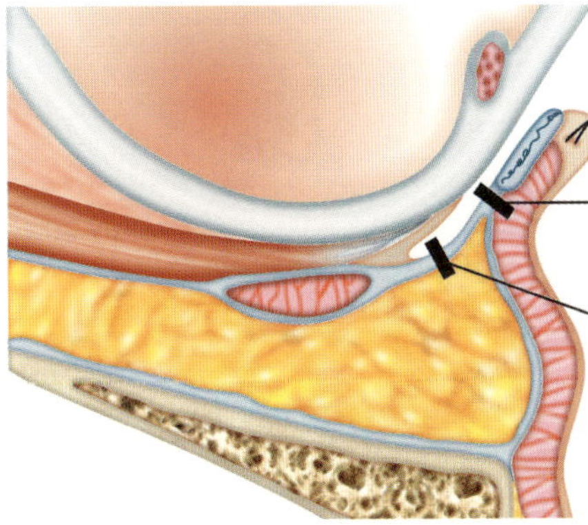

Fig. 6.16: Transconjunctival lower blepharoplasty can be performed either pre- or retroseptally. Preseptal dissection begins with an incision just below the inferior border of the tarsus and entering the preseptal plane. The retroseptal incision is made closer to the fornix and directly exposes the orbital fat pads

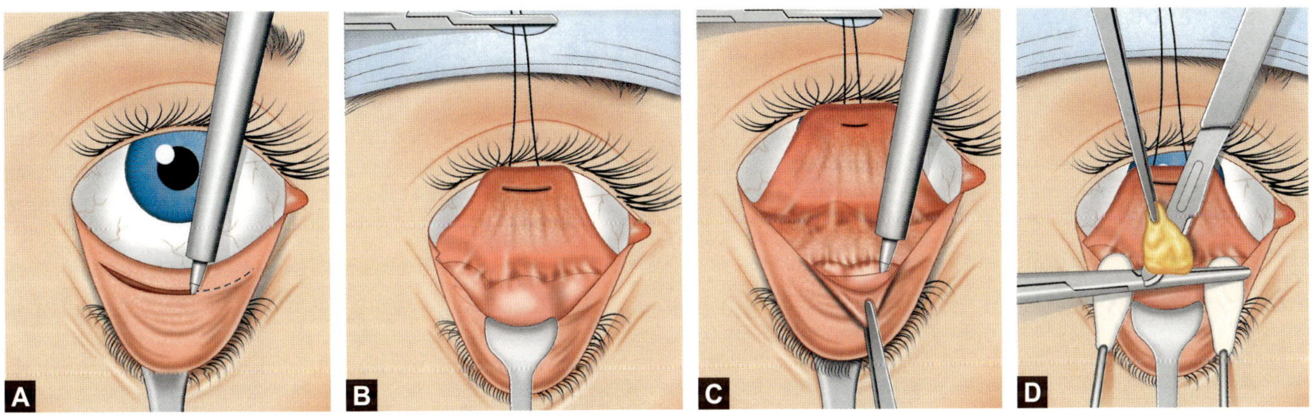

Figs 6.17A to D: If a preseptal dissection is performed, a transconjunctival flap can be developed and retracted superiorly to serve as a corneal protector

Local anesthetic is infiltrated into the conjunctiva at the level of the lower tarsal border if a preseptal approach is planned, or at the fornix if this approach is used. (It should be remembered that the transfornix approach, while more direct, may be associated with greater lower lid retraction postoperatively) (Fig. 6.16). The lower lid is retracted and everted with a wide double-hook and the lower border of the tarsus is identified. The conjunctiva in the midline is grasped with a 0.5 mm Bishop-Harmon forceps and cauterized with a small bipolar cautery. This tissue is then incised and sharp curved Iris scissors are used bluntly to dissect medially and laterally below the conjunctiva. The scissors are removed and one arm of the bipolar is advanced into the pocket. The conjunctiva is then cauterized as the bipolar forceps are withdrawn, and the tissue is then sectioned with the Iris scissors. This is done progressively both medially and laterally until the incision is complete. By grasping the lower edge of the incision with a forceps, a plane above (external to) the orbital septum is easily developed with a cotton-tipped applicator and followed down to the orbital rim (Figs 6.17A to D). A 5-0 Prolene is placed at the edge of the flap and clamped to the head drape superiorly to draw this lower conjunctival flap superiorly to cover the cornea.

Tissue Modifications

- *Excision*: After incision and elevation, the orbital septum should be identified and entered. In the skin-muscle flap and transconjunctival approaches, the septum is the deep surface of the dissection plane. In the skin flap approach, the orbicularis oculi must be incised and parted (or a strip excised) to expose the septum below. If muscle is hypertrophic, a strip can be excised at the lower border of the tarsal plate; if

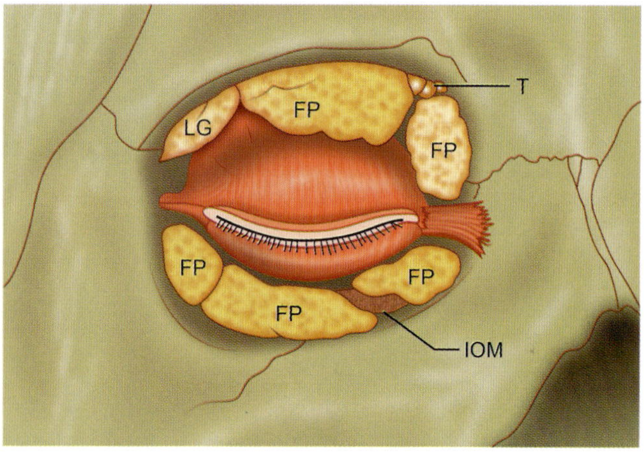

Fig. 6.18: Fat pads of the lower and upper lids. Note that the inferior oblique muscle (IOM) separates the nasal and central fat pads (FP) inferiorly

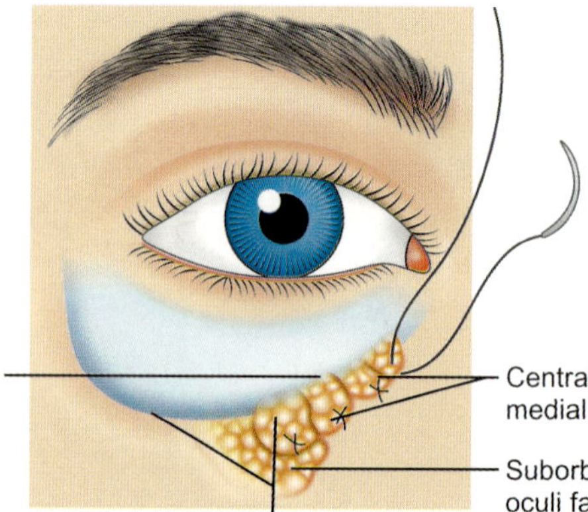

Fig. 6.19: Rather than resecting pseudoherniated orbital fat, it can be transposed and sutured to the periosteum below or through the skin above the tear trough

debulking is not necessary, the muscle is bluntly split. It is essential to obtain excellent hemostasis in each step to avoid hemorrhage and potential retrobulbar hematoma, and bleeding is meticulously controlled with fine bipolar forceps. The orbital septum is thus exposed. Gentle pressure on the upper lid and globe will better delineate the lower lid fat pads (Fig. 6.18). These are noted and the temporal fat pad is addressed first, as the temporal fat pad is often difficult to locate once the bulk of the central fat pad has been removed. The septum overlying the fat pad bulge is grasped with fine forceps, cauterized and incised. This is done sequentially deeper until all of the intervening layers of loose areolar tissue have been incised and the yellow orbital fat can easily be teased out with a fine forceps and a cotton applicator. Care is taken to cauterize and divide all layers of areolar tissue, or the fat will not fully mobilize. The base of the fat pad at the level of the orbital rim is then cauterized and cut with Iris scissors incrementally until only a thin connection remains. The base is then gently grasped with a forceps, avoiding traction on this tissue, which will be perceived by the patient as deep orbital pain. The connecting stalk is cauterized and cut, and then the stump is also cauterized to ensure exquisite hemostasis before allowing the stump to recede behind the septum. This process is then repeated for the central and nasal fat pads. Great care should be taken to avoid injury to the inferior oblique muscle, lying between the medial and central fat pads.

- *Suturing and tissue advancement*: Lower blepharoplasty has been criticized for overly hollowing the lower eyelid area. In reality, if properly performed, a lower lid blepharoplasty should not "hollow out" the lower eyelid. However, tear troughs and orbital hollowing from midfacial soft tissue atrophy and descent are often masked by pseudoherniation of orbital fat, and removal of orbital fat creates a wide, deep trough and a "hollow" appearance. In these cases, orbital fat can be transposed into the trough instead of resected. Once the fat has been fully mobilized, a 5-0 chromic suture is used to tack the fat inferiorly to the periosteum in the tear trough (Fig. 6.19). Alternatively, the suture through the fat can be passed through the skin at the appropriate location and tied over a bolster. The entire septum can be incised along the inferior orbital rim, "reset" inferiorly and sutured with 5-0 polyglactin 910 to the periosteum of the upper maxilla, allowing the orbital fat to prolapse inferiorly and fill the tear trough.
- *Skin excision and wound closure*: Once the orbital fat has been managed, skin resection is performed conservatively. For subciliary approaches, the lower lid is replaced into its anatomical position, and the skin (skin-muscle) flap is carefully redraped. If the surgery is performed under local anesthesia or light sedation, the patient is asked to direct his/her gaze upwards and the mouth is opened to put the eyelid skin on maximal stretch (Figs 6.20A and B). At this point, excess skin is marked and excised with scissors. If a transconjunctival approach has been used, skin excess is generally absent or minimal. However, a "pinch" excision can be performed if necessary, especially laterally. After the excess skin is marked and anesthetic infiltrated, the skin is grasped and pinched together at its base with a von Graefe fixation forceps or an Allis clamp; the skin is then excised at the base with iris scissors.

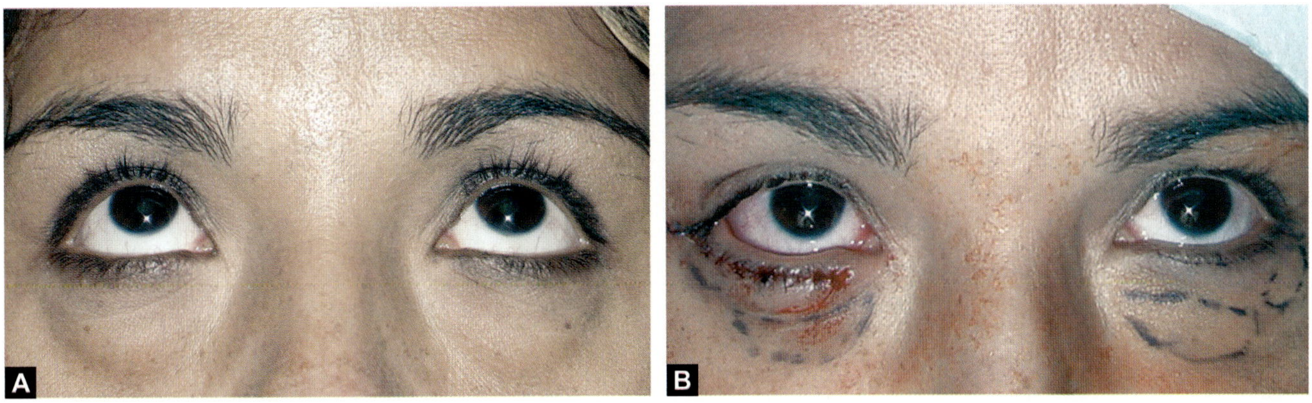

Figs 6.20A and B: (A) Preoperative and (B) intraoperative close-up view after blepharoplasty on the right eye was completed, with eyes directed upwards. Preoperatively, pseudoherniated fat pads are more easily seen in upgaze; postoperatively, skin resection is checked while the patient opens her eyes and mouth to put the lower skin on maximal tension. Note the mild right lower eyelid edema and slight intraoperative ectropion

- *Closure*: Wound closure is then performed, closing the subciliary incision by reapproximating the wound with interrupted 5-0 chromic sutures below the lashes, and the 5-0 polyglactin 910 dermal sutures followed by 6-0 polypropylene sutures for cutaneous closure lateral to the lateral canthus.

Dressings

No dressings are necessary, and all incisions are coated with ophthalmic antibiotic ointment. Cool compresses should be applied immediately.

TREATMENT OF THE LATERAL CANTHUS

Lateral Canthal Suspension

For patients with mild lower lid laxity, lateral retinacular suspension can be performed easily. This technique does not violate the lateral canthus and provides additional lower lid support but less lid shortening than a tarsal strip lateral canthoplasty. The condensation of the lateral portions of Whitnall's and Lockwood's ligaments, orbicularis oculi muscle and lateral canthal tendon form the lateral retinaculum. A 5-0 polypropylene suture is passed around the lateral retinaculum and sutured to the orbital rim superior and deep to the insertion of the lateral canthal tendon (Figs 6.21A and B). This is easily done if a four lid blepharoplasty is performed, but a small incision in the lateral aspect of the upper tarsal crease can provide sufficient access if the upper lid has not been violated; likewise, a small subciliary incision just medial to the lateral canthus is used if a subciliary blepharoplasty is not being performed.

Lateral Canthoplasty

Patients with significant lower lid laxity or horizontal lid excess can be treated with a lateral tarsal strip canthoplasty. After instillation of local anesthetic to the lateral ciliary margin of the lower lid, the lateral orbital rim at the lateral canthus and a pre-existing rhytid in the crow's feet area, a 5 mm skin incision is made in the crow's feet extending up to the lateral canthus. A straight hemostat is applied to crush the subcutaneous soft tissue and conjunctiva at the lateral canthus, and a canthotomy is performed by aligning straight Iris scissors along the skin incision and over the lateral canthus, directing the tips of the scissors laterally and away from the globe. The freed edge of the lower lid is then grasped, the scissors turned inferiorly and a cantholysis is performed. Complete cantholysis produces a freely mobile lateral lower lid. The lateral canthal tendon is then exposed by removing conjunctiva (deep) and skin (superficial). A double-armed 4-0 polytetrafluoroethylene (PTFE)-coated polyester suture (Polydek®) is then passed through the canthal tendon and anchored deep and superior to the natural site of the lateral canthal tendon insertion along the orbital rim (Fig. 6.22). A 6-0 chromic suture is placed to reapproximate the upper and lower lids at the grey line, and the crow's feet incision is closed with buried 4-0 polyglactin 910 sutures in the dermis and interrupted 6-0 polypropylene sutures for skin closure. Care should be taken to ensure good apposition of the lid to the globe and symmetric lateral canthi postoperatively.

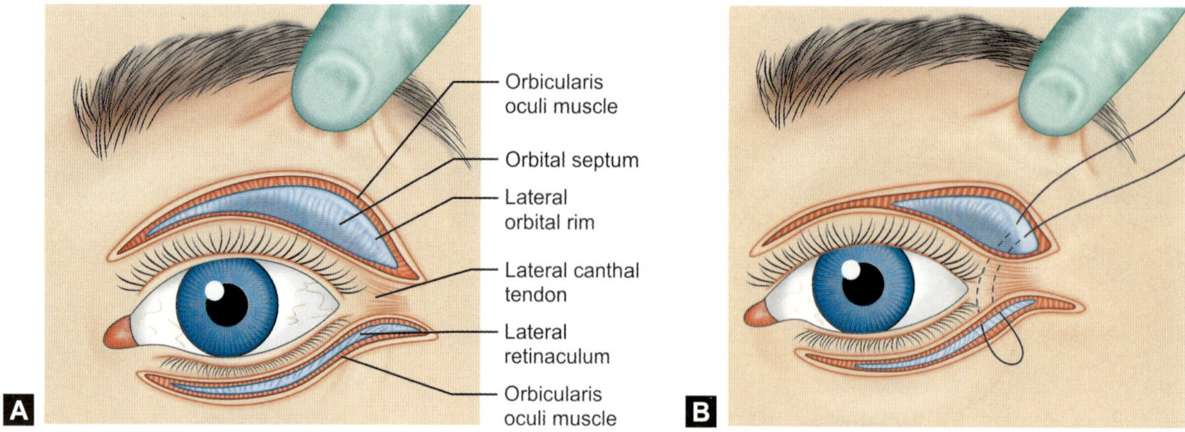

Figs 6.21A and B: Lower eyelid support can be enhanced with a lateral retinacular suspension

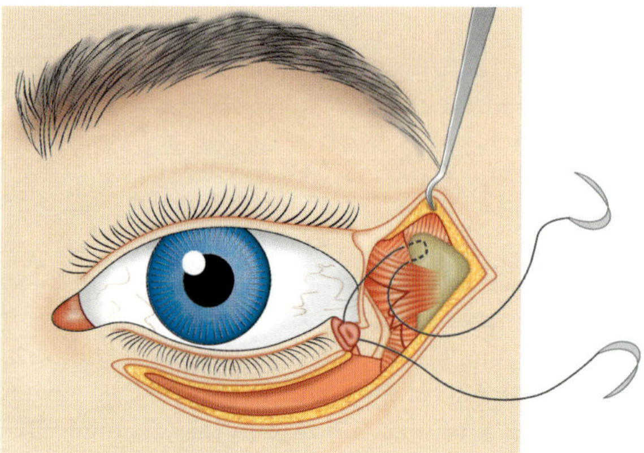

Fig. 6.22: Severe lid laxity is more effectively treated with a lateral canthoplasty

POTENTIAL COMPLICATIONS

Dry Eye Syndrome

Patients should be screened preoperatively for dry eyes with a Schirmer's test, and those with insufficient tear production should be referred to an ophthalmologist for evaluation. Postoperatively, mild dry eye complaints are not uncommon for the first 2–3 weeks. Patients with more persistent complaints or any patient with pain should be referred to an ophthalmologist.

Hematoma

Probably the most feared complication, retroseptal or retrobulbar hematoma generally occurs as a bleeding vessel retracts behind the orbital septum. As blood accumulates within retroseptal space, pressure on the central retinal artery can lead to ischemia and blindness. Although rare, this complication is catastrophic. Rapid diagnosis and aggressive management aimed at reducing intraocular pressure is essential. The head should be elevated, cold compresses applied, sutures should be removed and an ophthalmologist should be consulted as initial steps. Unless absolutely contraindicated, intravenous (IV) mannitol, acetazolamide and dexamethasone should be given. If these treatments fail to reduce intraocular pressure in short order, a lateral canthotomy with inferior cantholysis should be performed, and consideration is given to emergent orbital decompression.

Milia

These white nodules along the suture line occur when sebaceous glands become obstructed. They can be easily unroofed with a 30-gauge needle.

Asymmetry

Proper incision placement is essential in both the upper and lower eyelids. Especially in cases of senile ptosis, the upper eyelid crease may be indistinct. The surgeon should ensure that the incisions are symmetrical and lie 8–10 mm above the lash line. Subciliary incisions should also be symmetric, but lower lid asymmetry is more likely to result from asymmetric orbital fat pad resection. A common problem area is the temporal fat pad, as this can become more difficult to visualize unless resected first.

Infection

Infection is unusual, given the rich vascularity of the eyelid skin. If an infection is suspected, oral antibiotics (covering *Staphylococcus* and *Streptococcus*) should be initiated, and if there is no response within 48 hours, IV antibiotics should be given.

Ocular Injury

Errant needle tips can injure the globe, and the surgeon should always be aware of the needle tip's location. Injury during the surgery is also possible. The cornea should be protected with a corneal shield or with the conjunctiva (by keeping the upper lid closed during surgery or by draping the lower lid conjunctiva over the cornea) during dissection. The globe should be moistened with ophthalmic ointment and artificial tears throughout the surgery.

Extraocular Muscle Injury

The inferior oblique muscle can be injured during dissection of the nasal and central fat pads of the lower lid. Deep dissection in the upper lid could possibly injure the levator palpebrae superioris or its aponeurosis, leading to ptosis.

Chemosis

Conjunctival edema is generally limited but can cause temporary diplopia. Ophthalmic ointments and moisturizers should be applied liberally.

Blindness

Reportedly occurring in 1 per 20,000, postoperative blindness generally is thought to be related to retrobulbar hemorrhage with permanent blindness in 1 per 30,000 cases.

Malar Bags Persistence

Malar bags are not addressed by blepharoplasty and patients should be counseled as such preoperatively.

Diplopia

Most diplopia is temporary and due to perioperative edema. Permanent diplopia may be caused by injury to the inferior oblique muscle during resection of the nasal and middle lower lid fat pads.

Eyelid Malposition, Scleral Show, Ectropion

Rounding of the lower eyelid, exposure of the inferior limbus (scleral show) and frank ectropion with distraction of the lid away from the globe may occur because of lower lid laxity with or without excessive scarring. Skin resection in the lower lid should be conservative, and strong consideration is given to procedures that enhance lateral canthal support.

Epiphora

Epiphora may be transient or permanent. Immediately after surgery, edema may temporarily block lacrimal drainage. However, permanent epiphora may result from eversion of the lower lid or from scarring and obstruction of the inferior canaliculus.

Ptosis

In addition to levator muscle or aponeurosis injury, ptosis may "develop" after blepharoplasty. However, if mild ptosis exists preoperatively, patients may compensate with frontalis muscle hyperactivity; reduction of upper lid redundant skin reduces the need for accessory lid elevation using brow elevators, and as frontalis relaxes, the pre-existing true ptosis is "revealed". Preoperative evaluation should include an assessment of upper lid position with the brows in a neutral, unelevated position.

AFTERCARE

Cool compresses should be applied intermittently to the eyes for the first 24 hours. Ophthalmic ointments and artificial tears are applied over the first 7–10 days.

BIBLIOGRAPHY

1. DeMere M, Wood T, Austin W. Eye complications with blepharoplasty or other eyelid surgery. A national survey. Plast Reconstr Surg. 1974;53(6):634-7.
2. Fagien S. Algorithm for canthoplasty: the lateral retinacular suspension: a simplified suture canthopexy. Plast Reconstruct Surg. 1999;103(7):2042-53.
3. Hidalgo DA. An integrated approach to lower blepharoplasty. Plast Reconstr Surg. 2011;127(1):386-95.
4. Lee AS, Thomas JR. Lower lid blepharoplasty and canthal surgery. Facial Plast Surg Clin North Am. 2005;13(4):541-51.
5. McGraw BL, Adamson PA. Postblepharoplasty ectropion. Prevention and management. Arch Otolaryngol Head Neck Surg. 1991;117(8):852-6.
6. Rees TD, LaTrenta GS. The role of the Schirmer's test and orbital morphology in predicting dry-eye syndrome after blepharoplasty. Plast Reconstr Surg. 1988;82(4):619-25.

CHAPTER 7

Brow Lift

Anthony P Sclafani

OVERVIEW

The brow frames the upper portion of the periorbital area and the lower portion of the forehead. Brow position is frequently associated with, among other things, emotion, suggesting anger, sadness or surprise.

Esthetically, the position of the eyebrows should be assessed relative to the orbital rim and then lifted to an esthetically pleasing position, and the amount of elevation required should be noted. Ideally, the male brow runs fairly horizontally at or slightly below the orbital rim, while in women the brow should arch and peak a few millimeters above the rim at or just medial to the lateral canthus. The medial brow should begin along a vertical line drawn from the nasal ala through the medial canthus, while the lateral brow should end on a line running tangentially from the ipsilateral ala through the lateral canthus.

SPECIAL CONSIDERATIONS

Soft tissue anatomy of surgical facial rejuvenation includes the skin, superficial musculofascial layer, facial muscles and nerves. In the forehead, the fascial layer of the galea aponeurotica covers and envelops the frontalis muscle. Posteriorly, this layer continues into the occipitalis muscle fascia; inferiorly, the galea fuses with the periosteum about 2 cm above the orbital rim, while laterally the galea fuses with multiple layers of fascia just medial to the superior temporal line (superior-most attachment of the temporalis muscle). Anatomically, the galea becomes contiguous with the superficial musculoaponeurotic system (SMAS, a fascial tissue which covers and envelops the facial muscles) at the zygomatic arch, where they fuse with the periosteum.

The muscles which affect the brow and forehead include the frontalis muscle (brow elevator which originates posteriorly from the galea, coursing inferiorly to intermingle in the midline and with the orbicularis oculi muscles more inferiorly), orbital portion of the paired orbicularis oculi muscles (brow depressor), paired corrugator and depressor supercilii muscles (brow medializer and depressor, respectively originating from the superomedial orbital rim) and the midline procerus muscle (brow depressor originating from the nasal bones).

The facial nerve is the only motor nerve in the surgical field of forehead, face and neck rejuvenative procedures. After emerging from the stylomastoid foramen and branching at the pes anserinus, facial nerve branches become increasingly more superficial medially. The temporal branch runs superiorly to innervate the forehead and lateral orbicularis and corrugator muscles. The temporal branch crosses the zygomatic arch, usually in one to three branches, within the fusion of the SMAS and periosteum, and then runs on the undersurface of the temporoparietal fascia into the forehead. The supraorbital and supratrochlear nerves supply sensation to the brow and forehead anterior to the crown. These nerves emerge from notches or foramina along the superior orbital rim accompanied by arteries and veins, run posteriorly, branching and becoming more superficial peripherally. The supratrochlear nerve is generally found between 15 mm and 20 mm lateral to the midline, while the supraorbital nerve emerges approximately 23–26 mm from the midline.

ALTERNATIVES TO PROCEDURE

Botulinum toxin A (BTxA) blocks acetylcholine release into the neuromuscular junction. By treating brow depressors, the brow can be induced to elevate 2–3 mm. Soft tissue fillers, particularly hyaluronic acid derivatives, can be used to elevate the lateral brow by adding volume preperiosteally.

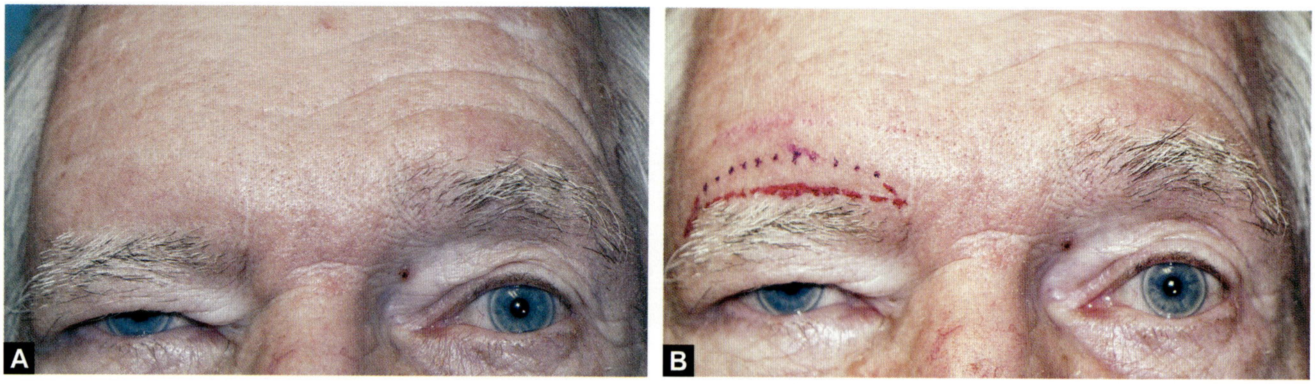

Figs 7.1A and B: (A) Patient with right brow ptosis after temporal tumor resection and sacrifice of the temporal branch of the facial nerve; (B) Direct brow lift planned. Lower limb of ellipse placed just above the brow hairs; upper limb marked by estimating the desired position of the top of brow in repose

TECHNIQUES

Direct Brow Lift

The direct brow lift is a simple procedure that can be performed under local anesthesia to reposition the lateral two thirds of the eyebrows.

Incision Placement

The incision is positioned at the superior-most hairs of the brow (Figs 7.1A and B). The brow is manually elevated to the desired position, and the excess skin is marked, generating an ellipse of skin for excision. A modification of this technique, the indirect brow lift, places the excisions in staggered, pre-existing horizontal forehead creases 1–2 cm above the brows.

Extent of Undermining

The upper border of the excision is undermined, exposing the lower frontalis muscle fibers.

Tissue Modifications

- *Excision*: The outlined ellipse of skin is incised down to frontalis muscle and removed; medially at the medial club head of the brow, the skin incision is more superficial, not penetrating muscle to avoid injury to the supratrochlear nerve (Fig. 7.2).
- *Suturing*: The fibers of the orbicularis oculi muscle at the inferior border of the excised ellipse are sutured superiorly to the frontalis muscle beneath the undermined superior skin edge with multiple 3-0 polyglactin 910 sutures. It is simpler to place all of these sutures first, tying them once all have been placed (Fig. 7.3).
- *Tissue advancement*: As these sutures are tied, the brow slides superiorly to rest at its new, elevated neutral position.

Wound Closure

A layered closure is meticulously performed, reapproximating dermis with multiple 5-0 polyglactin 910 sutures. Skin is closed with interrupted 6-0 polypropylene sutures (Fig. 7.4).

Midforehead Lift

The midforehead lift requires a visible midforehead incision in skin to develop the appropriate surgical planes in the central forehead. Ideal candidates for the midforehead lift are patients with a long forehead, fair skin and deep horizontal rhytids in the forehead. It is a reasonable choice in bald patients, but provides less effective lateral brow elevation.

Incision Placement

The midforehead lift utilizes a broken line incision in a mid-upper forehead crease in between the temporal crests (Fig. 7.5).

Extent of Undermining

A skin flap is raised off of the superficial surface of the frontalis muscle down toward the orbital rim in between the temporal crests (Fig. 7.6). The same plane is dissected superiorly to the hairline.

Tissue Modifications

- *Excision*: The frontalis muscle is incised between the left and right supraorbital nerves and inferior dissection below the galea is performed until the

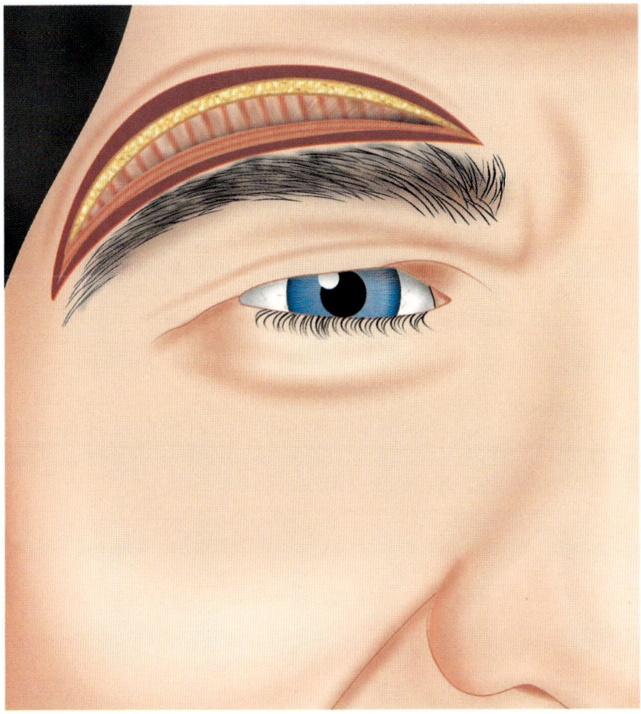

Fig. 7.2: After excision of the ellipse, frontalis (superiorly) and orbicularis oculi (inferiorly) muscle fibers noted laterally and centrally; medially, the dissection does not expose muscle in order to protect supratrochlear nerves

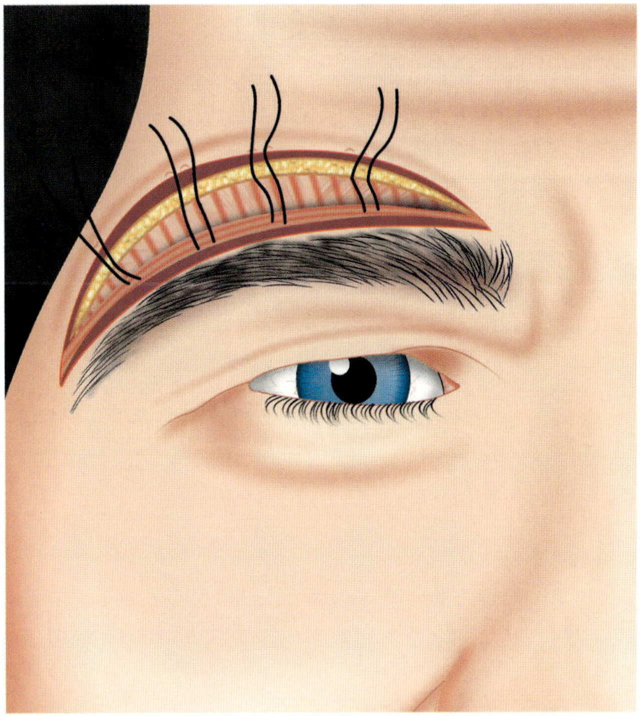

Fig. 7.3: Mattress sutures are placed between the orbicularis oculi and frontalis muscle fibers

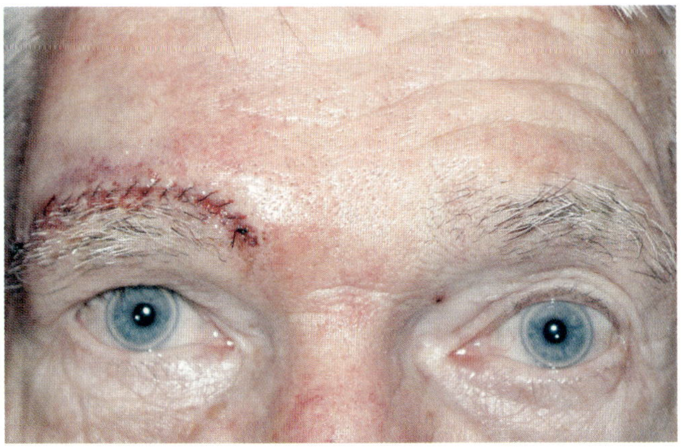

Fig. 7.4: Immediately after completion of the direct brow lift

corrugator supercilii and procerus muscles are identified at or near the supraorbital rim. These muscles are then divided and the stumps cauterized to smooth wrinkling in the glabella (Fig. 7.7).

- *Tissue advancement*: The frontalis muscle is then redraped superiorly until the brows approach an acceptable position (Fig. 7.8). Redundant muscle is excised and the muscle/galeal layer closed with interrupted 3-0 polyglactin 910. The brow position should be overcorrected by 50% to compensate for postoperative descent of tissues.

Closure

Meticulous hemostasis should be achieved with a bipolar cautery prior to skin closure, as multiple small vessels are transected during elevation of the skin flap. Skin is then redraped and excess skin is excised.

- *Layers*: Careful and accurate skin closure is then performed with 4-0 and 5-0 polyglactin sutures for dermal approximation and a running 5-0 polypropylene suture for cutaneous closure.

Dressing

A mildly compressive dressing on the forehead is placed and maintained with an elastic wrap for the first 24 hours.

Aftercare

Topical antibiotic ointment should be applied to the forehead sutures three to four times a day. Sutures are

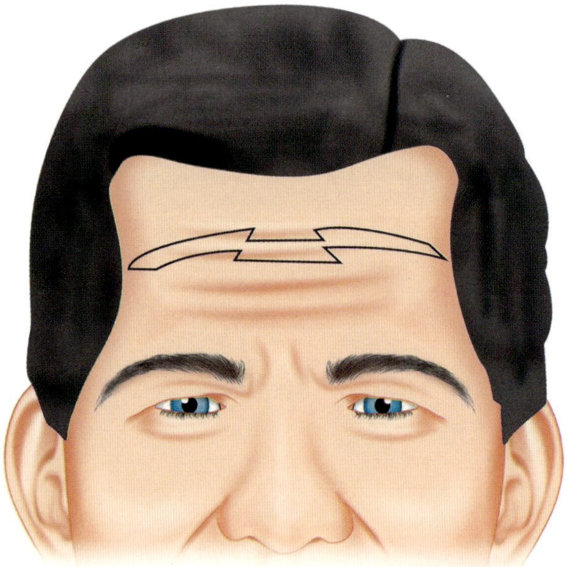

Fig. 7.5: Midforehead lift incision runs in pre-existing forehead creases with a staggered portion running in an adjacent crease

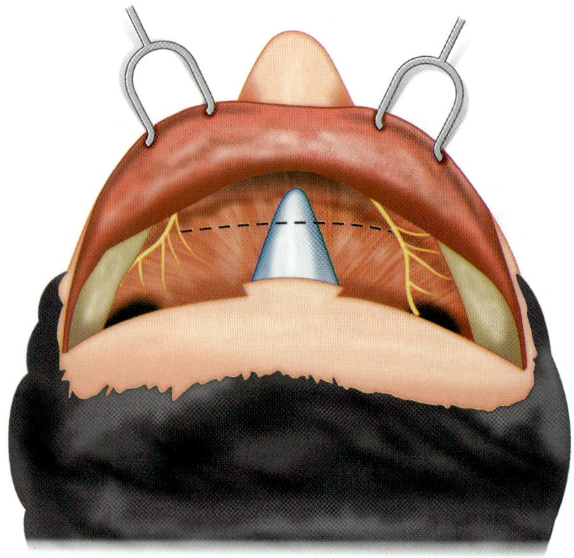

Fig. 7.6: A skin flap is sharply raised from the frontalis muscle, and an incision is made approximately 2 cm above the orbital rim and in between the supraorbital nerves

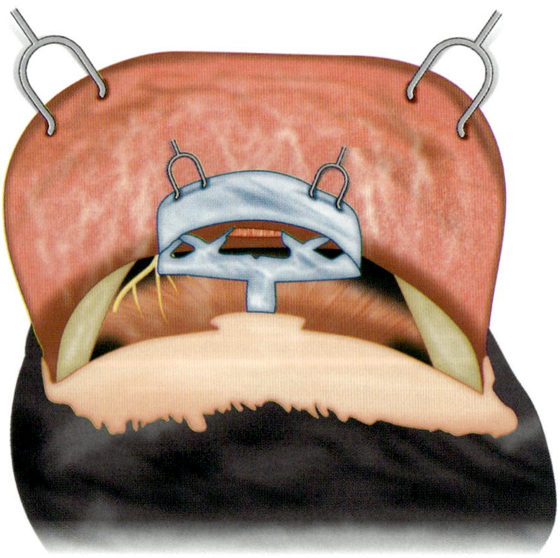

Fig. 7.7: A subgaleal plane is developed to the orbital rims, exposing the corrugator and procerus muscles which are carefully divided

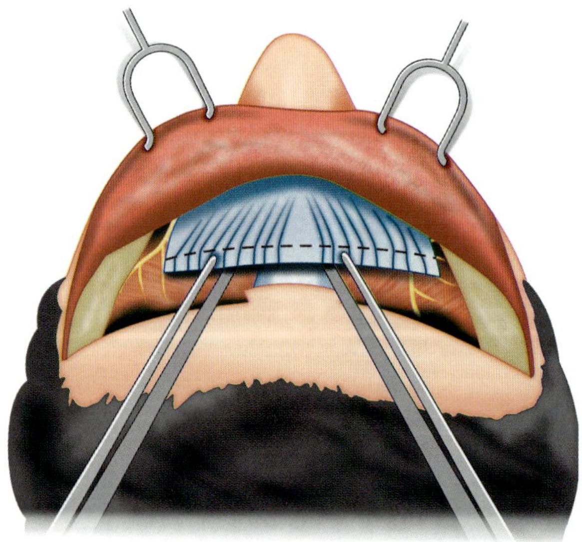

Fig. 7.8: The musculogaleal flap is retracted superiorly, resected and resutured, typically removing about twice the amount as brow elevation desired

generally removed 5–7 days after surgery, and patients are counseled to avoid sunlight for 2–3 months to limit or avoid hyperpigmentation.

Coronal Foreheadplasty

The coronal foreheadplasty employs an incision running over the crown from one helical root to the other. It provides wide access to the frontal bone, but requires significantly more dissection, is more subject to brow "settling" and has a longer recovery period than other more brow procedures. The coronal forehead lift is appropriate in cases with significant brow ptosis. Receding frontal hairlines or baldness is a contraindication to the coronal brow lift, since the long scar cannot be adequately camouflaged. Elevation of the temporal end of the brow requires a subtemporoparietal fascia dissection, which puts the temporal branch of the facial nerve at risk.

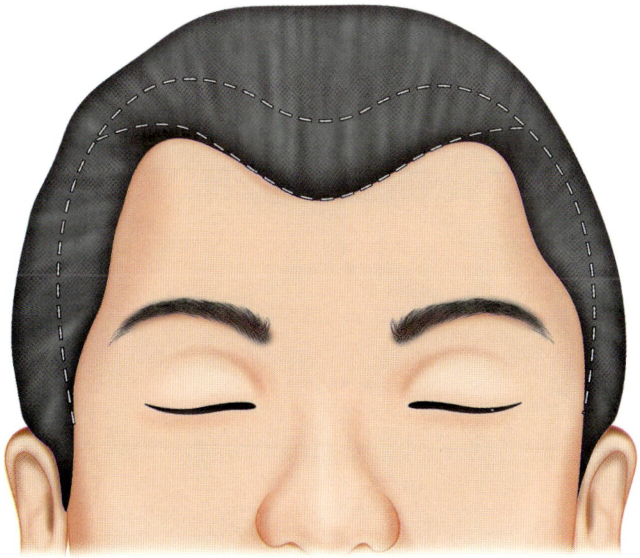

Fig. 7.9: The coronal brow lift incision begins above the auricle and runs across the forehead in a curvilinear fashion to continue into the contralateral temple, remaining at least 2 cm behind the frontal hairline. In any patient with a high forehead, a post-trichial incision will lead to an unacceptably high hairline, and instead the temporal incision continues as a trichophytic frontal incision

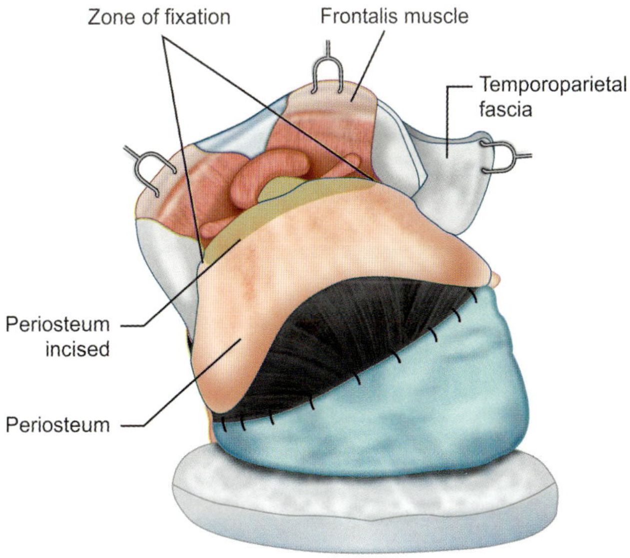

Fig. 7.10: The forehead flap is raised in a subgaleal plane centrally, a sub-temporoparietal fascia plane temporally and a subperiosteal place inferiorly. Dense adhesions just medial to the temporal crest are sharply divided

Incision Placement

The incision begins at the superior auricular root, and curves posteriorly as it proceeds superiorly, so that it lies behind the temporal hair trough. It then runs anteriorly, remaining at least 2 cm behind the frontal hairline. It then returns posteriorly, curving behind the contralateral temporal trough before curing down the temple to the opposite auricular root. In patients with high forehead requiring reduction, a trichophytic incision is made in an irregularly irregular fashion along the anterior central and temporal trough hairline, before returning to the temple (Fig. 7.9). The incision should be beveled parallel to the hair shafts to avoid follicular root injury and to promote maximal scar camouflage.

Extent of Undermining

In the temple, the TPF is identified and incised. Dissection is performed inferiorly in the plane between the deep temporal fascia (DTF) and the TPF and continued down to the lateral orbital rim, and medially until the dense attachments at the temporal crest are identified (Fig. 7.10). This dissection plane protects the temporal branch of the facial nerve, which runs within the leaves of the TPF. In between the temporal crest, the dissection place is in between the galea and periosteum, and as the central forehead plane is dissected, these dense attachments at the temporal crest are sharply divided all the way to the lateral orbital rim. The subgaleal plane is followed to a point approximately 2 cm above the orbital rim, at which point the periosteum is incised and a subperiosteal plane is completed onto the superior orbital rims.

Tissue Modifications

- *Excision*: The forehead flap is flipped forward and retracted to expose the corrugator and procerus muscles inferiorly. The corrugator muscle is dissected between the supratrochlear and supraorbital neurovascular bundles and a section of muscle is isolated between two hemostats. The intervening muscle is excised and the muscle stumps cauterized. The procerus muscle is transected horizontally and cauterized. The frontalis muscle is scored with cautery below the deepest transverse crease (Fig. 7.11).
- *Tissue advancement*: The forehead flap is then advanced superiorly sufficiently to elevate the brow to the desired position. The skin redundancy is noted and overcorrection is then perfomed, excising sufficient skin to overcorrect by 200–250% (Fig. 7.12).
- *Sutures*: Galeal edges are then reapproximated with interrupted 3-0 polydioxanone sutures.

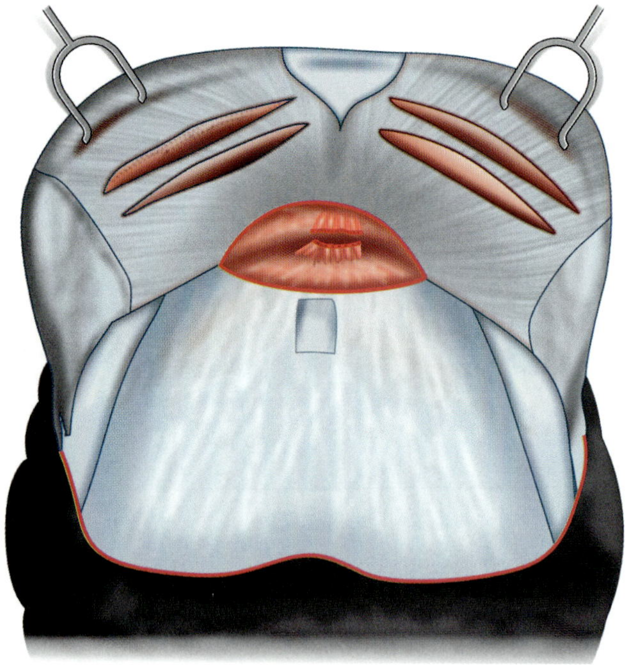

Fig. 7.11: Muscle modifications in the coronal brow lift include: myotomies of the frontalis below the two most dominant transverse forehead creases; transverse myotomy of the procerus; isolation, resection and cauterization of the corrugator muscles

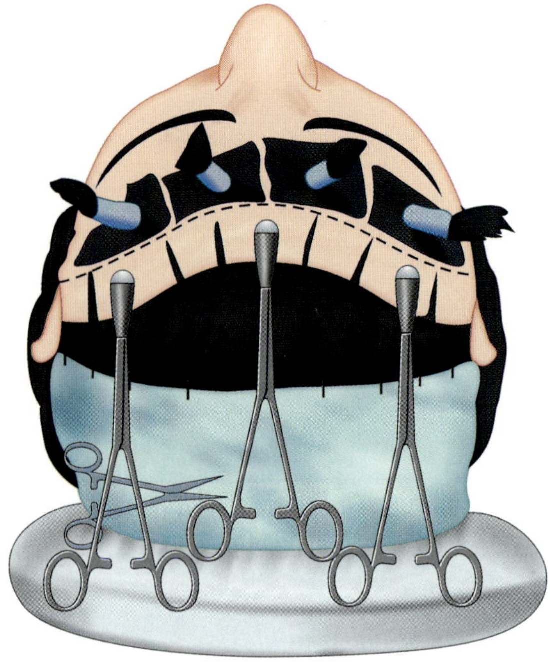

Fig. 7.12: The forehead flap is retracted superiorly and excess skin is noted and marked; generally, skin resection is 2.5–3 times the desired brow elevation

Closure

- *Layers*: The skin incision is closed in layers, with 3-0 polyglactin 910 for dermal reapproximation and surgical skin staples for cutaneous closure.
- *Drains*: A single flat, fluted drain is placed over the periosteum and brought out through a separate stab incision in the temple.

Dressings

A lightly compressive forehead dressing is applied and maintained for 24–48 hours.

Aftercare

The drain is removed when drainage decreases sufficiently (usually less than 5–10 cc/8 hours). Topical antibiotic ointment is applied to the skin staples until removed. Patients are counseled to avoid hot showers, since the forehead and crown may be numb for several weeks.

Temporal Lift

The temporal lift is essentially the temporal portion of the coronal foreheadplasty, and can be performed to elevate the tail of the brow.

Incision Placement

A skin incision in the temple is made sharply, with the blade parallel to hair follicles (Fig. 7.13).

Extent of Undermining

The TPF is identified and incised, and a dissection plane is developed inferiorly towards the orbital rim.

Tissue Modifications

- *Incisions*: The attachments at the superior temporal line are divided down to the orbit, releasing the orbital retaining ligament in this process (Fig. 7.14).
- *Tissue advancement*: The lateral brow is then pulled superolaterally.

Closure

- *Skin excision*: Extra skin is noted and marked, so that a 30–50% overcorrection is generated. The skin is then sharply excised.
- *Layers*: The wound is closed in two layers, with 3-0 polyglactin 910 sutures used to close the TPF and dermis, and surgical staples are used for cutaneous closure.

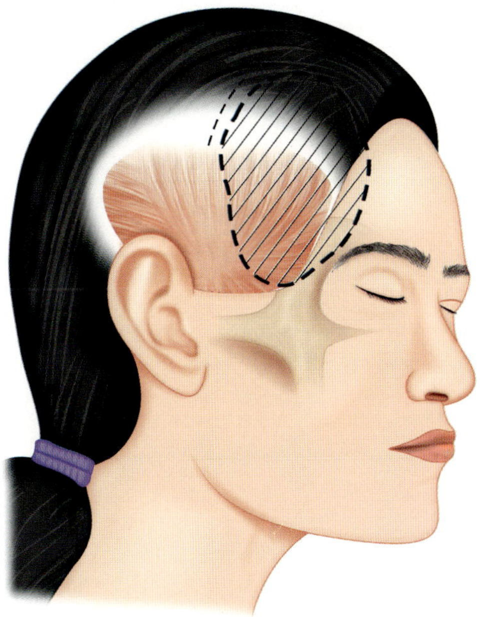

Fig. 7.13: The temporal lift requires a sub-temporoparietal fascia

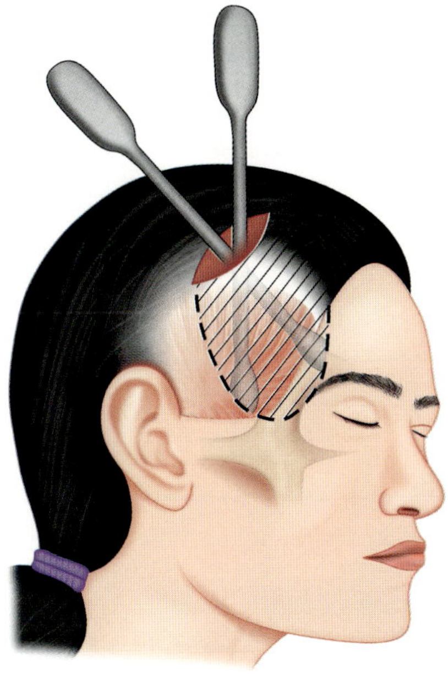

Fig. 7.14: Dissection is performed inferiorly to the orbital rim and medially beyond the temporal crest, with release of the dense attachments medially and inferiorly

Aftercare

Topical antibiotic ointment is applied to skin staples several times a day until the staples are removed.

Endoscopic Foreheadplasty

Endoscopic foreheadplasty combines a number of features of these procedures, but relies on a more functional understanding of brow dynamics. Endoforeheadplasty success is predicated on full release of brow retaining structures, division of the brow depressor muscles, preservation of the brow elevator muscle and stabilization of brow position until the elevated tissues have sufficiently readhered to underlying tissues.

Incision Placement

Three 1–2 cm sagittal incisions are made in the hair-bearing scalp in between the temporal lines: one midline, while the other two are above the midpupils. One additional incision is made in each temple, approximately 4 cm in length, parallel and posterior to the hairline (Fig. 7.15).

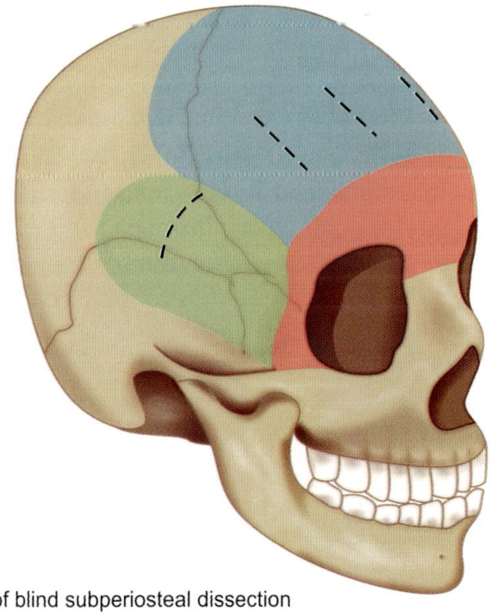

Fig. 7.15: Endoforeheadplasty can be performed through five remote incisions: two temporal incisions, allowing bilateral sub-temporoparietal fascial dissections, and one midline and two paramedian incisions allowing complete central subperiosteal dissection

Extent of Undermining

The author prefers to develop a subperiosteal plane centrally, although a subgaleal plane can be utilized alternatively. The skin incision is carried down through periosteum, and a Freer elevator is used to sweep the periosteum laterally to expose the calvarium. A monocortical hole is drilled beneath the inferior edge of the incision. The central forehead is then

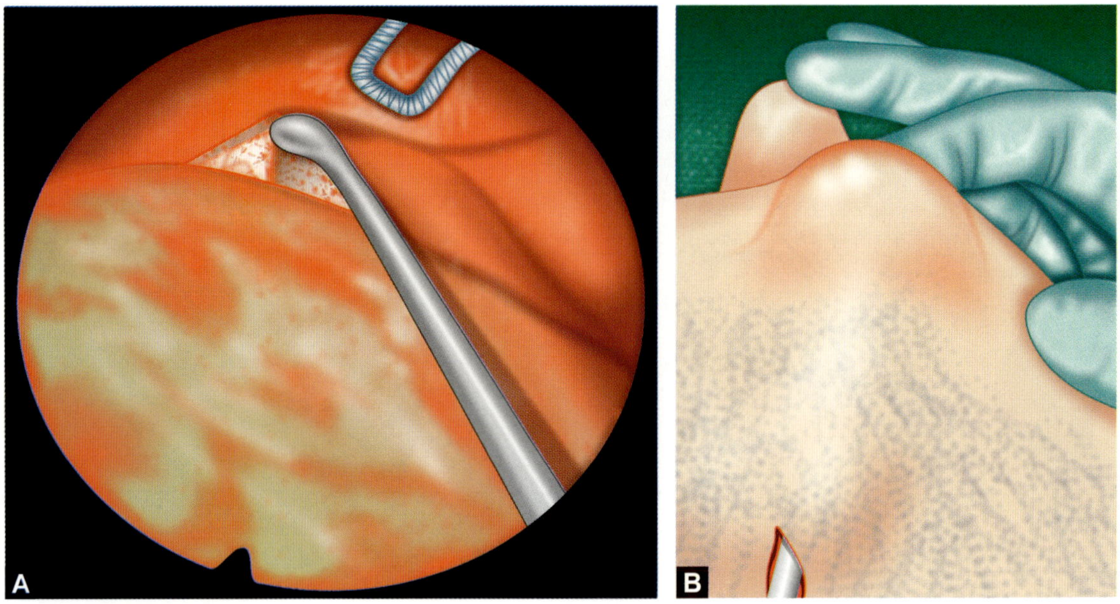

Figs 7.16A and B: (A) Inferior dissection under endoscopic guidance can be performed down to the orbital rim with exposure of the arcus marginalis; (B) Light external pressure can provide significant feedback as to the extent of dissection

dissected blindly between the temporal crests and from the crown down to a line approximately 2–2.5 cm above the orbital rim. A subperiosteal pocket is then dissected with the Freer elevator as well as specialized curved brow elevators down to the orbital rim and glabella under endoscopic exposure (Figs 7.16A and B). More highly curved elevators aid in dissection closer to the orbital rim. Laterally, the skin incision is extended through the TPF to expose the DTF. A small incision in the DTF is made directly below the incision to register the initial position of the incision. Beginning with a headlight, right angle retractor and Freer elevator (Figs 7.17A and B) and later using the endoscope (Fig. 7.17C), a sub-TPF plane is dissected medially toward the temporal crest and inferiorly towards the zygomatic arch and orbital rim. As the dissection progresses inferiorly, the surgeon should be alert for the presence of the zygomaticotemporal (sentinel) vein, bridging between the DTF and TPF, which is a good landmark for the temporal branches of the facial nerve coursing within the substance of the TPF above. If it is necessary to cauterize the vein, this should be done directly above the DTP with bipolar cautery.

Tissue Modifications

- *Incision*: With a spatulated elevator placed below the TPF and the endoscope in the midline central incision, the dense attachments at the temporal crest are divided. The elevator is pushed through these attachments with the blade pressed firmly against the calvarium under endoscopic visualization. The elevator is then angled to place its side edge against the bone, and the elevator swept superiorly and inferiorly to divide the rest of the attachments and connect the temporal and central pockets (Fig. 7.18A). This creates a wider dissection pocket, and allows better visualization of the inferior dissection (Fig. 7.18B). Periosteum is elevated until the entire orbital rim is visualized from one lateral canthus to the other, and is confirmed by visualizing the white condensation of the arcus marginalis. This requires division of the superior orbital retaining ligament.
- *Excision*: After the periosteum is opened, the brow depressor muscles are skeletonized and divided. A curved hook or spreading endoscopic forceps further splays open the periosteal incision, and the glabellar muscles are visualized. Branches of the supraorbital and supratrochlear nerves and vessels cross this area as well, as dissection should protect these structures. The muscles are then isolated, cauterized with insulated endoscopic forceps and divided, leaving the nerve fibers and vessels intact over a bed of fat (Fig. 7.19).
- *Tissue advancement*: Once the brow retaining ligaments and the brow depressor muscles are divided, the forehead flap is freely mobile and can be advanced superiorly as needed. While there are no longer any brow depressor forces at work, gravity will still lead to inferior descent of the brow, and the brow flap should be supported for a period of time sufficient for readherence of periosteum to

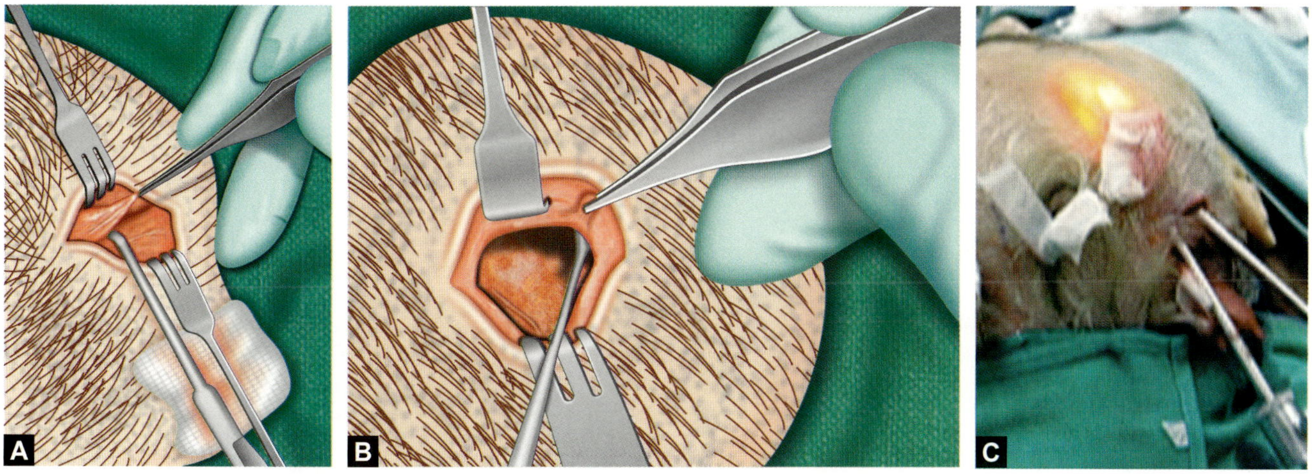

Figs 7.17A to C: (A) The temporoparietal fascia (TPF) is carefully identified and elevated under direct vision; once the fascia is identified, a plane directly above the underlying deep temporal fascia (DTF) is developed; (B) Under direct vision and (C) Later with an endoscope. The limit of the dissection is demonstrated by the extent of the transillumination of the skin

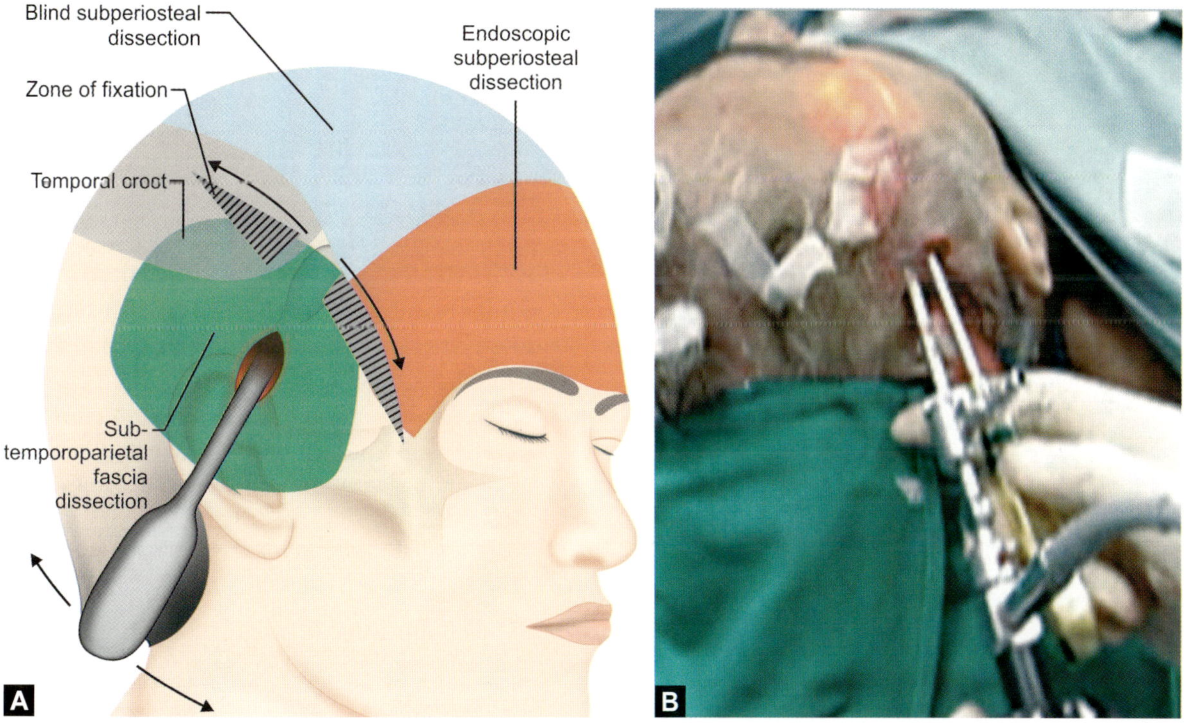

Figs 7.18A and B: (A) The zone of fixation, a dense confluence of multiple fascial layers densely adherent to the calvarium, is divided down to the lateral orbital rim, connecting the temporal and central pockets; (B) After the two pockets are connected, the endoscope can be advanced to the orbital rim

bone. The amount of desired brow elevation over the medial brow and midpupillary brow is then marked superior to the central and paramedian registration marks (Fig. 7.20), respectively. Monocortical holes are then drilled in these locations. Resorbable bone fixation devices (Lactosorb, Biomet Microfixation, Jacksonville, Fl) are then placed in these drill holes. A 3-0 polydioxanone suture is placed through the suture hole in these fixation screws, and the suture is then sewn to the periosteum and galea at the inferior edge of the incision (Fig. 7.21). Temporally, the TPF/skin flap is advanced posterosuperiorly the desired distance required to produce appropriate elevation of lateral brow elevation. A distance equal to the desired

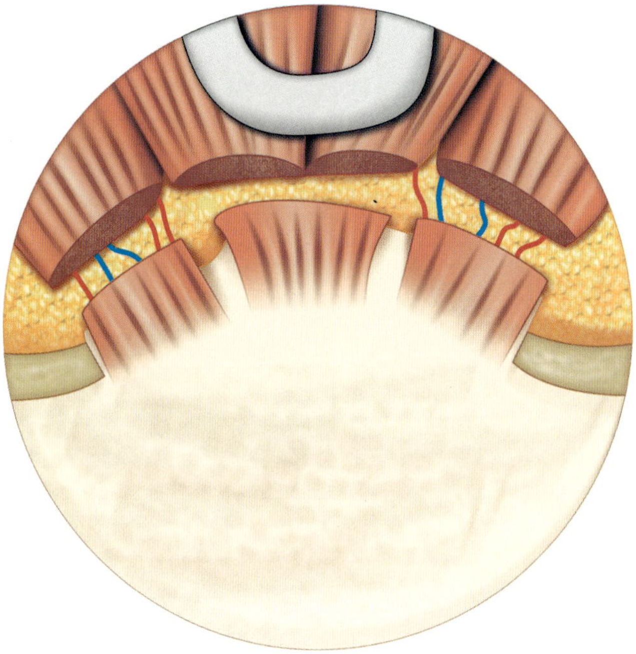

Fig. 7.19: The corrugator and procerus muscles are divided centrally, and the orbicularis muscle is separated laterally

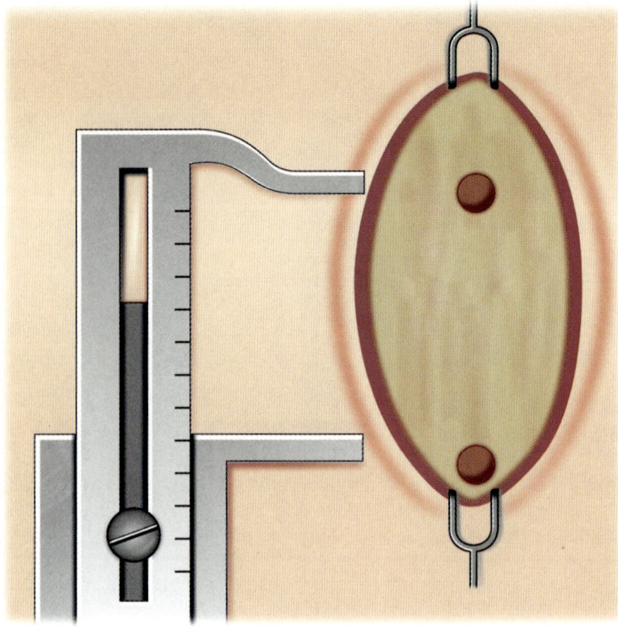

Fig. 7.20: The elevation desired is marked above the initial registration hole, and a monocortical hole is drilled at this point

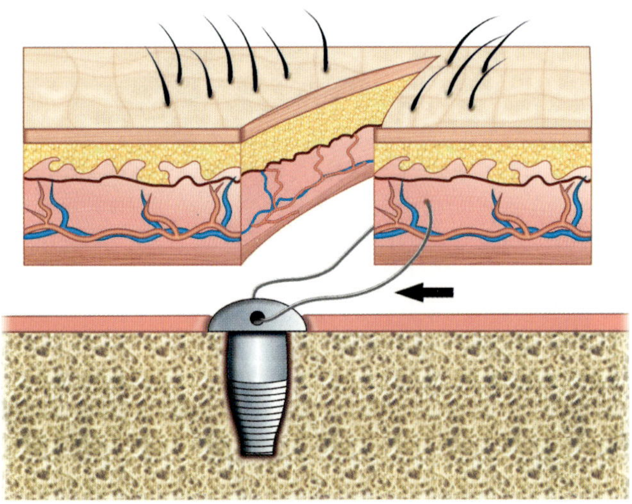

Fig. 7.21: A fixation device is placed in the upper hole and suture fixated to the lower edge of the incision

amount of lateral brow elevation is measured from the inferior skin edge and a 3-0 polydioxanone suture placed here. This is then sutured to the DTF 2–3 mm above the registration mark, elevating the lateral brow.

Wound Closure

- *Skin excision*: If skin redundancy is excessive, an ellipse of skin is resected from the superior edge of the temporal wound.
- *Layers*: The central forehead incisions are closed with one of two polyglactin 910 sutures in the dermis to ensure wound edge eversion. The skin is then closed with staples. The temporal incisions are closed similarly with sufficient polyglactin 910 dermal sutures to ensure skin eversion, followed by skin staples.
- *Drains*: If a drain is desired, it is placed over the bone in the upper portion of the dissection pocket, draped distally into the temporal dissection and exits the contralateral temporal dissection through a separate incision.

Dressing

A mildly compressive fluff gauze dressing is placed over the forehead and secured in place with a gauze wrap.

Aftercare

Cool compresses should be applied intermittently for the first 24 hours, and the head of bed kept elevated. The gauze wrap and drain are generally removed on postoperative day 1. Topical antibiotic ointment is applied to all staples three times a day until they are removed 1 week after surgery. Mild analgesics are generally necessary for only the first 1–3 days. Patient are allowed to shower on the first postoperative day, but are told to avoid hairdryer use for the first 10 days.

POTENTIAL COMPLICATIONS

Motor Nerve Injury

Injuries to the temporal branch of the facial nerve can occur during the temporal dissection of forehead procedures. Injury is best avoided by remaining in the appropriate surgical plane: below the TPF during dissection. Reported rates range from 1–3%. If nerve transection is identified intraoperatively, tensionless microscopic neurorrhaphy with 7-0 nylon sutures should be performed in order to maintain tone and (possibly) some muscular activity. Paralysis can only be assessed postoperatively after appropriate time is allowed to elapse for resolution of local anesthetic effects. Most nontransient postoperative paralysis is due to nerve pressure or traction, and will often improve spontaneously. Observation is wise and electric stimulation tests can be used to monitor for response.

Sensory Nerve Injury

Complete transection of either the supraorbital or supratrochlear nerves is uncommon during forehead procedures. However, small twigs of these nerves can be transected, especially during the midforehead lift; branches may also be cut during the endoforehead lift during the sectioning of the corrugator muscles. Focal areas of hypesthesia may be noted over the forehead and frontal scalp; these are typically small (< 1 cm) areas that may be permanent but generally get smaller over time.

Alopecia

Alopecia after forehead lifting not only is disconcerting but often causes the scars to be more visible. Generally, this is a transient effect (telogen effluvium), which usually recovers in 3–4 months. Permanent alopecia after foreheadplasty is related to the specific procedure performed. Coronal forehead lifting requires hair to camouflage the long scar; during skin incision, the scalpel blade should be held parallel to hair shafts to preserve the maximal number of follicles. Clinical hair loss has been reported in up to 30% of coronal forehead lifts, but if proper precautions are taken, is rarely a clinical significant entity. Alopecia around the endoscopic central forehead incisions can occur, but with resorbable fixation devices, alopecia occurs in only 1–3%.

Loss of Brow Elevation

This may occur if the depressor muscles are not fully divided or when the brow retaining structures, such as the lateral orbital retaining ligament, are not thoroughly divided.

Skin Slough

This is uncommon, but more likely with long skin flaps, especially in the midforehead lift.

Hematoma

Significant bleeding is uncommon, but as with any surgical procedure is possible.

Infection

Infection after a brow lift is rare, but is more is more common in patients with poorly controlled diabetes or pharmacologically immunosuppressed.

BIBLIOGRAPHY

1. Adamson PA. The forehead lift: refinements in technique. J Otolaryngol. 1986;15(2):89-93.
2. Booth AJ, Murray A, Tyers AG. The direct brow lift: efficacy, complications, and patient satisfaction. Br J Ophthalmol. 2004;88(5):688-91.
3. Brennan HG, Rafaty FM. Midforehead incisions in treatment of the aging face. Arch Otolaryngol. 1982;108(11):732-4.
4. Chajchir A. Endoscopic subperiosteal forehead lift. Aesthetic Plast Surg. 1994;18(3):269-74.
5. Pitanguy I. Indications for and treatment of frontal and glabellar wrinkles in an analysis of 3,404 consecutive cases of rhytidectomy. Plast Reconstr Surg. 1981;67(2):157-68.
6. Sclafani AP. Aesthetic surgery of the forehead and upper third of the face: Thomas Procedures in Facial Plastic Surgery. Shelton, Connecticut: People's Medical Publishing House; 2011.

CHAPTER

8 Midface Lift

Anthony P Sclafani

OVERVIEW

Aging of the midface occurs because a variety of factors occur to variable degrees. Particularly in the midface, bony resorption, fat redistribution and skin laxity will lead to skeletonization of the inferior orbital rim, development of the nasojugal groove and change in the shape shape of the midface, with less prominence over the malar eminence and loss of definition of the submalar area. The midface lift elevates descendent soft tissues to restore facial shape and volume in the midface.

SPECIAL CONSIDERATIONS

Facial analysis should demonstrate malpositioned soft tissue volume for a midface lift to achieve its goals, as the procedure should reposition volume; patients with significant soft tissue or bony atrophy will derive substantially less benefit from a midface lift than those with descended soft tissue. Hollows under the eyes can be corrected with a midface lift as long as there is sufficient soft tissue to be lifted; the same holds true for nasojugal troughs and malar flattening.

The condition of the lower eyelid is important, as this highly mobile structure can be easily distorted if appropriate steps are not taken. An elevated lateral canthus can be as aesthetically detrimental as rounding of the lower eyelid; in addition, frank ectropion can cause significant morbidity. Stabilization/protection of the lateral canthus is essential to avoid these complications.

ALTERNATIVES TO PROCEDURE

Alternatives to a midface lift include volumizing procedures, and while the midface lift redistributes existing volume, soft tissue fillers and fat transfer primarily can augment the desired areas. Additionally, malar or submalar implants can also be used to augment specific areas of the midface as needed.

TECHNIQUES

Midface Lift (Endoscopic)

The endoscopic midface lift rejuvenates the midfacial tissues by approaching the midface through a transtemporal approach over the zygomatic arch and inferiorly from the inferior orbital rim. Soft tissue elevation is in a superolateral direction.

Anesthesia

Supplementing either general anesthesia or intravenous sedation, local anesthetic with epinephrine should be injected subperiosteally over the forehead and along the orbital rim and subfascially in the temple.

Incision Placement

The endoscopic midface lift uses the same incisions as the endoscopic forehead lift: sagittal incisions behind the frontoparietal hairline (typically one midline and two paramedian) and an incision approximately 1 cm posterior to each temporal hairline, centered on a line running tangentially through the lateral canthus to the ipsilateral nasal ala (Fig. 8.1). These allow skeletonization of the orbital rim from the glabella to the lateral orbital rim and further.

Extent of Undermining/Dissection

The lower forehead is undermined in a subperiosteal plane with gently curve endoscopic periosteal elevators in between both temporal crests. The temporal dissection is begun by incising through the skin and temporoparietal fascia (TPF), identifying the deep temporal fascia. A fenestration is made in the deep temporal fascia, exposing the temporalis muscle, directly below the temporal incision. Dissection is then performed below the TPF up to the temporal crest, breaking through the zone of fixation

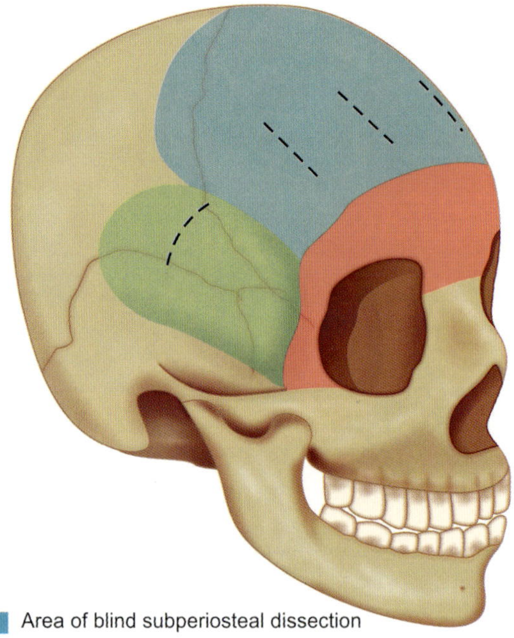

Fig. 8.1: Endoscopic midface lift is performed through temporal and frontoparietal incisions, similar to an endoscopic brow lift

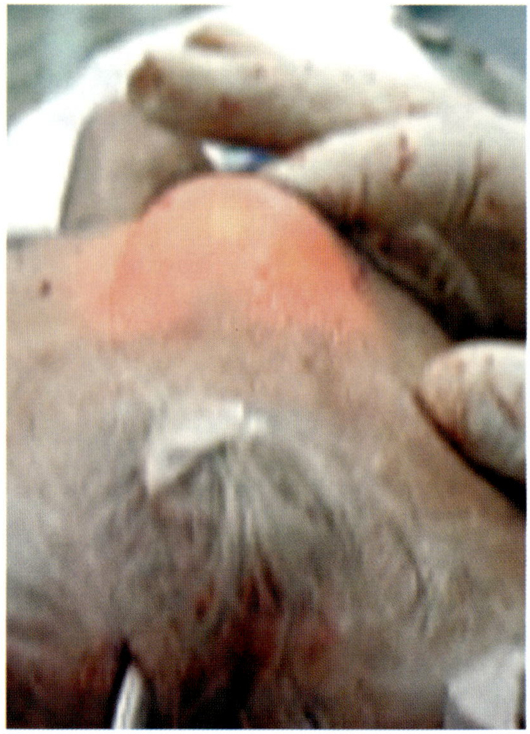

Fig. 8.2: Dissection is performed subperiosteally along the orbital rim. The index finger of the nondominant hand of the surgeon is placed at the rim to limit the extent of the dissection

just medial to the crest to join the temporal and central dissection pockets. Dissection then proceeds inferiorly along the superolateral orbital rim (Fig. 8.2), carefully avoiding disinsertion of the lateral canthal tendon, as well as following the deep temporal fascia inferiorly. During this dissection, a bridging "sentinel" vein may be encountered which runs in close proximity to the frontal branches of the facial nerve. If this vessel impedes access and dissection, it should be cauterized with bipolar cautery (staying close to the emergence of the vessel deep from the temporalis fascia) and transected with scissors. The dissection then proceeds along the inferior orbital rim and inferomedially, elevating the origins of the zygomaticus major and minor muscles and skeletonizing the malar eminence (Fig. 8.3).

Tissue Modifications

- *Suturing and tissue advancement*: Once the insertions of the zygomaticus major and minor are released, an expanded polytetrafluoroethylene (e-PTFE) suture is placed through the malar fat pad and anchored to the temporalis fascia in a (mostly) superior direction (Fig. 8.4). Too lateral a pull will increase the horizontal width of the face by adding excess soft tissue over the malar eminence. This suture is placed but is more easily tied after the central forehead sutures are placed. Long-term temporary fixation is important to prevent displacement of the composite flap inferiorly. Readherence of periosteum to bone is generally strong enough to support the flap after about 6 weeks; during the first 6 weeks postoperatively, the flap should be supported by some type of fixation. Multiple methods exist to stabilize the central forehead flap, including buried long-term resorbable or titanium screws or cortical tunnels, anchoring a suture from the periosteum below the anterior edge of each of the three central incisions to the outer table of the calvarium (Fig. 8.5). The author prefers resorbable screws placed in monocortical holes (Lactosorb, WL Lorenz, Jacksonville, Florida) secured with 3-0 polydioxanone sutures. Once these three sutures have been placed and tied, the e-PTFE midfacial elevation suture can be tied under tension, elevating the midface. For further stabilization and elevation of the lateral brow, the TPF is sutured superolaterally to the deep temporal fascia; the further the TPF is advanced past the registration incision, the more the tail of the brow will be lifted.

Closure

- *Layers/sutures*: The central forehead incisions are simply closed with 3-0 polyglactin 910 (Vicryl, Ethicon, Somerville, New Jersey) to close the incision in the

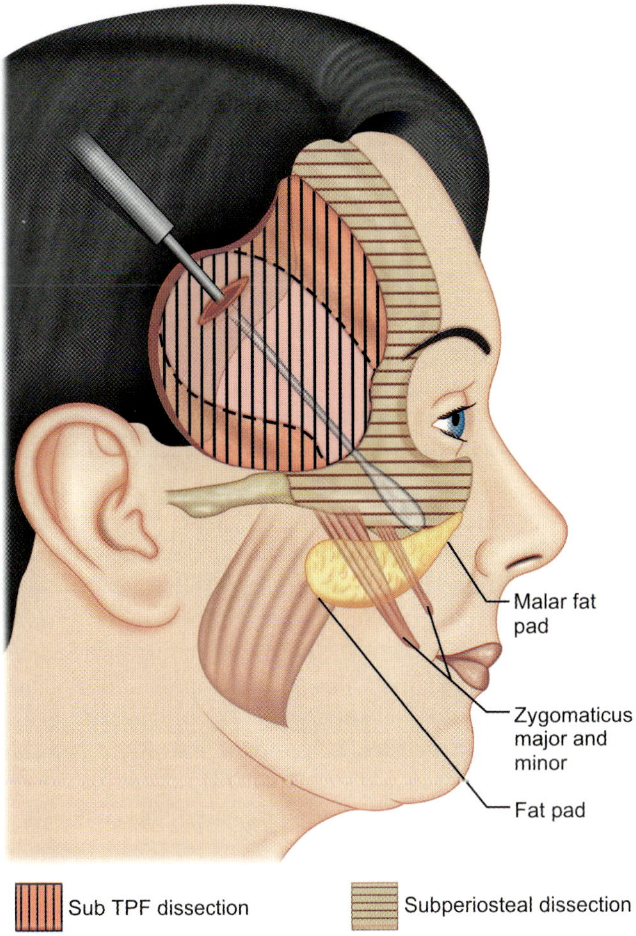

Fig. 8.3: Subperiosteal dissection is performed along the lateral and inferior orbital rim, disarticulating the origins of the zygomaticus major and minor muscles

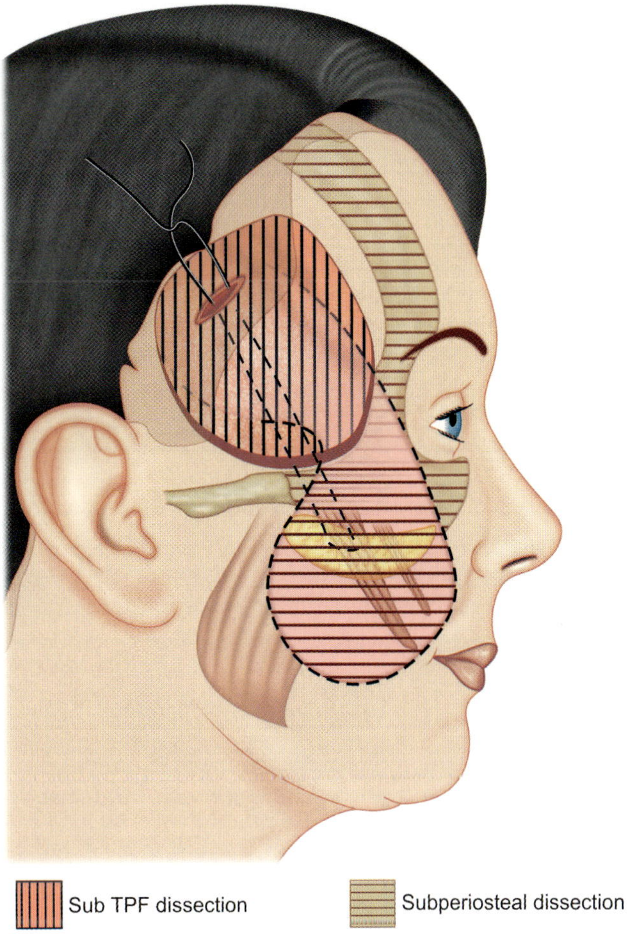

Fig. 8.4: A traction suture is placed through the malar fat, brought out through the temporal incision and tied on tension to the deep temporal fascia to elevate the midfacial soft tissues

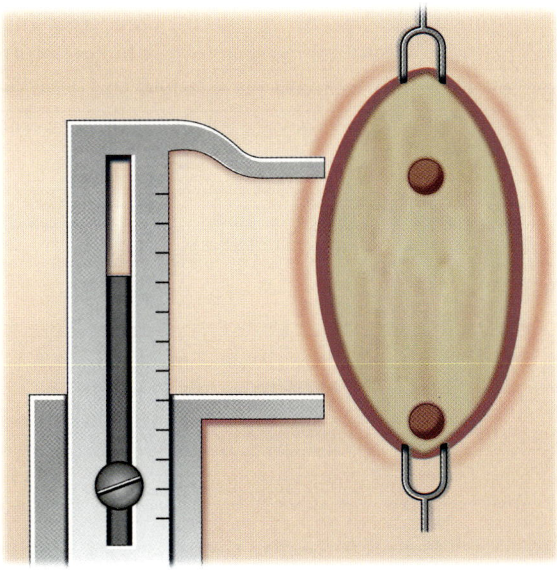

Fig. 8.5: Central incisions are closed after appropriate elevation of the central brows

periosteum and the frontalis, followed by staples for skin closure. The temporal incisions are similarly closed at a dermal level with 3-0 polyglactin sutures followed by skin staples.

- *Skin excision*: Skin excision is rarely necessary unless significant brow elevation is desired, when a small ellipse of skin may be removed prior to closure of the temporal incisions.
- *Drains*: Prior to closure, a drain may be placed over the calvarium in the central forehead and the deep temporal fascia laterally, but this is not always necessary.
- *Dressings*: A lightly compressive dressing is placed over the forehead for 12–24 hours to limit edema.

Potential Complications

Complications of the endoscopic midface lift are similar to those of the endoscopic forehead lift, with a few additions. Bleeding is rare, especially if the subperiosteal plane is dissected, although branches of the superficial temporal vein may be injured during the temporal dissection. Temporary hypesthesia of the forehead and scalp may result from stretching of the supraorbital and supratrochlear nerves, while cheek numbness will occur if the zygomaticofacial nerve is traumatized at its emergence near the malar eminence. Alopecia around the scalp incisions generally is temporary if it occurs, but patients with thinning hair may need to style their hair differently to camouflage the scars. Injury to the frontal branches of the facial nerve will cause an ipsilateral forehead paralysis, and can generally be caused by traction on the nerve or thermal injury from cautery use near the sentinel vein.

Aftercare

Postoperative care after an endoscopic midface lift is relatively simple. Antibiotic ointment is applied to the incisions until the skin staples are removed. Patients may need to use over-the-counter eye drops if they notice their eyes are dry or pruritic.

Midface Lift (Transpalpebral)

The transpalpebral midface lift approaches the midfacial tissues through a lower eyelid approach, and enables vectors of elevation more vertical than the endoscopic midface lift. This is useful for correction of nasojugal troughs, but potentially destabilizes and places more inferior pull on the lower eyelid.

Anesthesia

Like the endoscopic midface lift, the transpalpebral midface lift can be performed under intravenous sedation or general anesthesia, and if a subciliary incision is used, may also be performed after careful regional nerve block.

Incision Placement

The transpalpebral midface lift is performed either through a transconjunctival or a subciliary incision, depending upon the amount of redundant lower eyelid skin to be resected. In patients without significant lower eyelid skin redundancy, a canthotomy is performed by first making a small skin incision from the lateral canthus and extending 4–6 mm in an existing crow's feet rhytid. A straight clamp then straddles the lateral canthus down to the lateral orbital rim and the soft tissues clamped (Fig. 8.6). The clamp is then removed and cautery is used to incise the soft tissues down to bone (canthotomy). Curved Stevens scissors are then placed in the wound and directly inferiorly to divide the inferior limb of the lateral canthus (cantholysis) (Fig. 8.7). A transconjunctival incision is made approximately 3 mm below the lower tarsal border, and carried across to connect laterally to the canthotomy/cantholysis. The eyelid dissection then divides the orbital septum, inferior lid retractors and a preseptal dissection plane is developed (Figs 8.8A to C). This is followed to the inferior orbital rim (Fig. 8.9), and after preserving a 3–4 mm cuff of periosteum on the orbital rim, the periosteum is incised with a #15 blade and a subperiosteal plane developed.

Alternatively, a subciliary incision can be used if eyelid skin excision is planned. This is continued laterally until it meets the crow's feet incision. A suborbicularis oculi tunnel is created through blunt elevation with a Stevens scissors below the skin incision and the muscle divided on an angle (preserving an additional muscular sling inferior to the lower tarsus). The skin-muscle flap below this is then elevated to expose the orbital septum (see Chapter 6 for skin-muscle flap). Once the inferior orbital rim is reached, the periosteum is incised and the subperiosteal midfacial plane established and developed.

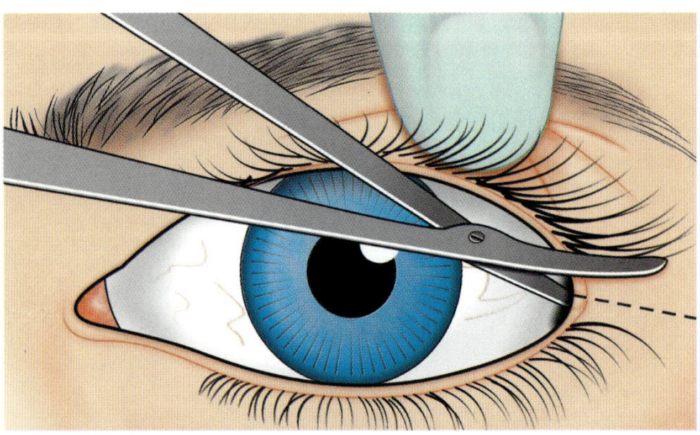

Fig. 8.6: The transpalpebral midface lift is facilitated by lateral canthal release. After incising the skin lateral to the canthus in a pre-existing skin crease, a straight clamp is introduced to crush the soft tissue to limit bleeding and then the tissue is divided (canthotomy)

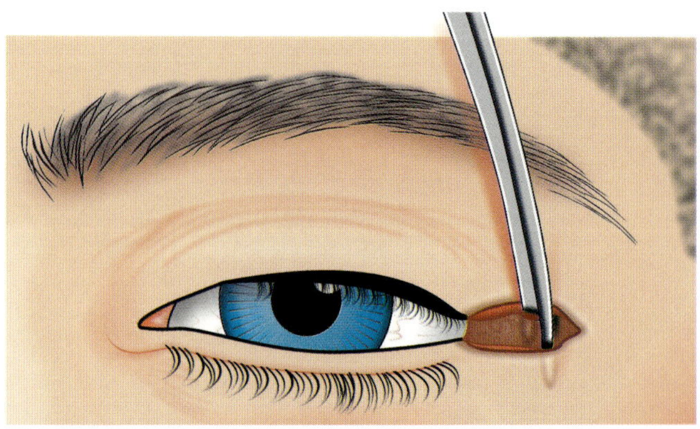

Fig. 8.7: Scissors are then used to divide the inferior limb of the lateral canthal tendon (cantholysis)

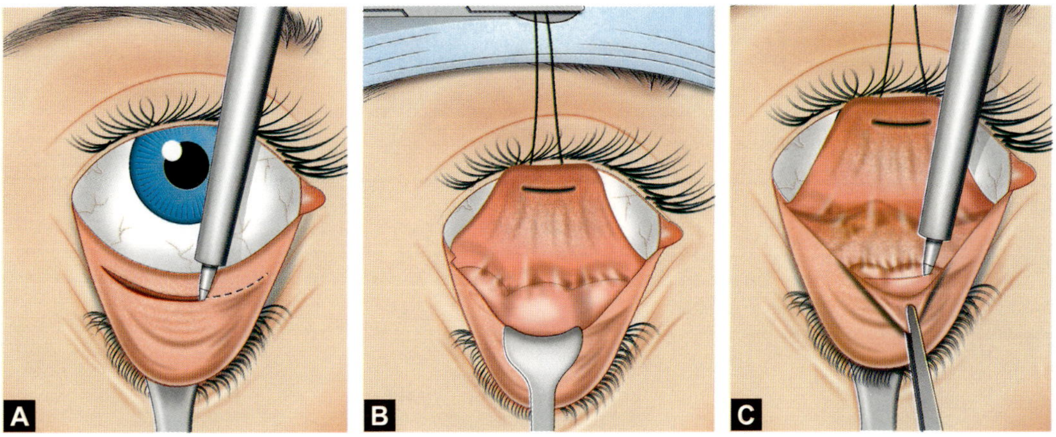

Figs 8.8A to C: A transconjunctival approach to the midface connects the eyelid dissection to the lateral canthal dissection. (A) Division of the conjunctiva and lower lid retractors and (B) Development of a conjunctival flap, which is retracted superiorly to protect the cornea. Further dissection then skeletonizes the inferior orbital rim and (C) Divides the periosteum several millimeters below the rim

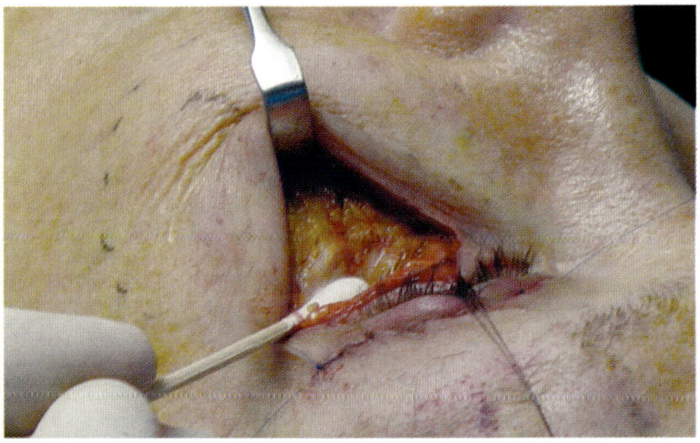

Fig. 8.9: Preperiosteal exposure of the orbital rim through a subciliary approach

Extent of Undermining/Dissection

The periosteum is then elevated off the face of the maxilla from the inferior orbital rim down to the gingivobuccal sulcus and between the malar eminence and medial insertion of the masseter muscle laterally to the nasal sidewall and pyriform aperture medially (Fig. 8.10). Care should be taken to completely skeletonize the infraorbital nerve (Figs 8.11A and B) as it emerges from the infraorbital foramen; both the infraorbital and the zygomaticofacial nerve (seen at the lateral extent of the dissection of the inferolateral orbital rim) should be preserved.

Tissue Modifications

- *Incision*: The periosteum at the inferior aspect of the dissection pocket, near the gingivobuccal sulcus, should be incised to provide full inferior release. This can be done with a #15 blade, and a clamp is then used to spread the incision open until fat is seen.

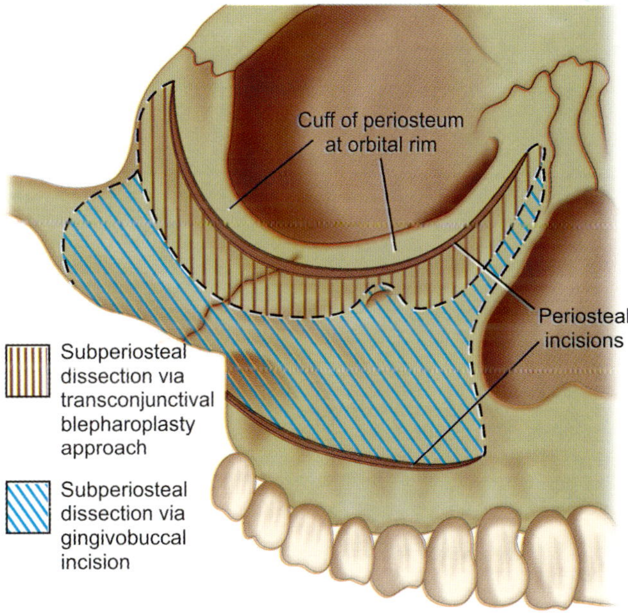

Fig. 8.10: Extent of periosteal dissection

- *Tissue advancement*: Once the midfacial tissues are fully mobilized, superior traction on the periosteum will elevate the midface without excessive force. If tissues are not sufficiently mobile, the dissection pocket should be reinspected and full periosteal elevation around the infraorbital nerve should be ensured. Additionally, soft tissues should be swept laterally until the masseter muscle origin is clearly seen. Finally, it is essential that the lateral orbital retaining ligament also be elevated to allow full midfacial mobilization.
- *Fixation*: It is essential that stable long-term fixation of the midfacial tissues in their elevated position be provided. A 3-0 polydioxanone or Mersilene suture

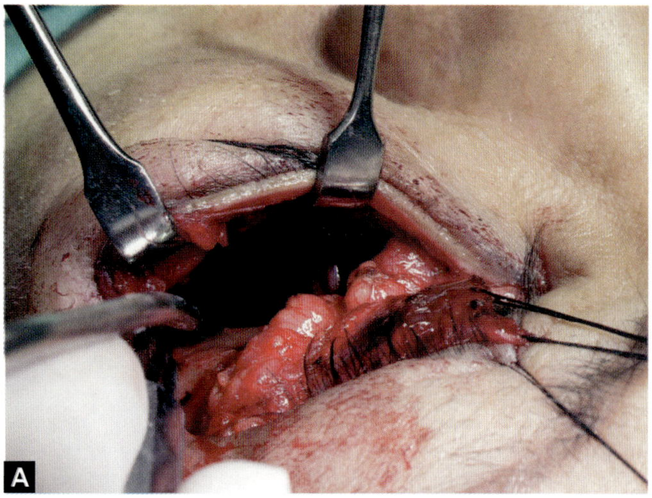

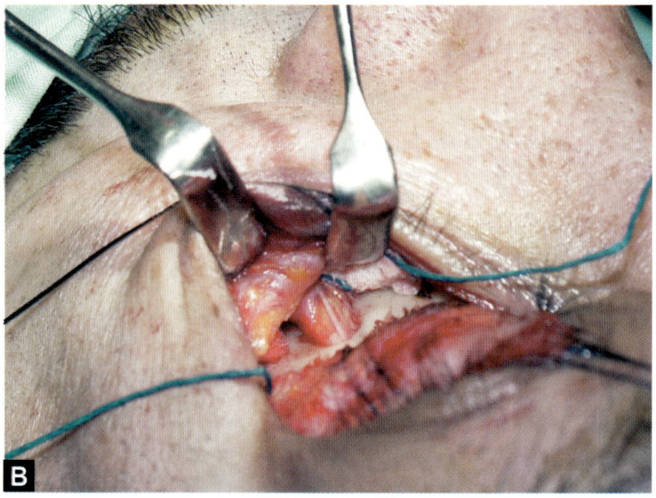

Figs 8.11A and B: (A) Inferior dissection exposes the infraorbital nerve; (B) Subperiosteal pockets are dissected lateral and medial to the infraorbital nerve and connected inferior to the nerve

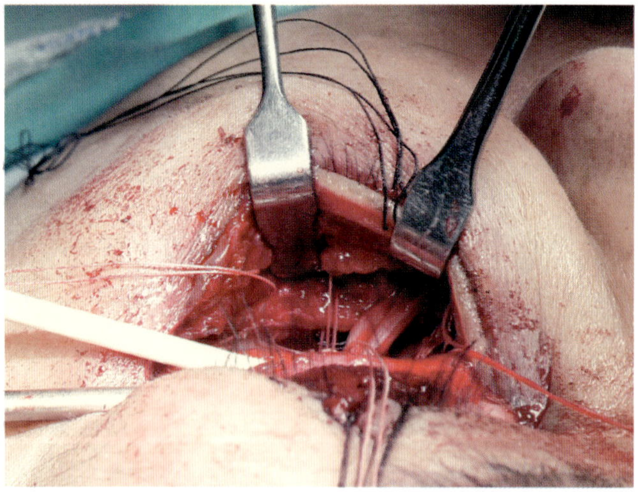

Fig. 8.12: Mersilene suspension sutures can be placed from the inferior cheek flap up to the periosteal cuff at the orbital rim

placed into the inferior periosteum may be placed medial or lateral to the infraorbital nerve and secured superiorly to the remaining cuff of periosteum at the infraorbital rim (Fig. 8.12). The periosteum near the inferolateral orbital rim tends to be thicker and holds sutures better, while medial periorbita is weaker and more flimsy. The soft tissues are elevated in the direction most necessary for aesthetic correction, so reliance on lateral rim sutures alone may prevent full correction of tear trough deformity. Bone anchored fixation devices, such as the Endotine Midface B implant (MicroAire, Charlottesville, Virginia) or the Mitek 2.0 TACIT anchor (DePuy Synthes, Warsaw, Indiana), can successfully maintain elevation of the soft tissues of the midface (Figs 8.13A to D). The implant tines pierce the lower periosteum, and the implant "tail" is pulled superiorly and fixed in position to the bone just below the orbital rim with a resorbable screw. Sutures to the medial inferior orbital rim periosteal cuff are then placed to gently drape soft tissue volume into the nasojugal trough (Fig. 8.14). Sutures to the lateral orbital rim provide additional stabilization (Fig. 8.15).

The lateral canthus is then reconstructed, placing a 4-0 e-PTFE suture from the lateral edge of the of the lateral canthal tendon to the internal aspect of the lateral orbital rim approximately 2–3 mm above the original site of the lateral canthal tendon insertion. If lower lid skin has been resected, as part of a lower blepharoplasty, the lateral canthal tendon is shorted and resuspended slightly higher to prevent lower lid retraction postoperatively (Figs 8.16A and B).

Closure

Orbicularis oculi muscle at the lateral canthus is then closed with a buried 4-0 Vicryl suture, and a 6-0 fast absorbing chromic suture reapproximates the upper and lower lids at the gray line. Lateral skin is then closed with a 6-0 fast absorbing gut suture. The conjunctival incision does not need to be closed, but the wound edges should be gently and carefully aligned; if the incision is closed, 6-0 fast absorbing chromic sutures should be used without everting wound edges. If a subciliary approach has been used, skin resection should be conservatively performed while the patient gazes superiorly with mouth

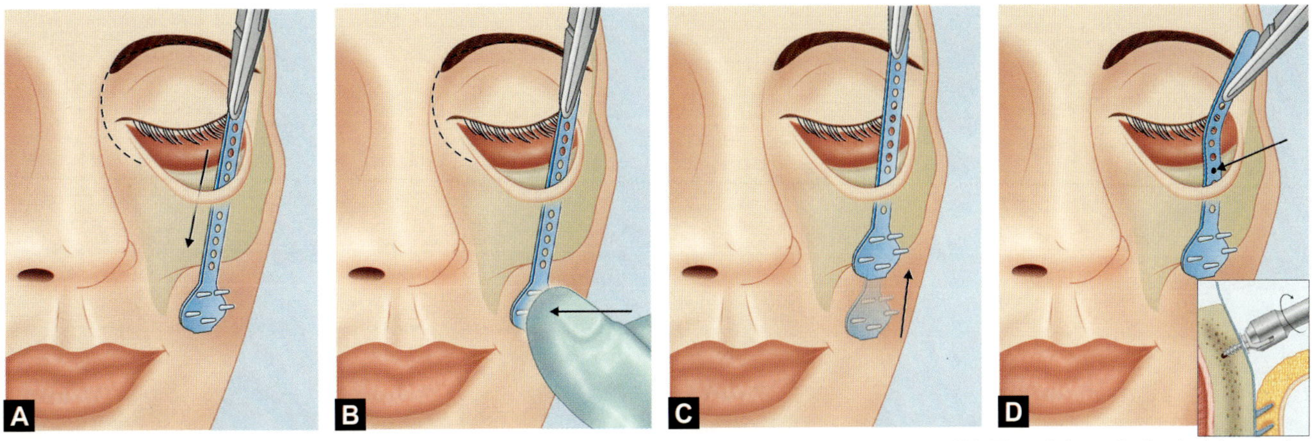

Figs 8.13A to D: Alternatively, fixation devices such as the Endotine Midface B can be used and (A) Placed through the incision to the location of desired soft tissue elevation; (B) With gentle finger pressure, fixation tines are impaled on the soft tissue; (C) The device is retracted superiorly until the desired tissue elevation is produced and (D) A hole is drilled at the appropriate location near the orbital rim and a resorbable screw placed (inset). Excess device is then removed

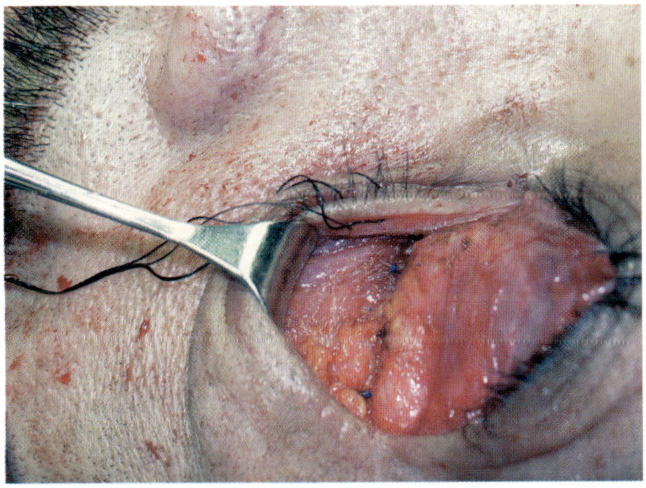

Fig. 8.14: Additional soft tissue fixation along the rim is performed medially and laterally as needed to further efface any soft tissue volume deficit

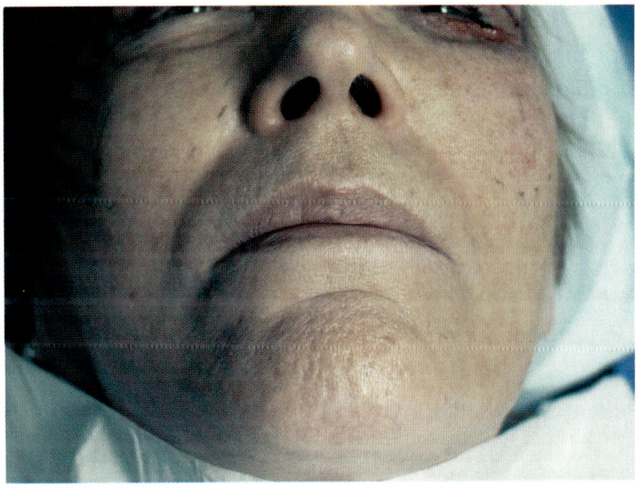

Fig. 8.15: Intraoperative photo showing the degree of elevation achieved (patient's left) compared to (right) unoperated side

open. Any slight skin excess present postoperatively can be treated with a skin pinch excision once postoperative edema has subsided. The skin is then closed with interrupted 6-0 chromic sutures.

Dressings

Cool compresses can be applied to the eyes and cheeks, but no dressings are required.

Potential Complications

Temporary midfacial hypesthesia is very common, but typically resolves within several weeks. Permanent numbness is rare as long as care is taken during dissection around the infraorbital nerve. Focal hypesthesia at the inferiolateral orbital rim and malar eminence can be permanent if the zygomaticofacial nerve is damaged during dissection. Hematoma is rare but should be evacuated if observed. Most significantly, lid malposition can occur if fixation of elevated tissues is inadequate. A lateral canthoplasty, or at a minimum a canthopexy, should always be performed along with the transpalpebral midface lift.

Aftercare

Care after transpalpebral midface lift is rather simple. Cool compresses are continued intermittently for the

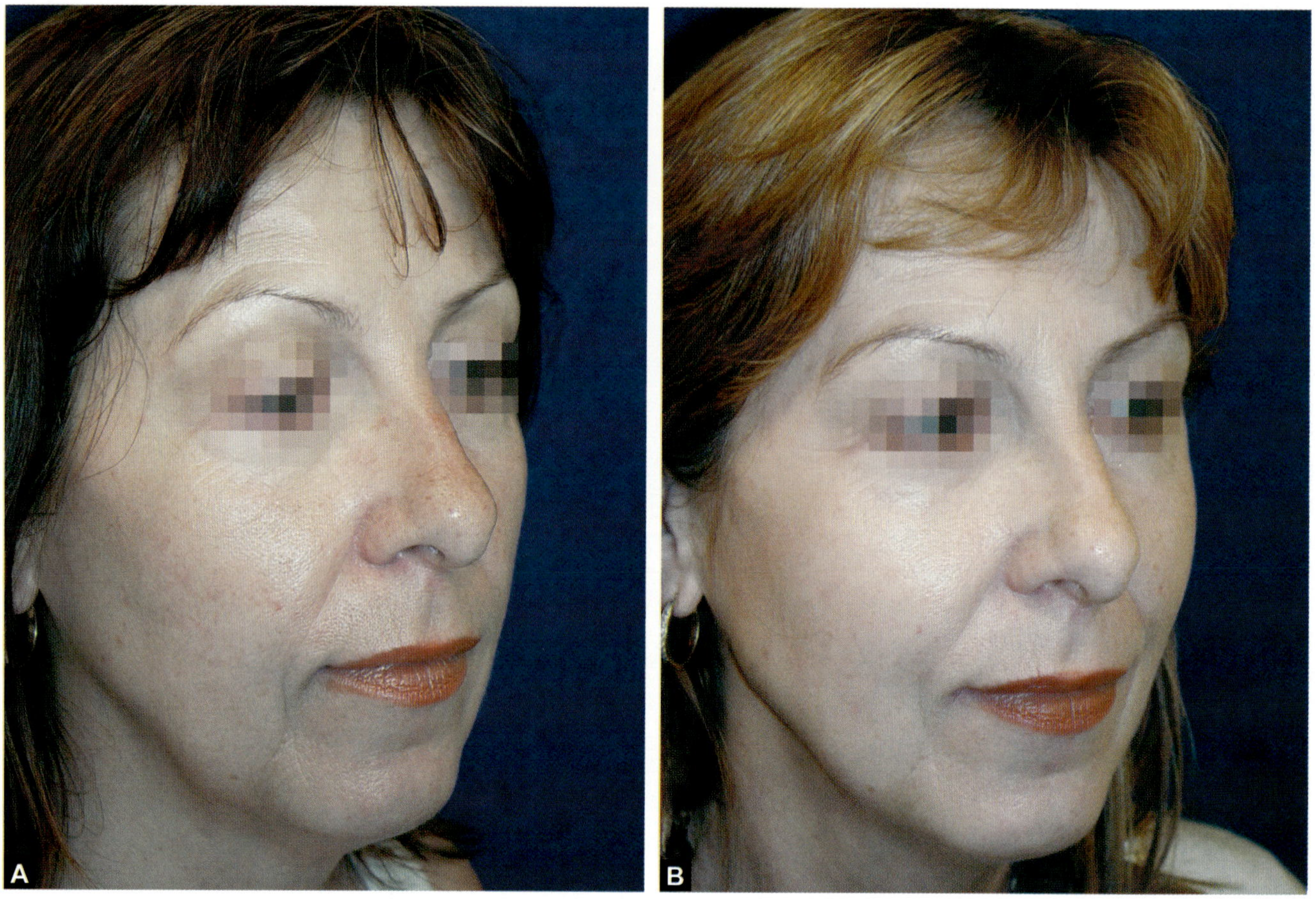

Figs 8.16A and B: Transpalpebral midface lift. (A) Preoperative view; (B) Postoperative view

first 24–36 hours. Eye lubricants, such as artificial tears and basic ointments, can be applied during the first postoperative week. Sutures are removed from the lateral canthal area 5–7 days after surgery.

BIBLIOGRAPHY

1. Codner M. Modifying the subperiosteal cheek lift. Aesthet Surg J. 2003;23(3):203-4.
2. DeFatta RJ, Williams EF. Midface lifting: current standards. Facial Plast Surg. 2011;27(1):77-85.
3. Hoenig JF, Knutti D, de la Fuente A. Vertical subperiosteal mid-face-lift for treatment of malar festoons. Aesthetic Plast Surg. 2011;35(4):522-9.
4. Marotta JC, Quatela VC. Lower eyelid aesthetics after endoscopic forehead midface-lift. Arch Facial Plast Surg. 2008;10(4):267-72.
5. Sclafani AP. Comprehensive periorbital rejuvenation with resorbable endotine implants for trans-lid brow and midface elevation. Facial Plast Surg Clin North Am. 2007;15(2):255-64.

CHAPTER 9

Rhinoplasty

Anthony P Sclafani

OVERVIEW

Rhinoplasty involves the reconfiguration of the nose for aesthetic reasons, functional improvement, or both. From its beginnings as a purely reconstructive procedure designed to repair nasal damage for trauma or infection, rhinoplasty has become a method of improving nasal aesthetics and/or function. While there are many excellent texts covering the nuances of rhinoplasty, this chapter is intended to provide an overview and description of the common techniques of rhinoplasty.

SPECIAL CONSIDERATIONS

Rhinoplasty reshapes, resects or augments the natural bony, cartilaginous and soft tissue structures of the nose. The final result occurs when the natural fibrotic and contractile forces of wound healing no longer alter the structure of the nose. While most changes are apparent early after surgery, many (particularly those in the nasal tip) are thought to take as long as 12–18 months, with final changes often occurring many years later. The key to establishment of a stable long-term result is maintenance of the integrity of the natural support structures of the nose. In the upper nose, the periosteal attachments of the nasal bones should be maintained to the greatest degree possible. In the middle vault, over resection of the upper lateral cartilages (ULCs) should be avoided and the internal nasal lining not violated. In the nasal tip, the major and minor support structures of the tip (Table 9.1) should be respected and protected to the greatest degree possible. Changes to tip contour, rotation and projection after alterations of these structures can be predicted based on the "tripod concept" of the nasal tip (Fig. 9.1).

Nasal obstruction that presents preoperatively or can be anticipated to occur postoperatively secondary to surgical maneuvers should be managed pre-emptively. Correction of a deviated septum and/or inferior turbinate hypertrophy should follow standard techniques and principles. Pre-existing (natural or surgically related) nasal valve collapse must be prevented/managed for any rhinoplasty to be considered successful.

ALTERNATIVES TO PROCEDURE

Camouflage techniques (so-called "medical" or "injection" rhinoplasty) can be used to alter the appearance of the nose. Soft tissue fillers (e.g. hyaluronic acid derivatives, calcium hydroxylapatite) can be injected carefully to recontour the nose. A low dorsum or concavities (particularly postoperatively) can be treated by restoring volume with soft tissue fillers. More aggressive techniques, such as altering tip shape, can also be managed with fillers, although less viscous fillers should be used to avoid vascular occlusion or pressure necrosis of the nasal tip skin. Botulinum toxin A can assist in managing nasal tip ptosis in many cases by causing temporary paralysis of the depressor septi muscle. However, none of these techniques can provide the stable, safe, functional and long-term results gained by a well-performed rhinoplasty.

TECHNIQUES

Approach

Access to the anatomical structures of the nose is gained via one of two basic methods: the intranasal (closed) approach or the external (open) approach. An intranasal closed approach hides all incisions within the nasal vestibule, may be more direct and may require less extensive dissection. The external approach, on the other hand, requires a transcolumellar incision and generally requires more dissection, but more fully exposes the lower lateral cartilages (LLCs). Both are useful and safe approaches if performed properly, and the particular approach should be chosen based on which approach most enhances the surgeon's ability to perform the required cartilage modifications.

Table 9.1: Major and minor tip supports

Major tip supports	*Minor tip supports*
Length, strength and integrity of the LLCs	Interdomal ligament
Attachment of the ULCs to the LLCs	Nasal spine
Fibrous attachment of the medial crural footplates to the caudal septum	Attachments of LLCs to overlying skin
	Dorsal and caudal septum
	Skin
	Membranous septum
	Sesamoid cartilages

(LLC: Lower lateral cartilage; ULC: Upper lateral cartilage)

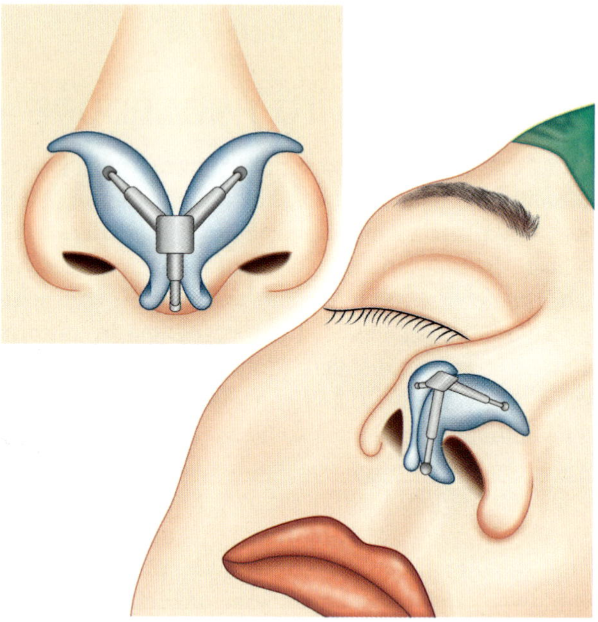

Fig. 9.1: The "nasal tripod" model of nasal tip support

Anesthesia

Rhinoplasty is generally performed under intravenous sedation or general anesthesia for patient comfort and by surgeon preference. Except in cases under general anesthesia (where its use can lower the seizure threshold), 4% cocaine on pledgets will yield excellent topical intranasal anesthesia and vasoconstriction. It is possible, however, to perform rhinoplasty under regional blockade and oral anxiolysis. Infratrochlear, dorsal nasal, infraorbital, nasopalatine and sphenopalatine nerve blocks can provide adequate anesthesia, and are useful in reducing parenteral medication needed in sedation and general anesthesia cases as well. Preperiosteal and preperichondrial infiltration of local anesthetic over the nasal dorsum and ascending processes of the maxillae facilitate dissection, but the volume used should not distort the nose.

Incision Placement

Intranasal Approach

- *Intercartilaginous incision*: The intercartilaginous incision (Fig. 9.2A) transects the soft tissue attachments between the cephalic border of the lateral crus of the LLC and the caudal margin of the ULC, an area fibrous attachment where the LLC rests external to the ULC (the "scroll region"). This incision is useful in providing access to the upper two-thirds of the nasal dorsum as well as in delineating the lateral crus of the LLC during tip delivery. A wide double hook or short Vienna nasal speculum is used to telescope the lateral crus cephalically over the caudal end of the ULC (Fig. 9.2B). A #15 blade incises the mucosa just above the caudal edge from the medial edge of the pyriform aperture laterally up to the anterior septal angle medially (Fig. 9.3A). Further dissection cephalically to the caudal border of the pyriform aperture is performed either sharply with a scalpel blade or bluntly by spreading dissection with a Stevens scissors. Dissection is directed over the nasal dorsum and connects to the dissection from the contralateral incision (Fig. 9.3B). Dissection of the lower nasal dorsum generally requires conversion of the medial aspect of the incisions to a partial or full transfixion incision to expose the anterior septal angle and allow full release of the supratip area.
- *Transcartilaginous incision*: In cases where a cephalic portion of the lateral crus will be resected, the incision can be brought more caudally to a position where the new cephalic border of the lateral crus will be located (Fig. 9.4A). The incision is first made only through the mucosa. An angled converse tip scissors is used to dissect the vestibular mucosa off the lateral crus cephalic to the mucosal incision, up to the cephalic border of the LLC (Fig. 9.4B). Next, a scalpel blade incises the lateral crus at the same point as the mucosal incision. Converse tip scissors then dissect

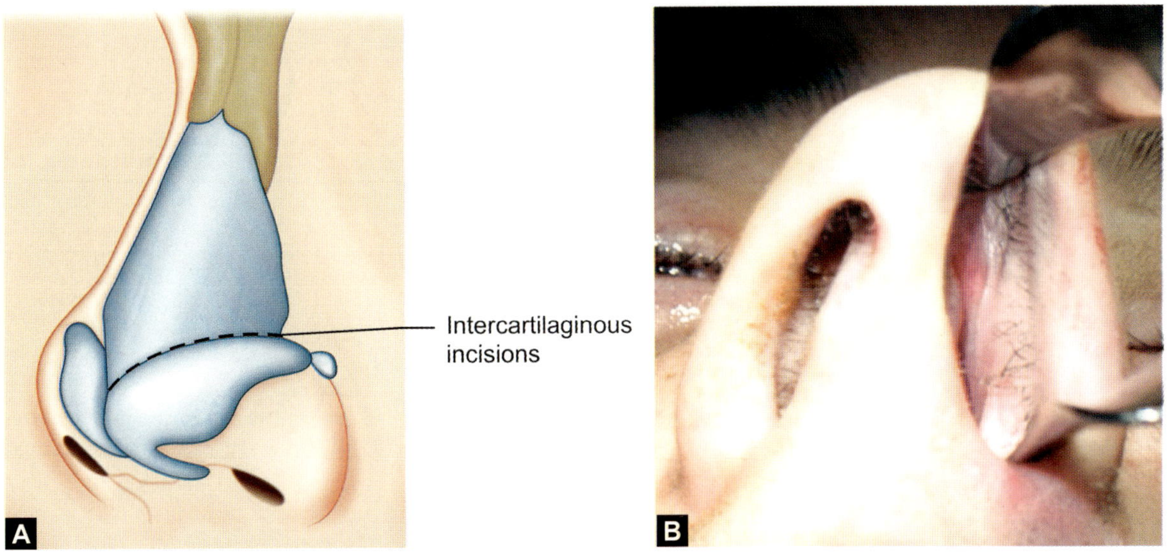

Figs 9.2A and B: (A) The intercartilaginous incision is placed at the junction of the upper lateral cartilages (ULCs) and lower lateral cartilages (LLCs); (B) By retracting the ala cephalically, the caudal edge of the ULC is shown

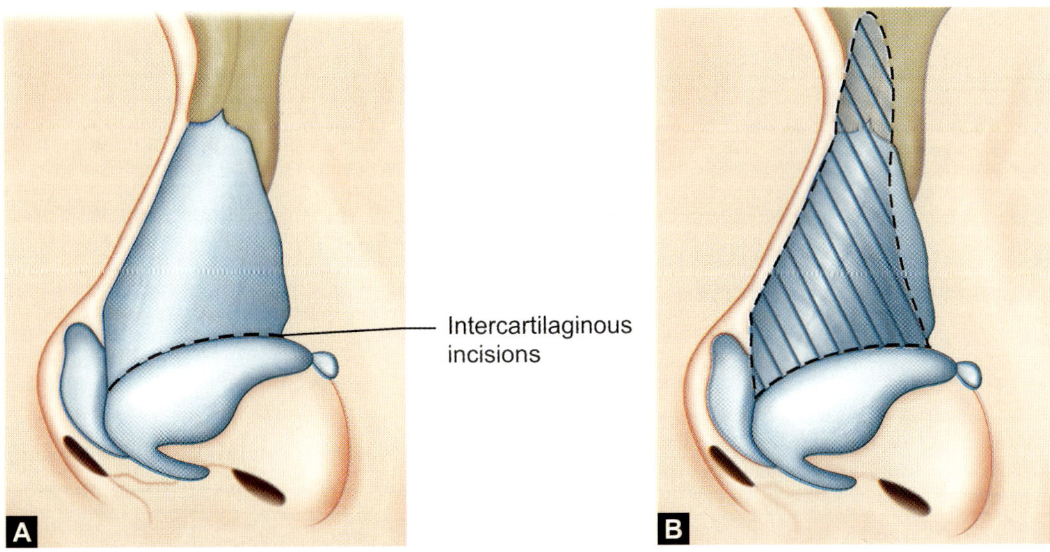

Figs 9.3A and B: (A) The intercartilaginous incision runs from just medial to the pyriform aperture to the anterior septal angle; (B) Undermining is performed in order to create a common plane with the contralateral dissection

the cephalically delineated cartilage away from attachments to the overlying soft tissue until this strip of cartilage to be excised is attached only laterally and medially (Fig. 9.4C). Scissors are then used to excise the outlined cephalic strip of cartilage. At this point, what had been a transcartilaginous mucosal incision is now an intercartilaginous incision.

A slight modification of this technique is the intercartilaginous incision with retrograde lateral crus dissection. The intercartilaginous incision is made first. The lateral crus is the everted with external finger pressure. Converse tip scissors are used to dissect deep and superficial to the cephalic portion of the cartilage, staying in a preperichondrial plane (Fig. 9.5). An assistant gently retracts the vestibular mucosa to expose the cephalic edge of the crus, which is then excised with either tip scissors or a #15 blade (Fig. 9.5). As with the transcartilaginous incision, mid-dorsal dissection is performed through the incision.

- *Marginal incision*: The marginal incision runs along the caudal margin of the LLC. This is most easily accomplished grasping the vestibular edge with a

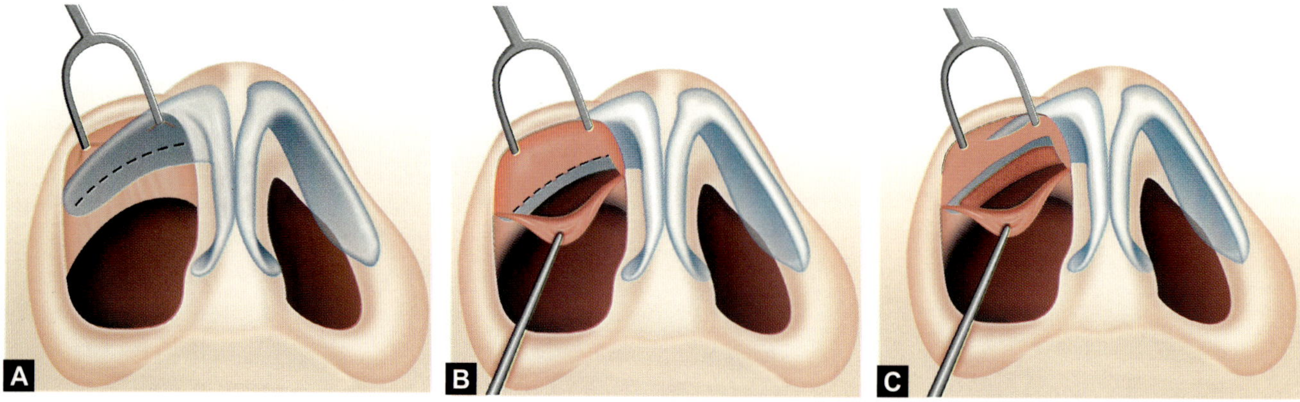

Figs 9.4A to C: (A) The transcartilaginous incision is placed directly at the site of the planned cephalic resection of lateral crura; (B) Vestibular mucosa is dissected off cephalic edge of the lateral crus to be resected; (C) After the cartilage is incised, it is dissected free from the soft tissue attachments on its external surface and resected cephalically

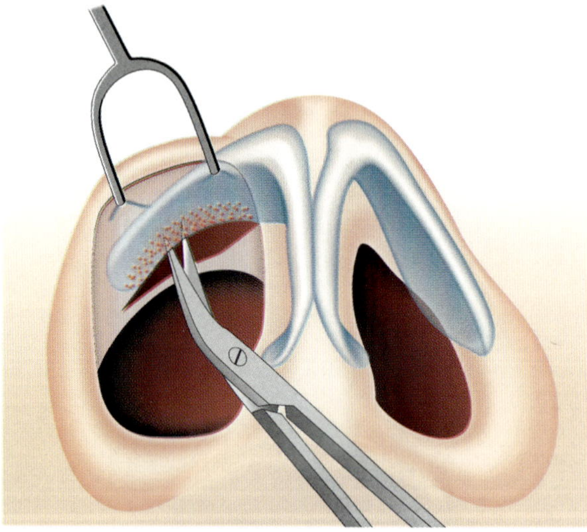

Fig. 9.5: After the intercartilaginous incision is made, the mucosa is dissected in a retrograde fashion, exposing the cephalic edge of the lateral crus. With the mucosal flap retracted, the cephalic edge of the cartilage is excised

sharp double hook and everting the ala with finger pressure (Fig. 9.6A). It is important to follow the caudal edge of the cartilage, which does not run along the alar rim, to avoid unnecessary transection of soft tissue of the alar rim; disturbance of this tissue risks significant soft tissue alar retraction, especially in the soft tissue facets. When delivery of the LLC is planned, the marginal incision continues down the side of the columella to a point just above the medial crura footplate. Sharp and blunt dissection with Converse scissors proceeds just above the perichondrium and below the nasal superficial musculoaponeurotic system (SMAS) until the marginal incision is completely connected to the intercartilaginous incision above the LLC, and the LLC forms a bipedicled flap (Fig. 9.6B). By simultaneously retracting the alar skin cephalically and the LLC caudally, the LLC is "delivered" out of its pocket within the nasal tip and widely exposed (Fig. 9.6C). Modifications, such as removal of a cephalic strip (Fig. 9.6C) or placement of an interdomal or transdomal suture, are facilitated by this exposure; however, the LLC is destabilized by the extensive dissection, and LLC asymmetries and relationships are more difficult to appreciate, since the cartilage is placed on stretch.

External Approach

- *Marginal incision*: The same marginal incision used in the delivery technique is made, ending at the midlevel of the medial crura. Again, the soft tissues of the ala just above the perichondrium are carefully dissected free and elevated using the Converse tip scissors. Performing this dissection first reduces traction on the nasal tip skin during elevation.
- *Transcolumellar incision*: A broken-line (commonly an inverse gull-wing or stair-step) incision is then made across the midportion of the columella. It is important to place the incision midway between the dome and the convexity of the medial crural footplate, as the skin rests directly against the cartilage in this location and the scar cannot retract through soft tissue as it would if made higher (near the soft tissue facets) or lower (below the medial crural footplates). Connecting the marginal and transcolumellar incisions creates a continuous incision across the caudal margins of the LLCs and allows elevation of a widely based skin-soft tissue flap (Fig. 9.7A).

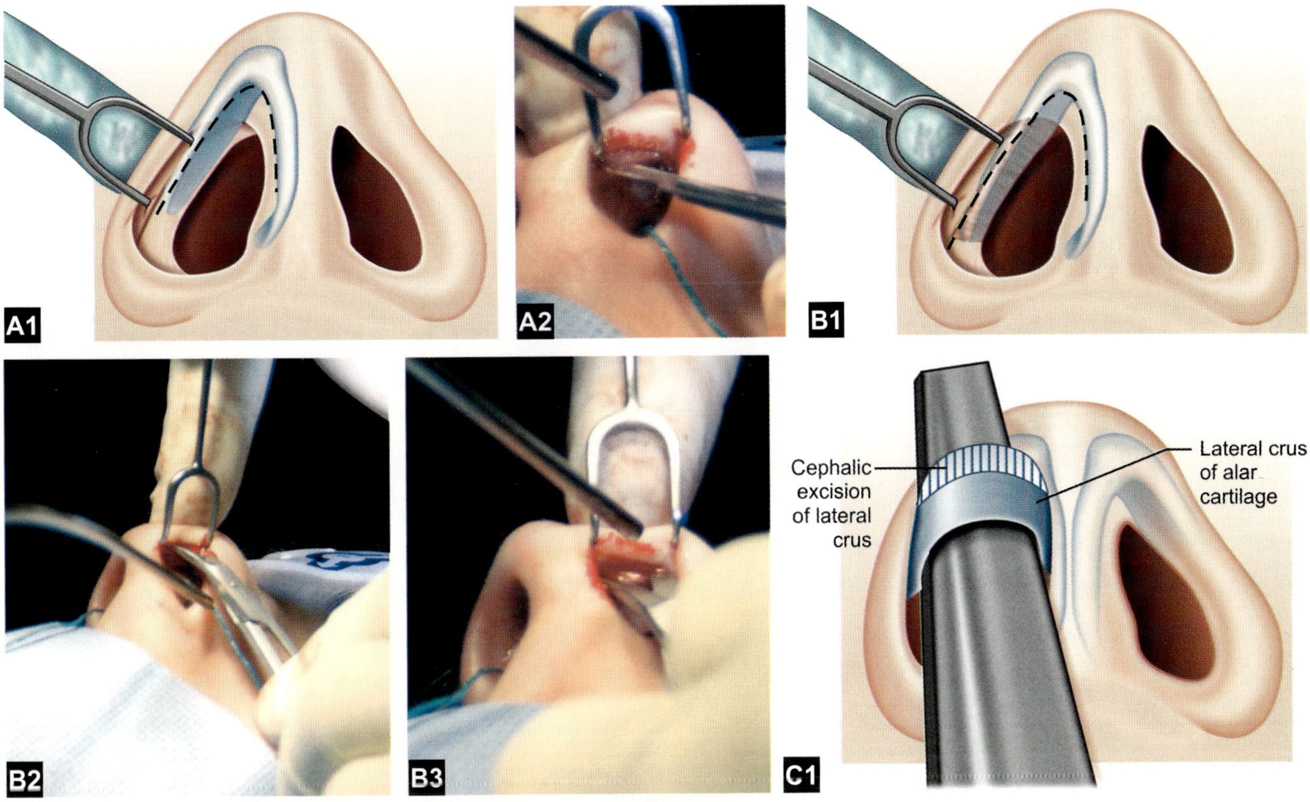

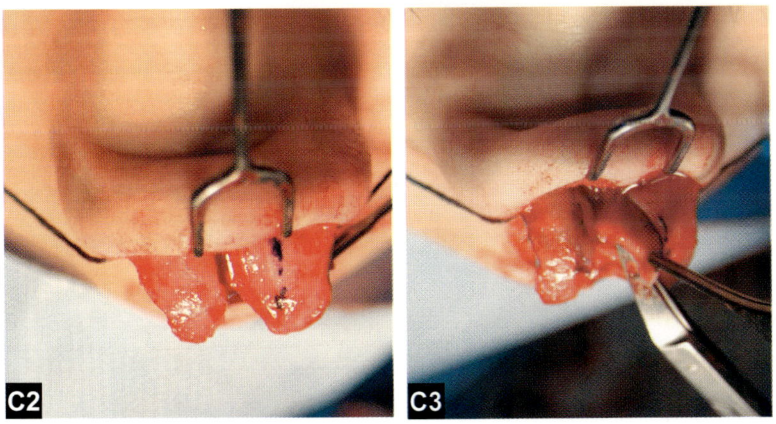

Figs 9.6A to C: (A1) Diagram and (A2) Photograph of the marginal incision, running along the caudal edge of the lower lateral cartilage (LLC); (B1) Delivery technique requires dissection to isolate the lower lateral crus as a bipedicled flap; (B2 and B3) Photographs of dissection through the marginal incision directly above the perichondrium of the LLC; (C1) Delivery of the flap provides access for modification of the cartilage; (C2 and C3) Cephalic strip of LLC marked and dissected (shown here during an open approach, for clarity)

Extent of Undermining/Dissection

If dissection of the soft tissue from the LLC was thorough after the marginal incisions, the columellar skin flap elevates easily. Initially, one tine of a double hook is placed in each nasal sill for inferior traction, while a single hook helps to elevate the columellar flap, as the soft tissue over the cartilage can generally be swept cephalically with a cotton tip applicator (Fig. 9.7B). The double hook is then used to retract the skin flap as separate single hooks stabilize each soft tissue facet. All soft tissue is removed from the LLCs laterally to the areas of the hinge. Blunt dissection with a cotton tip applicator or Stevens scissors helps to expose the anterior septal angle and cartilaginous dorsum (Fig. 9.7C). A periosteal elevator is used to elevate the dorsal periosteum from the caudal end of the nasal bones to the nasal root (Fig. 9.7D). If lateral osteotomies are planned, stab incisions are made at the lateral pyriform aperture just below the insertion of the inferior turbinate. A Joseph elevator is used to tunnel subperiosteally along the planned course of the lateral osteotomy (Fig. 9.8).

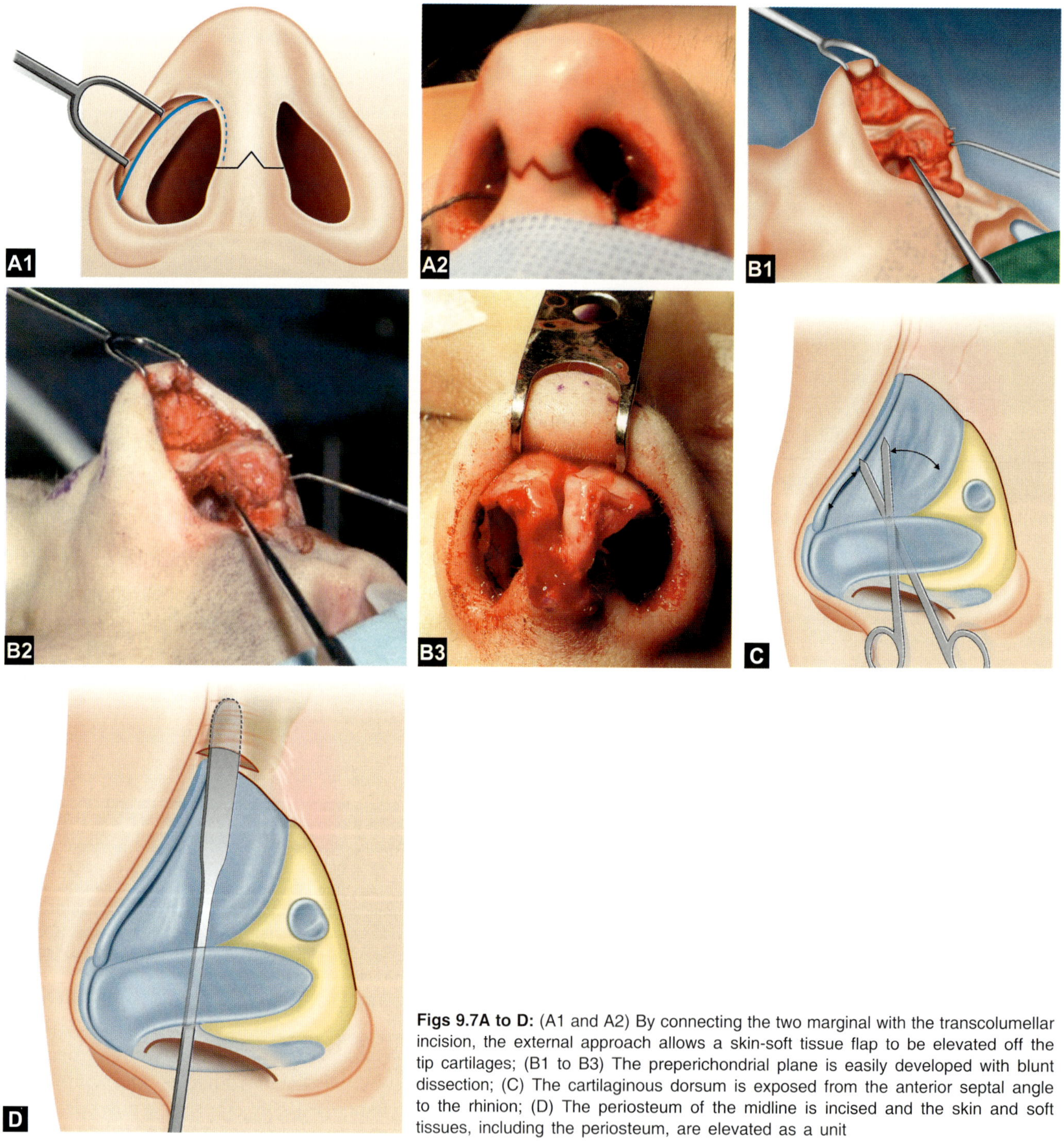

Figs 9.7A to D: (A1 and A2) By connecting the two marginal with the transcolumellar incision, the external approach allows a skin-soft tissue flap to be elevated off the tip cartilages; (B1 to B3) The preperichondrial plane is easily developed with blunt dissection; (C) The cartilaginous dorsum is exposed from the anterior septal angle to the rhinion; (D) The periosteum of the midline is incised and the skin and soft tissues, including the periosteum, are elevated as a unit

Dorsal Tissue Modifications

Dorsal Reduction

The height of the nasal dorsum can be lowered if necessary. After an Aufricht retractor is placed to expose the nasal dorsum, the cartilaginous portion of the dorsum is lowered by incrementally shaving the cartilage (Fig. 9.9). Especially when significant dorsal reduction is performed, it is essential to avoid violation of the nasal mucosa. If this is exposed, the mucosa should be dissected free from the cartilage with a Cottle elevator so that only cartilage is resected. The skin flap is redraped and the surgeon runs his finger along the dorsum to ensure a smooth and even dorsum. If irregularities are noted, the tip of the Aufricht retractor is placed up to the site of interest and the irregularity exposed and refined.

The bony dorsum can be reduced using either osteotomies or rasps. Large bony humps can be removed with unguarded (Rubin) or double-guarded (Fomon or Cinelli) osteotomes (Figs 9.10A and B). It is important to maintain the plane of the cutting blade parallel to the desired plane of the dorsum. Edges of the osteotomies can be smoothed with fine rasps. Minor bony excess can be incrementally removed with coarse or fine rasps. As with the cartilaginous dorsum, periodically, the skin is redraped and the contour of the dorsum is palpated with a finger, and any remaining irregularities addressed. It is important to palpate the nature of these, especially in the "keystone" area at the bony-cartilaginous junction. In this area, the cartilaginous septum runs below the caudal nasal bones; as these are lowered by rasps, the septal cartilage will be exposed. Injudicious rasping further will depress the dorsal septum, leaving its height unchanged, while the rasp will continue to lower the nasal bones. Occasionally, a high radix needs to be reduced with a glabellar push rasp (Fig. 9.11). If an "open roof" deformity (discontinuity of the nasal bones over the dorsum) develops after dorsal reduction (Figs 9.12A and B), osteotomies are necessary to mobilize the nasal bones and close the defect.

Dorsal Augmentation

The under-projected dorsum can be augmented with a number of materials, natural or synthetic.

- *Septal cartilage grafts*: The most common graft is septal cartilage, harvested through a standard septoplasty approach. To provide greater augmentation, pieces can be stacked, sutured together and carved to fit over the nasal dorsum.
- *Conchal cartilage grafts*: Conchal, unlike septal, cartilage is not is the operative field during rhinoplasty. Additionally, conchal cartilage is generally concave and better suited to alar grafts (see below). Dorsal grafts, however, can be created, especially if opposing conchal segments are sutured together for additional height and to neutralize curvature and warping tendency. Through either a posterior (centered over the postauricular crease) or anterior (located on the conchal wall side of the antihelix) incision (Fig. 9.13), the perichondrium is incised and elevated from the conchal cartilage as far medially as the external auditory meatus. Generally, only the horizontal portion of conchal cartilage is harvested, as a cartilage incision is made at the junction of the horizontal and vertical portions of the conchal bowl cartilage. If it is necessary to remove more cartilage, this incision can be placed at varying distances up the conchal

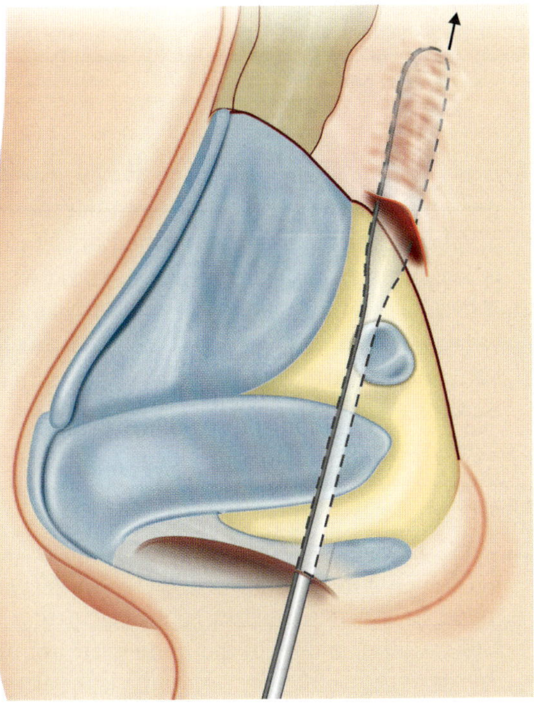

Fig. 9.8: Subperiosteal tunnels are also created along the lines of planned lateral osteotomies

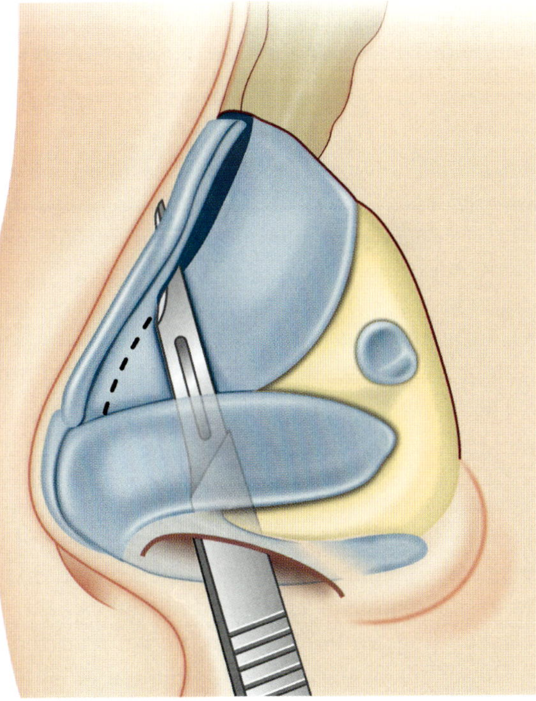

Fig. 9.9: The cartilaginous dorsum is reduced by shaving portions of cartilage with a scalpel

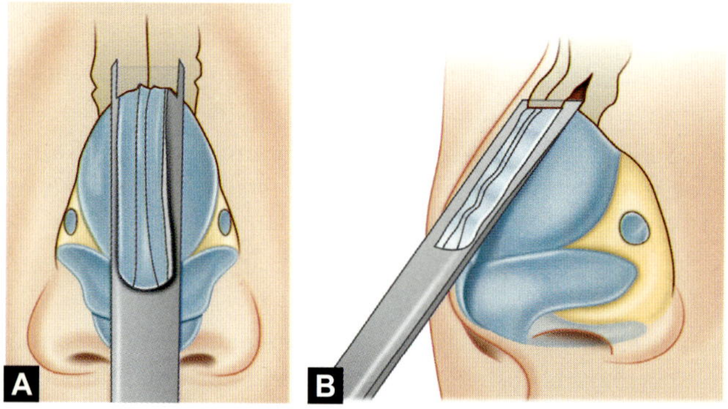

Figs 9.10A and B: Bony humps are removed using 8–10 mm wide osteotomes. Small bony dorsal humps are reduced with rasps

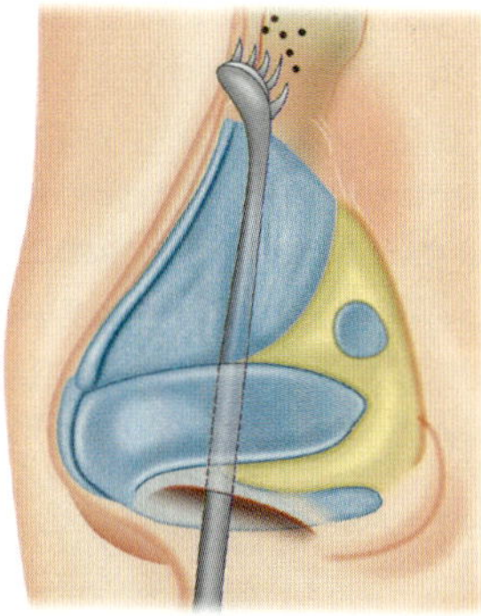

Fig. 9.11: A glabellar "push" rasp can be used to deepen a high radix

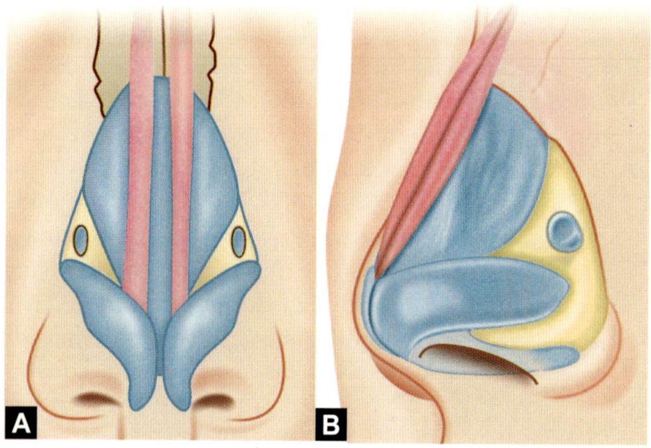

Figs 9.12A and B: Failure to correct an open roof deformity with lateral osteotomies may leave a widened, "ridged" dorsum

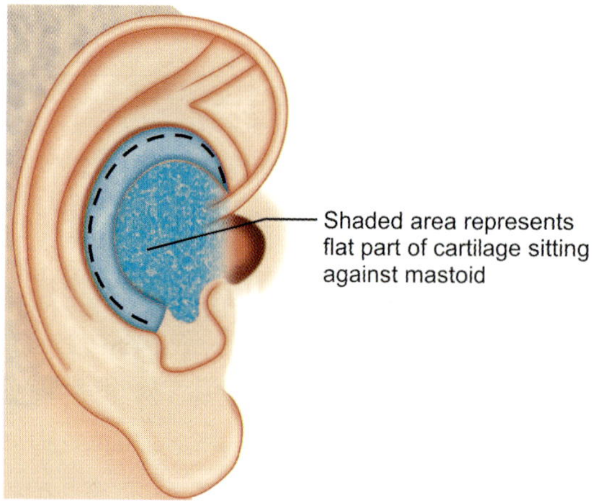

Fig. 9.13: Conchal cartilage can be harvested through an anterior (dotted line) or posterior incision, and can easily utilize the portion of cartilage adjacent to the mastoid

bowl wall, but patients should be informed of and have accepted auricular medialization preoperatively. The cartilage is then dissected free from the opposite perichondrium. The incision is then closed with a running 4-0 chromic suture, and mattress sutures of 4-0 chromic are placed between the medial and lateral aspects of the auricle to eliminate surgical dead space.

- *Rib cartilage grafts*: Larger grafts can be formed from harvested costal cartilage. A 5 cm anterior chest/inframammary incision is made and intercostal muscles are divided with electrocautery until rib is exposed. The perichondrium is incised and dissected from the cartilage circumferentially using a Freer elevator (Figs 9.14A to C), and can be facilitated using a Doyen rib stripper. A 5 cm segment of cartilage is harvested by cutting through the ends of the segment while an elevator is held between cartilage and posterior perichondrium. The wound is then irrigated, a Valsalva maneuver is performed and if no air leak is noted, the muscles are reapproximated with 3-0 Vicryl, a 7 mm Jackson-Pratt drain is placed and the wound closed in layers with 3-0 and 5-0 Monocryl sutures. The cartilage is then carved symmetrically to minimize warping.
- *Split calvarial bone grafts*: Split calvarial bone grafts are typically harvested from the parietal bone lateral to the sagittal sinus. The skin incision is carried down to the periosteum and a Weitlaner retractor used to maintain exposure. A U-shaped incision is made in the periosteum, a periosteal flap is raised and the dimensions of the bone graft are marked in the calvarium. Staying just outside of these marks, a cutting burr is used to drill a trough around the

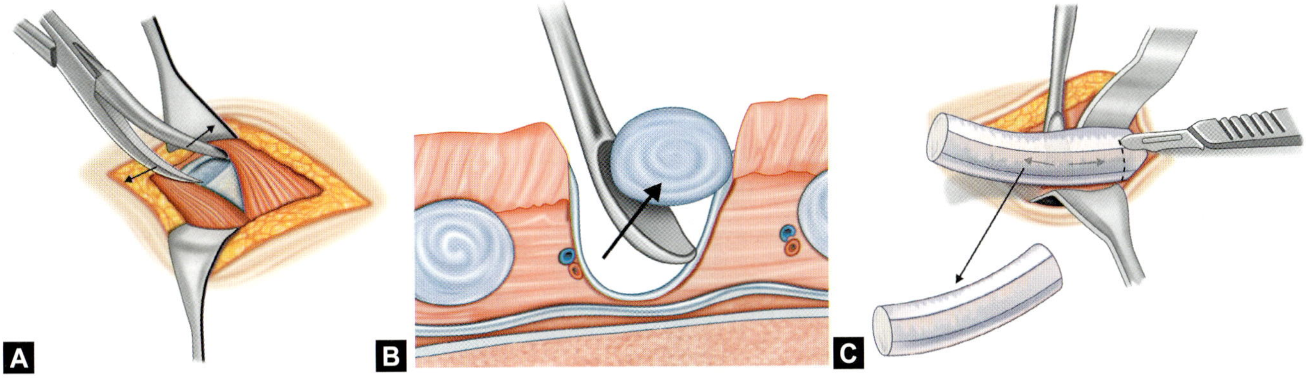

Figs 9.14A to C: Costal cartilage grafts are harvested after carefully elevating the periosteum

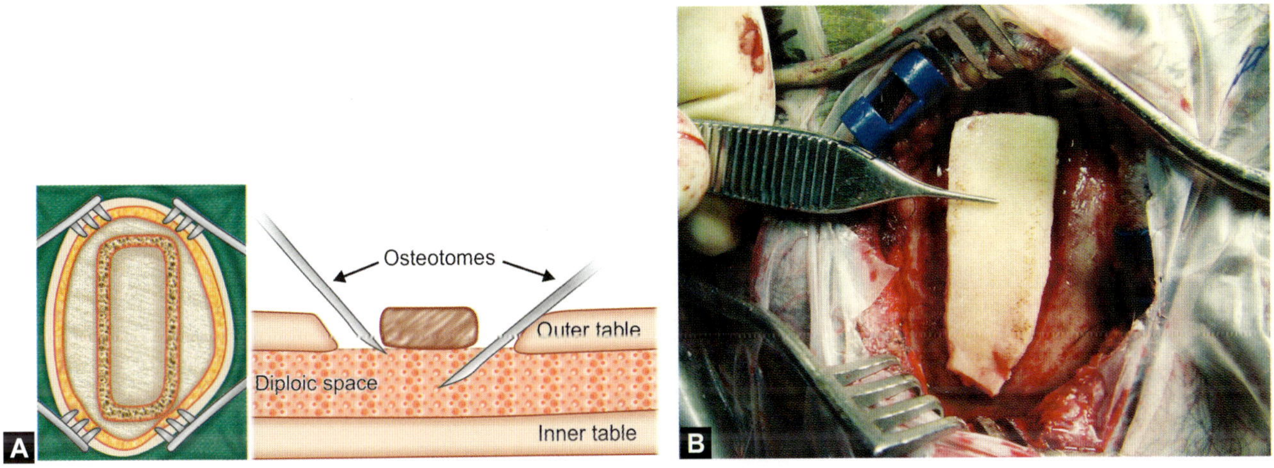

Figs 9.15A and B: (A) Split calvarial bone graft harvest requires identification of the diploic space level, followed by division of the diploae with gently curved osteotomes; (B) Split calvarial bone graft

intended bone graft through the outer table until the diploic space is encountered. While the edge of the bone graft remains sharp, the outer edge of the trough is saucerized. This allows a bone chisel to be placed in the diploic space at an angle sufficient to avoid deep penetration of the inner table while dividing the diploic space below the graft, as the osteotome is advanced incrementally as it is moved circumferentially (Figs 9.15A and B). Once the graft is isolated, bleeding from the donor site can be controlled with bone wax. The periosteal flap is then replaced and secured in place with 4-0 Vicryl sutures, and the skin incision is closed in layers with 4-0 Vicryl sutures and skin staples. The graft itself is then contoured to the appropriate size and shape, and is generally secured in place as a dorsal graft with a titanium screw.

- *"Turkish Delight" grafts*: In cases in which dorsal augmentation is desired and the quantity/quality of available harvested cartilage is poor, a diced cartilage graft may be used. Small (1–2 mm) pieces of cartilage saturated with whole blood are wrapped in an oxidized cellulose mesh in a cigar shape. The graft is then placed over the nasal dorsum and the held in position by the overlying skin flap and dressing. Subtle contour changes are possible in the early postoperative period by massaging the graft.
- *Homografts*: Decellularized dermal grafts can be used to provide minor degrees of dorsal augmentation. These are limited by their thinness, as well as partial graft loss during the initial period of revascularization. They are especially useful in camouflaging minor dorsal irregularities.
- *Alloplasts*: Traditional teaching is that alloplastic implants are generally inferior to natural materials in most cases. However, many patients lack sufficient remaining septal and conchal cartilage and refuse more invasive harvesting sites such as rib or calvarium. Alloplastic implants can provide significant bulk if

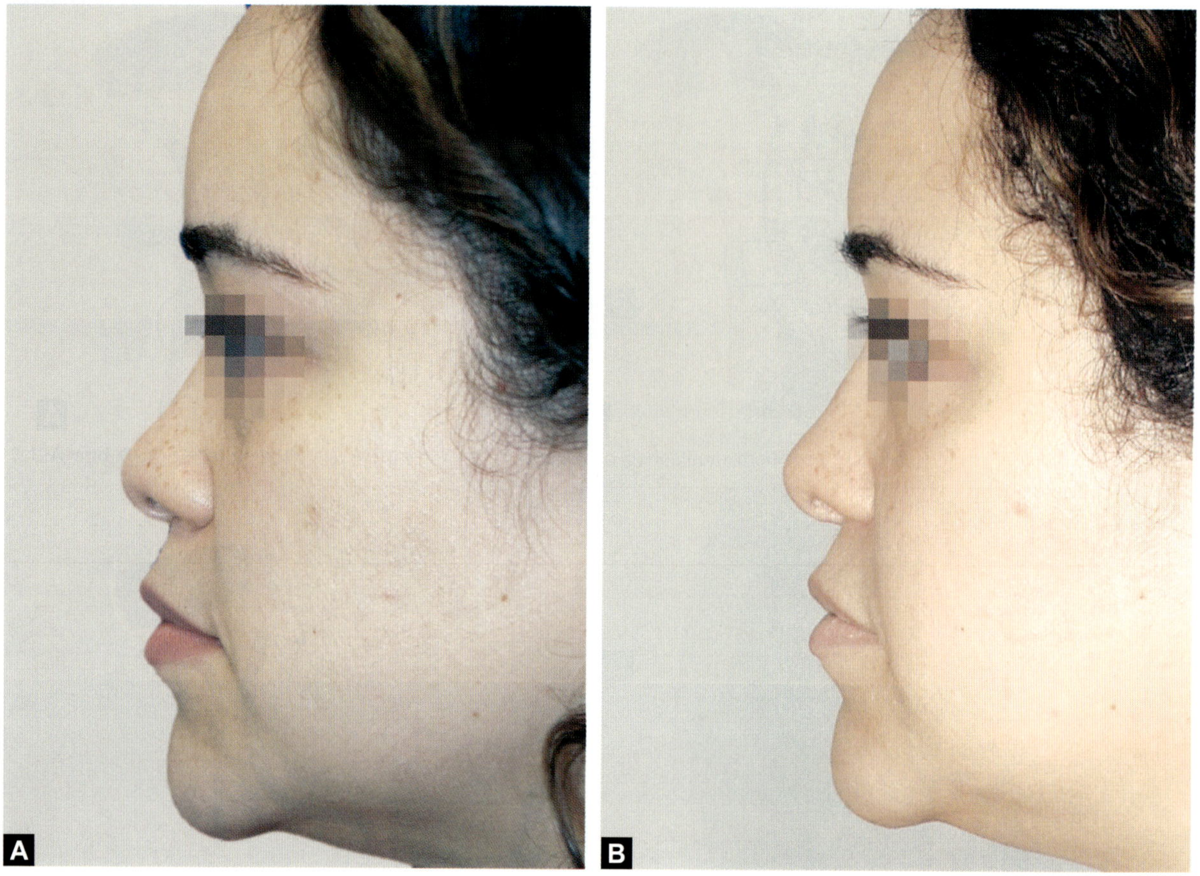

Figs 9.16A and B: Alloplasts such as expanded polytetrafluoroethylene (e-PTFE) and porous high density polyethylene (PHDPE) can provide reliable dorsal augmentation. (A) Preoperative and (B) postoperative views after alloplastic dorsal augmentation

used judiciously. Dorsal augmentation is the most common nasal use for alloplasts. Silicone, expanded polytetrafluoroethylene (e-PTFE) or porous high density polyethylene (PHDPE) implants generally are quite safe and effective for dorsal augmentation if the local vasculature is relatively intact (Figs 9.16A and B); however, alloplasts should not be used in patients with septal perforation or connective tissue disorders as these circumstances may raise the risk of infection.

For most grafts (other than calvarial bone grafts), creation of a tight, symmetric, "precise" pocket is preferred, and graft is placed and the incisions closed; however, if the dissection pocket is significantly larger, the graft should be sutured in place.

Generally, the entire dorsum is augmented from the radix to the supratip. Occasionally, a deep radix exists with either a high or normal dorsum, and discrete augmentation of the radix is necessary. A piece of cartilage, lightly morselized with the tines of a Brown-Adson forceps, is trimmed to the size needed. Both ends of a double-armed 5-0 chromic suture are passed from the deep to superficial side of the graft. Ink marks are made on the radix skin in locations corresponding to the sites of suture passage through the cartilage. Each needle is then passed under the skin flap elevated by an Aufricht retractor and through the flap directly through the corresponding skin mark. Using Bayonet forceps, the cartilage graft is passed into the radix as the sutures are pulled (Fig. 9.17). Once the cartilage is properly seated in the radix, the retractor is removed and the suture ends loosely tied, securing the graft in place.

- *Spreader grafts*: In cases of significant dorsal reduction (with its attendant risk of nasal valve collapse), when internal nasal valve collapse already exists or when there is significant deviation of the dorsal septum or depression of the ULC, a spreader graft can be placed between one or both medial border of the ULC and the dorsal septum. Dissecting a pocket in between these two cartilages is essential to successful placement of a spreader graft. This is facilitated by continuing the submucoperichondrial dissection of a septoplasty to the dorsum, where the Cottle

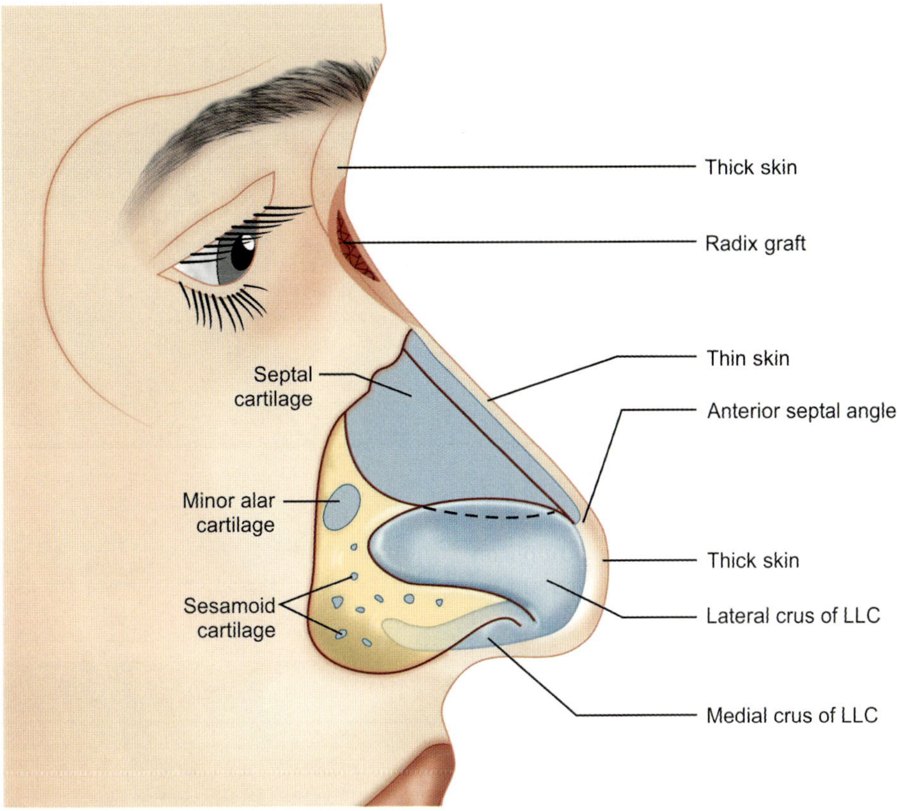

Fig. 9.17: Small radix grafts can be secured in place with a transcutaneous suture

elevator can gently divide the fusion of the ULC with the septum; once this is done, the Cottle elevator sweeps the mucosal attachments to the medial ULC laterally. A 3 cm × 5 mm × 5 mm piece of cartilage is carved and placed in this pocket (beginning at the caudal nasal bones and extending to or beyond the anterior septal angle), secured with 5-0 Nylon sutures caudally and cephalically (Figs 9.18A to C). Undesired caudal extension is then trimmed with scissors or scalpel. While spreader graft placement is simplified with an external approach, it can also be performed endonasally.

- *Osteotomies*: Nasal bone osteotomies are performed to reposition or reshape the nasal bones. There are three basic locations (medial, intermediate and lateral), two approaches (endonasal or percutaneous) and two styles (perforating or continuous) of osteotomies (Fig. 9.19). Medial osteotomies are performed adjacent to the nasal midline, lateral osteotomies are performed at the nasofacial junction [through the ascending (nasal) process of the maxilla] and intermediate osteotomies are performed somewhere in between these two (through the nasal bone itself). Endonasal approaches are performed through incisions within the nose, while percutaneous approaches are typically performed through keyhole skin incisions along relaxed skin tension lines or existing creases and folds near the nasal sidewalls. Perforating osteotomies are performed in a "postage stamp" interrupted fashion, leaving small intact bridges of bone and periosteum in between (the weakened bone is subsequently broken with external manual pressure while the periosteal bridges remain intact), while continuous incisions are carried through the bone in a linear fashion. While the choice of which approach and style is generally a matter of surgeon preference, endonasal approaches hide scars better while percutaneous approaches allow for more discrete osteotomy. Continuous osteotomies provide more complete mobility of the bone segment, while perforating osteotomies, by preserving "bridges" of periosteal and skin attachment, lessen the risk of flail bone segments.
  - *Medial osteotomies*: Medial osteotomies (Fig. 9.20) are performed to eliminate fixation of the nasal bones medially. If bony dorsal reduction has already been performed, a portion of the caudal nasal bone attachment has already been removed.

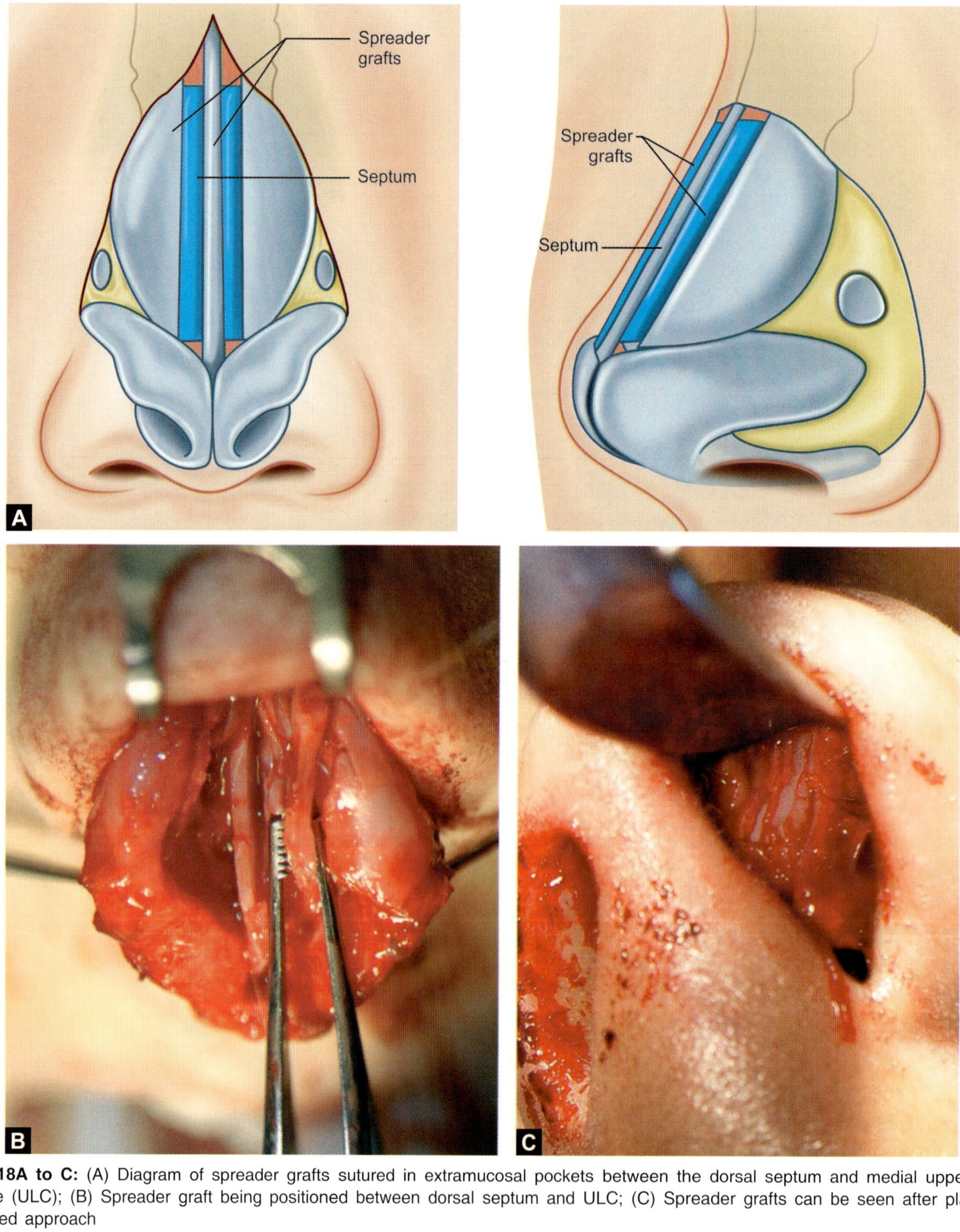

Figs 9.18A to C: (A) Diagram of spreader grafts sutured in extramucosal pockets between the dorsal septum and medial upper lateral cartilage (ULC); (B) Spreader graft being positioned between dorsal septum and ULC; (C) Spreader grafts can be seen after placement via closed approach

A single guarded osteotome (with the guard placed superficially as an indicator of osteotomy progression) is placed along the dorsal nasal septum and advanced cephalically until stiff bony resistance is met. By gently tapping the osteotomy with a mallet, the osteotomy is taken superiorly in a straight fashion just off the midline until the duller sound of the osteotome hitting the nasal process of the frontal bone is heard. Alternatively, a "fading medial" or "medial oblique" osteotomy

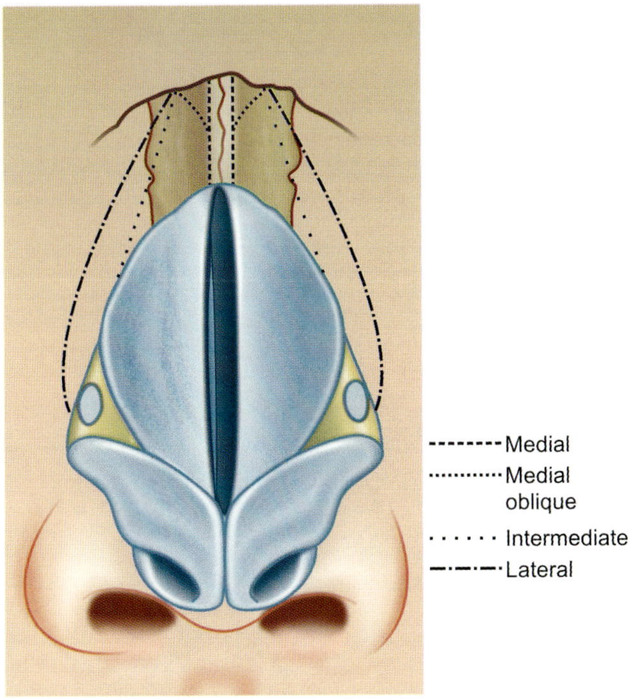

Fig. 9.19: Osteotomy locations

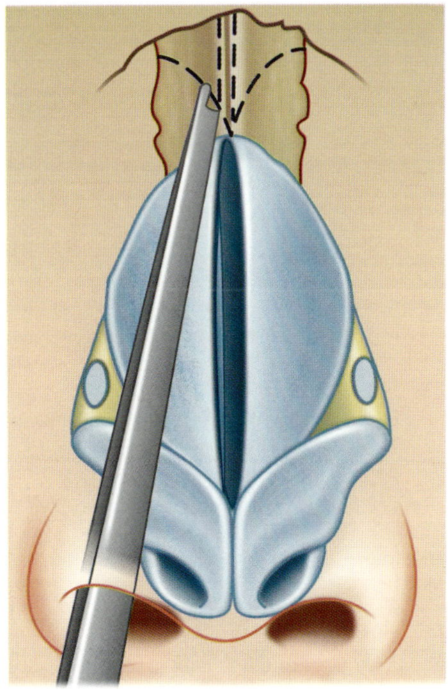

Fig. 9.20: Medial osteotomies are performed just off the midline

can be performed. It is simpler to perform this type of osteotomy when the Anderson-Nievert curved osteotomes are used. The osteotome is placed in the same fashion as in the medial osteotomy. However, the osteotomy path is allowed to follow the curvature of the blade, and the osteotome encounters the nasal process slightly more laterally. This position facilitates complete mobilization of the nasal bone by making it possible to connect the medial and lateral osteotome lines.

– *Intermediate osteotomies*: Intermediate osteotomies (Fig. 9.21) are useful when there is significant asymmetry or significant convexity/concavity of the nasal bones, and can be performed unilaterally or bilaterally. Combined with medial and lateral osteotomies, the intermediate osteotomy divides the nasal bone into two segments that can be manipulated to change the lateral contour of the bony arch. After the medial osteotomy, but prior to the lateral osteotomy, the nasal bone is still fixed laterally. A stab incision at the lateral perform aperture is made just lateral to the anterior end of the inferior turbinate with a #15 blade. A Joseph periosteal elevator is used to elevate a tunnel of periosteum along the planned line of the lateral osteotomy. The curved Anderson-Nievert osteotomy is then introduced into the wound and advanced until the bone of the pyriform is engaged. The osteotomy is then advanced medially along the caudal edge of the nasal bone until it rests at the desired point of medial osteotomy; usually, the intermediate osteotomy is midway between the medial and lateral osteotomies, but this is individualized to each case and is at the point of maximal convexity/concavity. The osteotomy is gently tapped with the mallet and the osteotomy continued in a gentle curve to meet the cephalic end of the medial osteotomy. The osteotome is then gently withdrawn to the level of the caudal nasal bone, swept laterally and positioned properly for the lateral osteotomy.

– *Lateral osteotomies*: If intermediate osteotomies have not been performed, the steps outlined above are performed to position the curved Anderson-Nievert osteotome at the lateral aspect of the pyriform aperture (Fig. 9.22). Once the tip of the osteotome rests on bone, the osteotome is swept medially so that the tip rests approximately 6–8 mm medial to the lateral extent of the pyriform. In most cases, a “high-low-high” lateral osteotomy will be chosen. From this position, the osteotome tip is initially directed and advanced laterally, toward the nasomaxillary junction. This maintains a small portion of the lateral pyriform

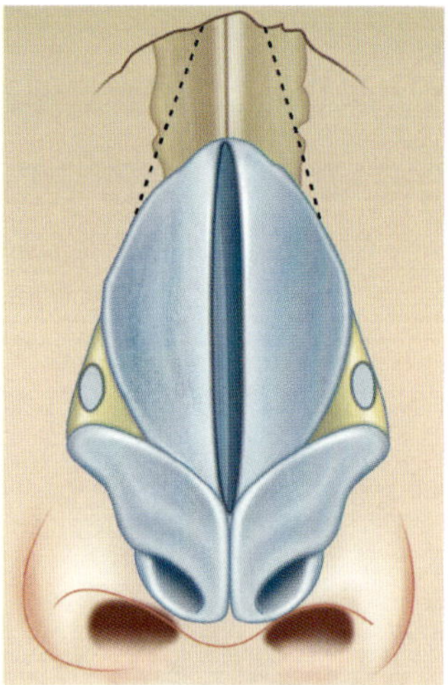

Fig. 9.21: Intermediate osteotomies are located in between the medial and lateral osteotomies, and can be used to correct nasal bone asymmetries

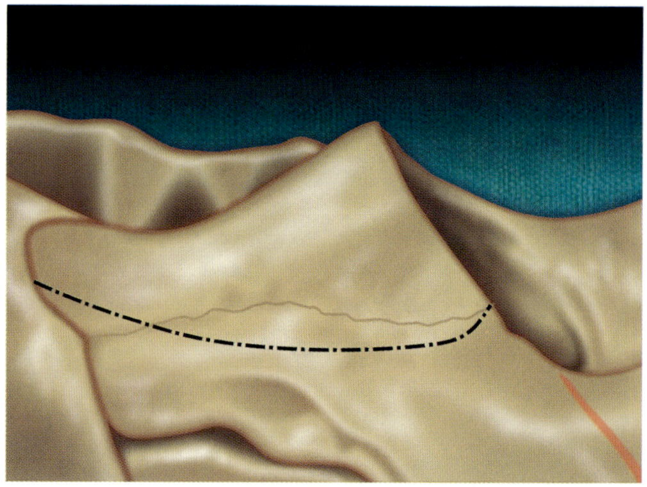

Fig. 9.22: Lateral osteotomies generally run, in some part, along the nasomaxillary groove and may preserve a triangle of bone at the lateral pyriform aperture to prevent medial alar collapse

bone (Webster's triangle) intact caudally, which serves to prevent excessive medial collapse of the ala. The osteotome is driven superolaterally for 6–8 mm and then allowed to curve more medially as it courses superiorly. The osteotomes are guided along the ascending process of the maxilla and allowed to follow the curvature of the osteotome medially and run medial to the lacrimal crest and up to the nasal process of the frontal bone, again eliciting a dull "thud" as the denser frontal bone is encountered. By following this curved path, the lateral meets the medial osteotomy, completely freeing the nasal bone. With splayed and widened nasal bones, this may not be performed, and a "low-low-high" osteotomy may be chosen to maximally narrow the bony dorsum. Once both bones are freely mobile, they are manually manipulated into a midline and symmetric position; if the nasal bone is noted to be too medial, a Goldman elevator is placed endonasally and used to elevate and position the nasal bone appropriately. Stability of the nasal bones is fostered by maintaining as much soft tissue attachment to the bones as possible as well as avoiding over resection of bone.

Tip Tissue Modifications

Conceptually, tip reduction may appear quite simple, and reduction tip plasty is one of the more common maneuvers in rhinoplasty. However, careful attention to symmetry and a firm understanding of the tripod concept is essential to achieve consistently good results. The natural curvatures of the LLCs and soft tissues of the nasal tip should be assessed, and support of the nasal tip position should be assessed. Incisions and excisions are the most potent methods of tip modifications, but also may be the most difficult to control.

Excision

The basic tip excisional maneuver is the cephalic strip. While a cephalic strip excision can be performed using either a transcartilaginous, intercartilaginous or delivery approach, excellent and symmetric exposure is required. A minimum of lateral crus should remain intact in order to maintain support to the lateral limb of the tripod; typically, between 6 mm and 8 mm of lateral crural width is preserved, depending on the tensile strength of the crus and its relative contribution to tripod support (Fig. 9.23). When resecting tip cartilage, each cartilage is assessed and measured first, and the adage, "measure twice, cut once" applies. The cut, made with a fresh #15 blade, should be beveled to slope gently from the cartilage into the intercartilaginous space to avoid a sharp step-off, and the resected cephalic portion carefully dissected from the underlying vestibular mucosa; this is best done using an angled Converse tip scissors. Similar amounts of cartilage are resected from each side, and while historically the resected specimen was compared for symmetry, the remaining cartilage is what must be symmetric. The removal of a portion of the width of the lateral crus both weakens the lateral limb of the nasal tip tripod but also creates a dead space between the upper and LLCs. The

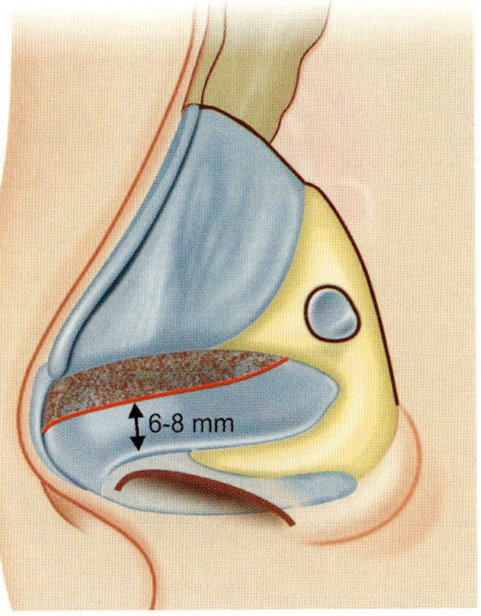

Fig. 9.23: Cephalic strip excision generally preserves 6–8 mm width caudally

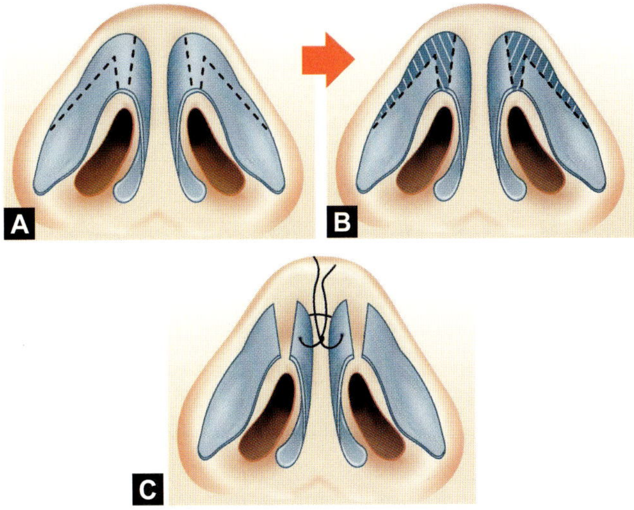

Figs 9.24A to C: Hockey stick excision of lateral crus

combination of these two weakens the span of the lateral crus, allowing it to fall inward towards the nasal inlet, while simultaneously allowing lateral crural cephalic retraction with tip rotation and retrodisplacement.

More dramatic changes can be gained in selected cases with the interrupted strip, in which an angled, "hockey stick" resection is performed (Figs 9.24A to C), which includes a portion of the remaining lateral crus laterally in additional to the cephalic strip resection. As one would imagine, significantly more inward collapse and tip retrodisplacement and rotation occur. In general, it is always best to re-establish linear continuity of the lateral and medial crura if cartilage is excised with 5-0 monofilament permanent or semipermanent sutures.

Similar to lateral crural segmental resection, the medial crus can also be shortened (the Lipsett procedure) (Fig. 9.25). Carefully measured segments of medial crura can be excised or transected and overlapped in order to shorten the medial tripod limb. The crura should be incised just below the intermediate crura, below the domes, to avoid affecting the shape of the cartilage domes. Care should be taken to affect equal changes bilaterally. Again, the underlying mucosa should be dissected free from the cartilage, and continuity re-established with sutures. A columellar strut is sutured in place between the shortened medial crura for enhanced stability.

Another cartilage excision, dome truncation (Figs 9.26A to C), can be performed to narrow and deproject a nasal tip with otherwise good rotation. After the vestibular mucosa is dissected off of the undersurface of the cartilage of the domes, a domal suture is passed

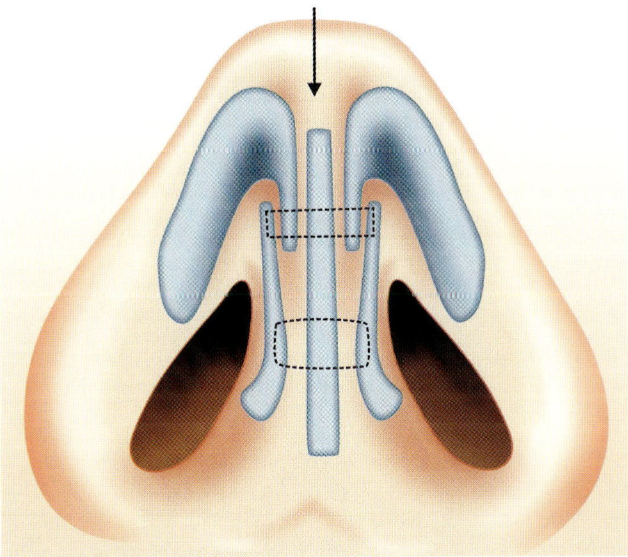

Fig. 9.25: Medial crural resection retrodisplaces and counter-rotates the tip

across both medial and both lateral crura, just below the desired height of the tip. The excess height of the LLCs is then resected; the cut edges of cartilages are best camouflaged with a cap or shield graft.

Incision

The classic incisional technique of the nasal tip is the Goldman tip, named after Irving Goldman. In this technique, the vestibular mucosa and the LLC are transected at the dome and allowed to heal secondarily. As one would imagine, the compromise of the integrity of

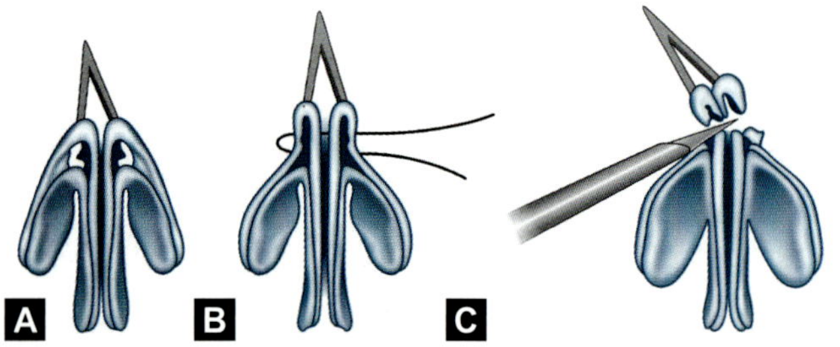

Figs 9.26A to C: Dome truncation resects equal amounts of medial and lateral crura, decreasing projection but not changing rotation

the nasal tip tripod support is significant, and contractile forces will pinch and over rotate the nasal tip, while the transected mucosa may heal with webs and create a nasal valve stenosis.

Simon's modification, the vertical dome division (VDD), is a potent technique that allows significant tip changes while re-establishing the nasal tripod support (Figs 9.27A to C). As with the Goldman tip, the VDD transects the LLC; however, there are several important differences. In the VDD, the vestibular mucosa remains intact, preventing stenosis. The location of cartilage transaction is chosen based on the desired effect. If no increase in tip projection is needed, the cartilage is transected at the dome. In patients requiring increased tip projection, the incision is brought 2–4 mm laterally onto the lateral crus, and the medial segments are sutured together to "steal" lateral crus and add height to the medial crus while shortening the lateral segment of the tripod. These changes increase tip projection and rotation. The cephalic ends of the lateral crura are also secured to the new medial segment, thus re-establishing continuity of the LLC and integrity of the lateral limb of the tripod. As one would imagine, great care must be taken to resuture the lateral crural segments, as significant caudal-cephalic changes can be made when the LLC is divided.

More focally, the lateral crural overlay (Figs 9.28A to E) can be used to treat the overly-long lateral crus. After the vestibular skin is undermined and separated from the undersurface of the lateral crus, a full-width incision is made perpendicularly from the caudal to cephalic edges of the midportion of the lateral crus. The medial segment is then sutured in an overlapped position to the lateral segment of cartilage.

Suturing

There are a multitude of tip suture techniques that have been described. These can be used to reposition the nasal tip, change the contour of the medial or lateral crura or to

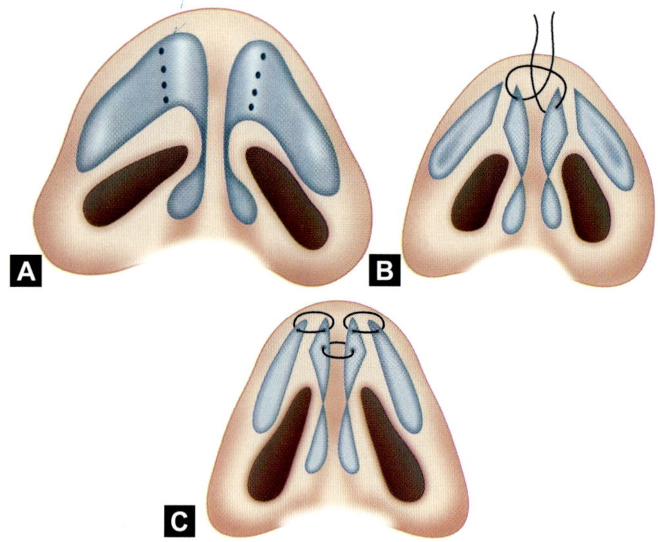

Figs 9.27A to C: Vertical dome division

reinforce or stabilize the LLC. While there are numerous suture techniques, this chapter will describe only the more germane ones. A few basic tenets apply to all of these. First, fine sutures of 5-0 monofilament should be used. While polydioxanone sutures maintain strength long enough to develop secure fibrosis, the author's preference is for clear nylon sutures, and no problems of suture granuloma, exposure or extrusion associated with the nylon have been observed. Secondly, wide undermining in the areas affect by the suture is necessary, relieving any restrictive forces that might otherwise hinder the effect of the suture. Thirdly, the integrity and support of the cartilage should be taken into account. Excessively rigid cartilage may resist suture sculpting and require weakening by cephalic strip excisions, scoring or direct incisions. Finally, suture knots should be placed in hidden areas, such as between two segments of cartilage when possible or at least between cartilage and vestibular skin.

- *Transdomal sutures*: Transdomal sutures (Figs 9.29A and B) are used to narrow the angle formed by the intermediate crus. The bulbosity of the nasal tip and flare of the ala can be addressed with this simple suture. Any cephalic resection of the lateral crus should be performed first, as this will also affect the intermediate crural angle. A horizontal mattress suture is then placed symmetrically around the dome, so that equal lengths of medial and lateral crura are drawn together, and there is no change in tip projection. Sutures should be placed at least 2–3 mm from both the cephalic and caudal edges of the cartilage to prevent pinching or flaring. In patients requiring added tip projection

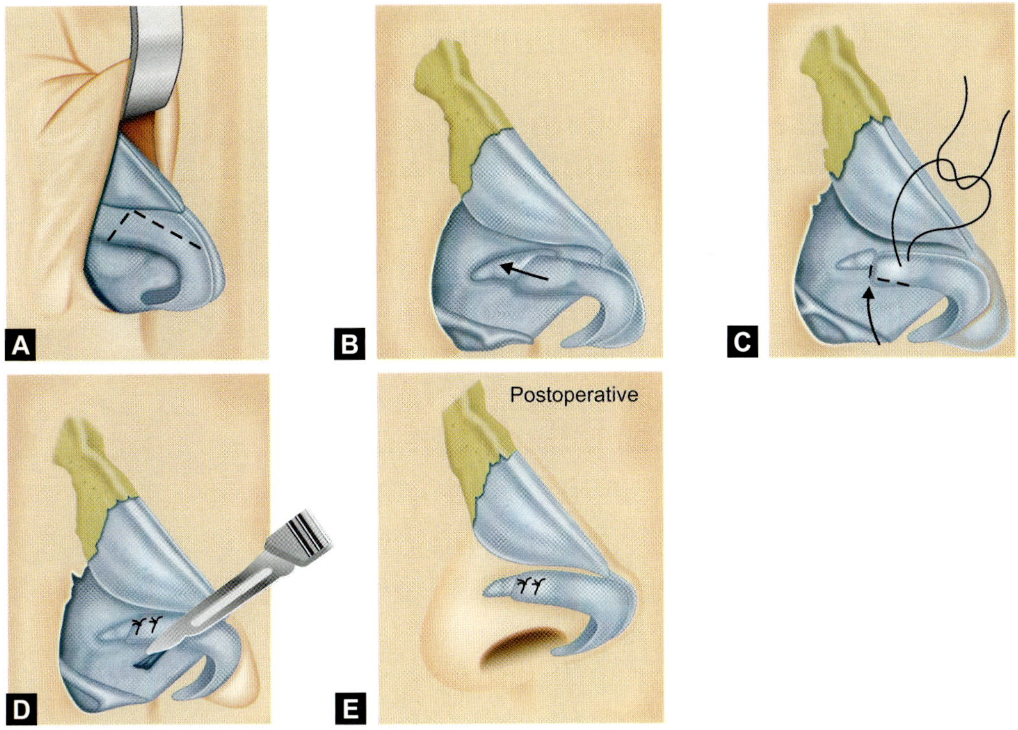

Figs 9.28A to E: Lateral crural overlay

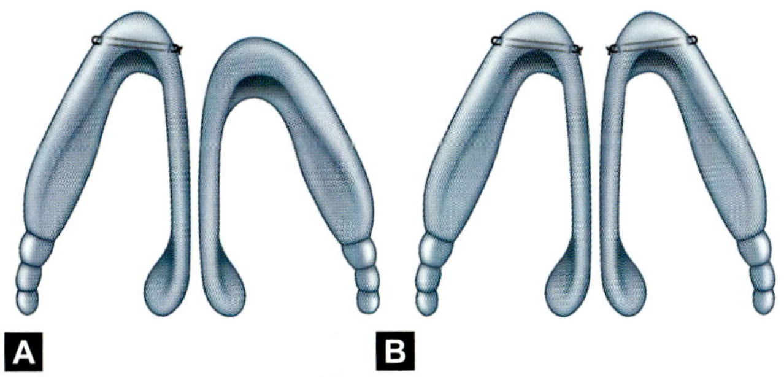

Figs 9.29A and B: Transdomal sutures straddle the dome of each lower lateral cartilage (LLC) to narrow this portion of the tip

and rotation, a lateral crural "steal" procedure (Fig. 9.30) can be performed to recruit lateral crural cartilage into the intermediate crus. Once the degree of required additional projection is determined, the position of the new dome is marked and the vestibular mucosa is additionally dissected free of the cartilage. The cartilage in the region of the new planned dome is lightly morselized with a Brown-Adson forceps to allow it to bend and assume its new shape. A transdomal mattress suture is then placed symmetrically about the new dome and tied. Likewise, decreased projection and rotation can be affected in a similar manner, as the dome is shifted to a more medially along the LLC. Often, a columellar strut is placed to reinforce the strength of the medial limb of the nasal tip tripod in these cases.

- *Interdomal sutures*: Interdomal sutures (Fig. 9.31) are placed to unify nasal tip cartilages. Broad and bulbous tips may have widened distances between the domes that may be filled with soft tissue. After removing this soft tissue, an interdomal suture is placed through the medial crus to the lateral crus, then back through the lateral crus and the medial crus; the suture is then similarly passed through the contralateral medial and lateral crura at locations identical to the first side and tied in the intercrural space.
- *Lateral crural sutures*: Excessively concave or convex lateral crura can be contoured as needed with lateral crural sutures (Figs 9.32A to C). The vestibular mucosa should be elevated from the entire segment of the lateral crura to be spanned, and mattress sutures placed across the span of excessive curvature. For externally convex lateral crura, the longitudinal span of the suture runs on the external crural surface, while for concave crura, the longitudinal length of the suture runs on the nasal side of the cartilage. Alternatively, a lateral crural strut graft can be used (vide infra).

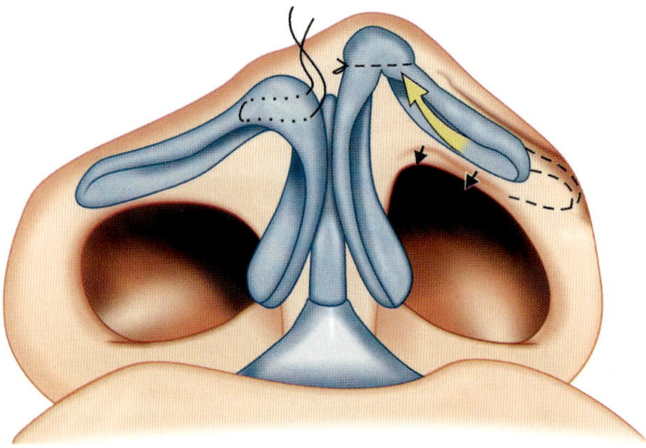

Fig. 9.30: Lateral crural steal procedure advances lateral crural cartilage into the medial segment, increasing projection and rotation of the tip

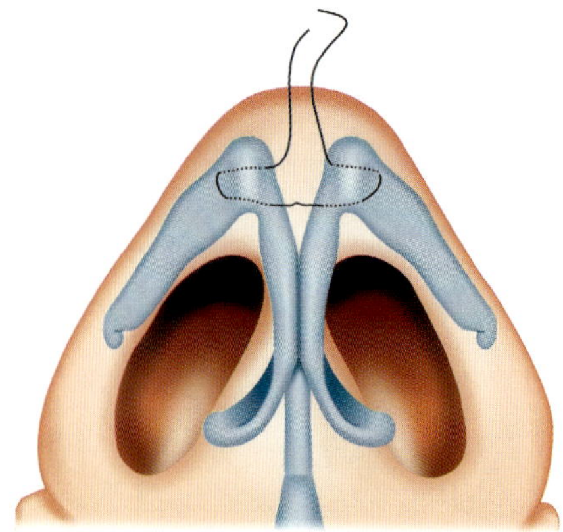

Fig. 9.31: Interdomal sutures can be used to stabilize the medial segment of the tripod, as well as narrow widely placed tip defining points

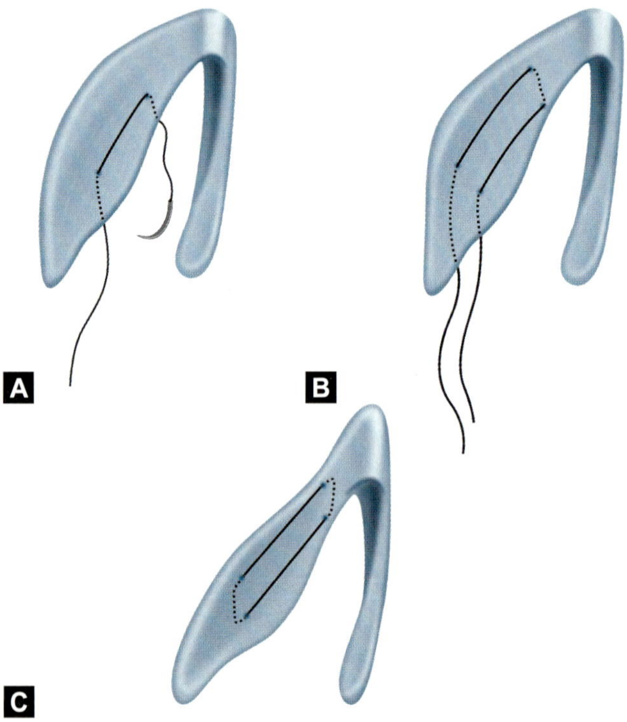

Figs 9.32A to C: Lateral crural sutures can be used to adjust the convexity of the lateral crura

- *Lateral Crural Spanning Sutures*: Appropriately curved but weak or flail lateral crura can be supported with a lateral crural spanning suture. A suture is passed through a portion of one lateral crus at its weakest point and then through a portion of the other lateral crus at an analogous point and tied over the dorsal septum (Figs 9.33A and B). Similarly, an ULC spanning suture can also be placed to help widen a narrow or flail internal nasal valve.

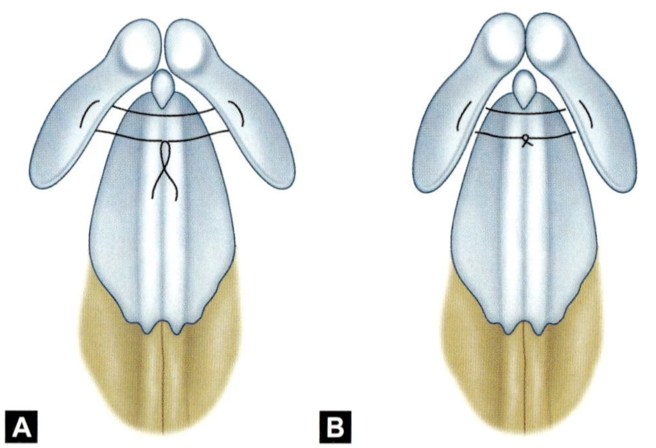

Figs 9.33A and B: Lateral crural spanning sutures are used to stabilize internal nasal valves weakened by flail lateral crura

- *Tip Projection Control Sutures*: Nasal tip projection can be relatively directly affected with the use of tip projection control sutures (Figs 9.34A to D), as described by Tebbitts. A suture can be placed through the cephalic sides of the medial crura just below the dome and through the caudal septum. Depending on where this suture is placed on the caudal septum, the entire medial limb of the nasal tripod can be projected or deprojected. It is important to free the attachments of the medial crural footplates to the caudal septum to allow full mobilization. With significant deprojection, the footplates will flare laterally and should be addressed to prevent postoperative nasal obstruction.

Grafts

Grafts are a potent way to reshape and reinforce the nose, and can be placed in anatomical or nonanatomical

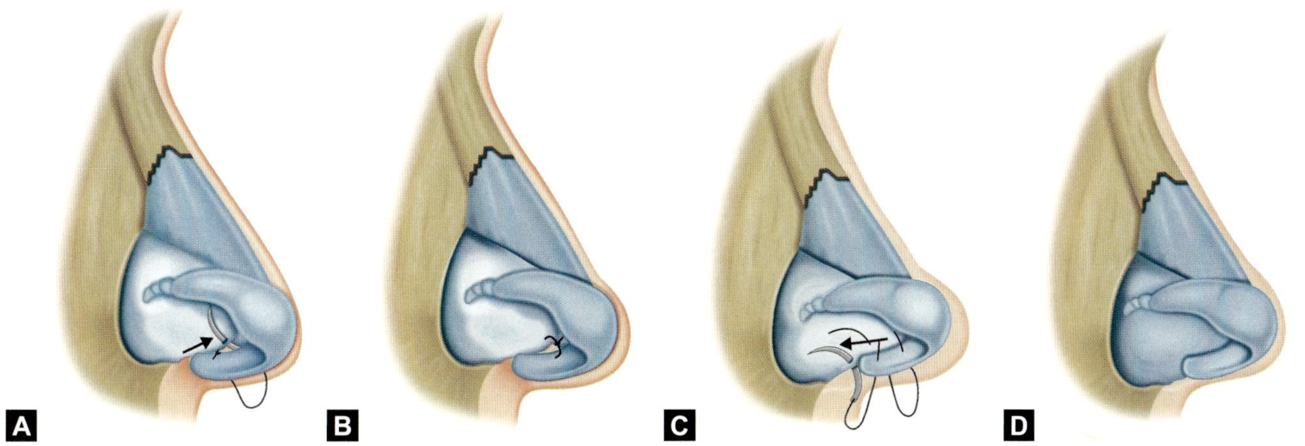

Figs 9.34A to D: Tip projection control sutures advance the tip anteriorly or posteriorly along the caudal septum, depending on their exact placement

positions. Septal cartilage is readily available in most cases, and is generally the preferred source. However, conchal cartilage can be used and is especially useful when curvature is desired. Finally, costal cartilage can be harvested but typically requires more contouring than costal cartilage.

- *Columellar strut*: A strut of cartilage can be placed in the columella between the medial crura. As a basic function, the strut will allow reinforcement of the medial tripod leg strength, and also can be used to straighten irregularities of the medial crura. A rectangular piece of cartilage approximately 3–4 mm wide and long enough to span from just above the anterior nasal spine to above the domes is carved from harvested cartilage. A pocket is dissected in between the medial crura inferiorly, leaving a modest amount of soft tissue over the bone. The strut is placed into this pocket and the medial crura sutured together through the strut in at least two locations, one of which is located at the junction of the medial and intermediate crura (Fig. 9.35). Strut cartilage extending beyond the domes is excised with a #11 blade. A number of variations of the basic strut graft exist and can be used to modify tip position. For an under-projected tip, the medial crura are advanced dorsally as they are sutured through the strut, effectively increasing tip projection. For derotation of the tip, the strut can be trapezoidal in shape, wider dorsally; this portion is sutured to the caudal septum near the anterior septal angle, rotating the tip downward. A columellar strut can be incorporated into a septal extension graft, which is significantly wider and is sutured to the posterior nasal spine, as well as to caudal septum with extended spreader grafts. This graft combination can be used to address a retracted columella.
- *Shield graft*: The shield graft is used primarily to add definition to the nasal tip. It is especially useful in thick-skinned noses, as well as revision noses with tip irregularities. The shield graft is aptly named, wider at the top than the bottom. It is important to bevel the edges of the graft to better blend the contour. The top of the graft rests 1–2 mm above the domes and helps to define the tip. Inferiorly, the graft is sutured to the intermediate crura and medial crura (Fig. 9.36). The basic shield graft can be modified to provide enhanced apparent rotation or to widen a deep nasolabial angle. A "stacked" shield graft can be constructed by suturing a second, smaller piece of cartilage to the backside of the shield graft superiorly. When this layered graft is sutured in place, the graft "tilts" downward simulating lengthening of the nose. Alternatively, by extending the inferior portion of the graft, a deep nasolabial angle can be improved.
- *Cap graft*: A cap graft is sutured in place between the tip defining points and used to soften the nasal tip, especially in patients with thin skin, but generally does not provide significant tip projection. Lightly crushed cartilage or temporalis fascia can be used for a cap graft.
- *Umbrella graft*: When a greater degree of projection than provided by a cap graft is needed, an umbrella graft can be used (Figs 9.37A and B). Combining a columellar strut with an onlay graft, tip support is strengthened and projection is enhanced.

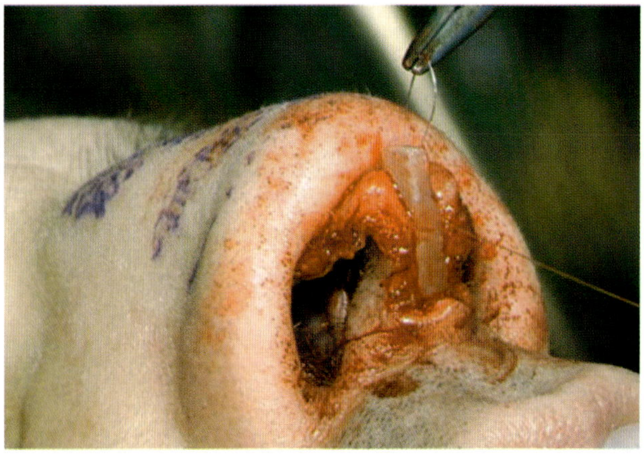

Fig. 9.35: Columellar strut grafts can stabilize the medial nasal tip support

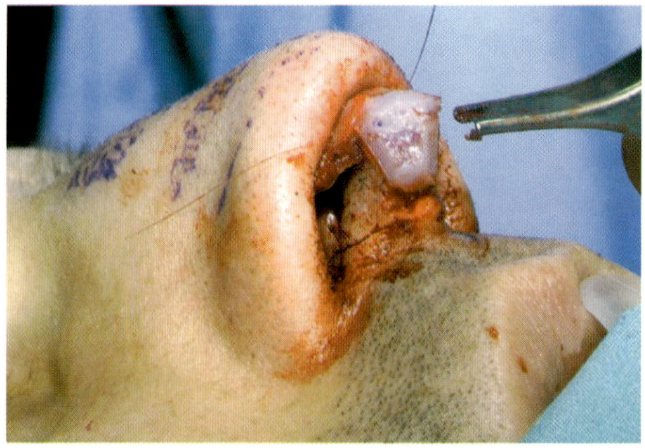

Fig. 9.36: A shield graft can define the tip and infratip lobule

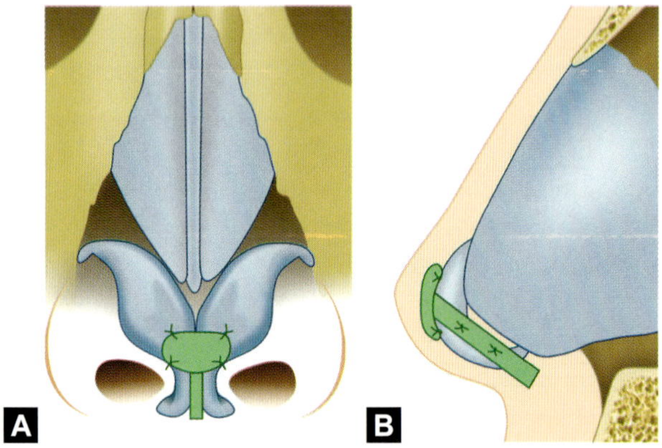

Figs 9.37A and B: Tip support and definition can be enhanced with an umbrella graft

- *Premaxillary grafts*: Small (1–2 mm) pieces of diced cartilage can be placed anterior to the nasal spine in order to correct an acute nasolabial angle (Figs 9.38A and B).
- *Lateral crural strut grafts*: Lateral crural strut grafts can be used to straighten and strengthen the lateral crura. 2–3 mm wide grafts can be sutured directly to the underside of the lateral crura in multiple locations with interrupted sutures. Grafts should be placed in the midportion of the lateral crus, and should extend from the intermediate crus laterally to the pyriform aperture. The lateral ends of these grafts are placed into pockets over the pyriform aperture (Figs 9.39A and B).
- *Alar batten grafts*: Alar batten grafts are placed at the junction of the ULCs and LLCs to support the internal nasal valve area. Lenticular grafts wide enough to overlap the upper and LLCs are placed to span from the pyriform aperture to the dorsal septum (Fig. 9.40). The graft is placed in a tight pocket over the pyriform laterally, and secured to the dorsal septum with sutures. The cephalic edge of the lateral crus (and if necessary, the caudal edge of the ULC) is sutured to this spanning structure.
- *Lateral crural spanning graft*: A lateral crural spanning graft can be used to open a deficient internal nasal valve. The graft is draped over the dorsal septum and sutured laterally into pockets created between the lateral crura and the underlying vestibular mucosa (Fig. 9.41). The resilience of the cartilage draws the nasal valve outward.
- *Rim grafts*: Rim grafts are used to correct retracted alar margins. Grafts of appropriate length and 2 mm × 2 mm in size are placed in pockets along the alar rim caudal to the lateral crus (nonanatomically) to advance the alar skin inferiorly (Figs 9.42A and B). Precise pockets which are just large enough to accept the grafts obviate the need for suturing the grafts in place.

Closure

Rhinoplasty closure is quite simple, but requires careful attention to detail. All incisions should be closed to prevent excessive soft tissue retraction from healing by secondary intention.

- Transfixion and intercartilaginous/transcartilaginous incisions should be closed with interrupted 4-0 chromic sutures. Simple end to end closure without eversion should be performed.

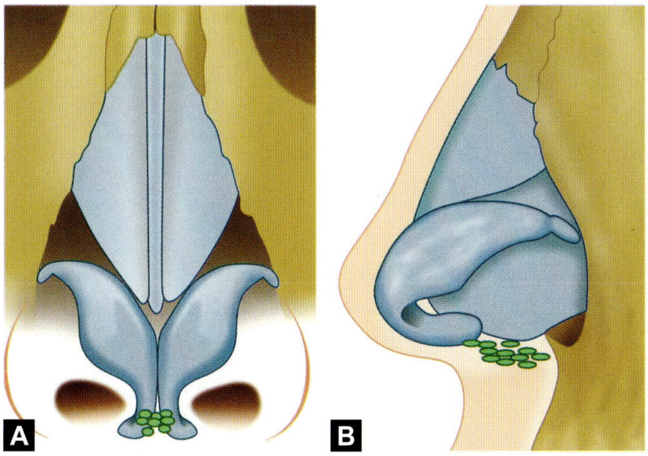

Figs 9.38A and B: Premaxillary plumping grafts are small pieces of cartilage placed (through either a transfixion or transcolumellar incision) into the soft tissue anterior to the nasal spine to open an acute nasolabial angle

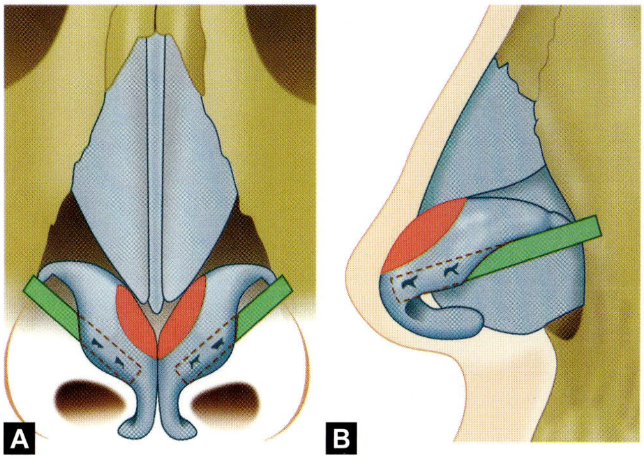

Figs 9.39A and B: Weak or misshapen lateral crura can be reshaped or supported with lateral crural strut grafts. Placed between the lateral crural cartilage and underlying mucosa, these grafts are sutured to the crura and placed into precise pockets over the pyriform aperture

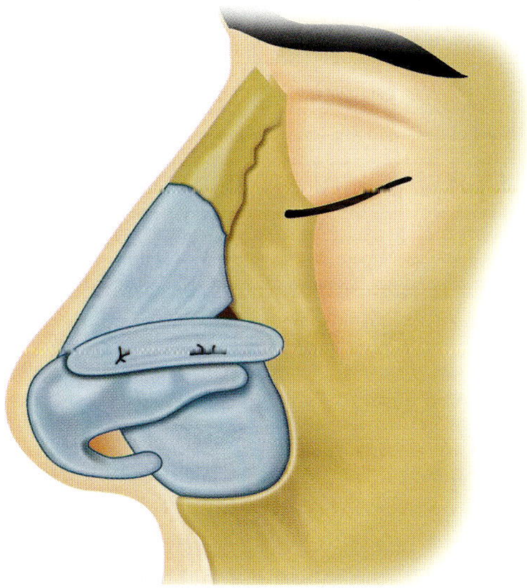

Fig. 9.40: Alar batten grafts span from the dorsal septum medially to precise pockets over the pyriform aperture laterally, and are centered over the cephalic lateral crus/caudal upper lateral cartilage (ULC)

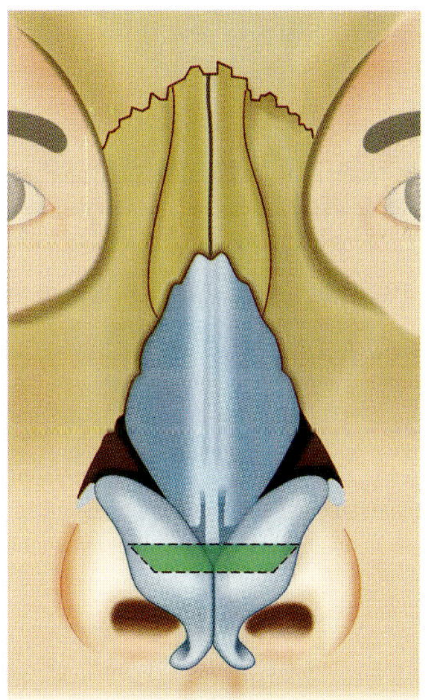

Fig. 9.41: A piece of cartilage spans over the dorsal septum and is pocketed bilaterally below the lateral crura. Lateral crural spanning grafts take advantage of the natural resiliency of cartilage

- The transcolumellar incision is closed with interrupted 6-0 monofilament sutures (polypropylene or nylon).
- Access incisions used in the case of external perforating osteotomies are closed with single 5-0 plain gut sutures.

Dressings

A critical component of rhinoplasty is the dressing and cast. Elevation of the nasal skin creates a potential space which can easily be filled with postoperative fibrosis and ruin an otherwise well-performed procedure. The nasal dorsum (from radix to supratip) should be secured in place with paper tape. Especially in cases of significant nasal tip changes or if the open approach has been used, the nasal tip is also taped snugly. If osteotomies have been performed, a splint of thermoplastic material is placed over the upper two-thirds of the nose.

POTENTIAL COMPLICATIONS

Epistaxis

Postoperative epistaxis is uncommon but may be troublesome when it occurs. Patients should be told to discontinue antiplatelet and other anticoagulant drugs,

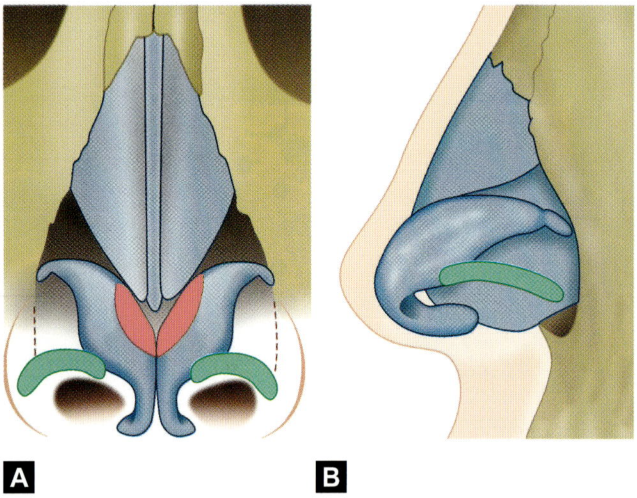

Figs 9.42A and B: Rim grafts are placed in soft tissue pockets along the malar margin and are designed to correct soft tissue retraction

unless medically contraindicated. If continuous pressure against the maxilla just lateral to the alae for 15 minutes fails to stop the bleeding, gentle anterior packing may be necessary. Blood clots are evacuated with suction and the nose examined. Turbinate bleeding may be cauterized. Gelfoam or Surgicel packing moistened with a topical decongestant (1% phenylephrine or 0.05% oxymetazoline) can be applied. More significant (expandable foam or balloon) packing may be necessary, but care should be taken to avoid, if possible, lateral displacement of the nasal bones. Significant hemorrhage may require operative intervention.

Septal Hematoma

Rarely, a septal hematoma can develop and should be drained emergently. Clinically, lateral bulging if the septum is noted; palpation with a cotton tip applicator can help to distinguish a hematoma from simple postoperative edema or a recurrent septal deviation. The septal wound closure should be opened and the clot evacuated. The flaps are then imbricated with a 4-0 chromic suture and soft silicone septal splints are sewn in place trans-septally and maintained for 2 weeks.

Infection

Postoperative infection is uncommon. Most significant is the development of toxic shock syndrome. Fever over 102°F, sunburn-like rash, nausea and vomiting are common initial presenting complaints; progression of the infection can lead to rapid renal and cardiovascular collapse. Packing should be removed immediately, the patient hydrated and treated with parenteral antistaphylococci and streptococci antibiotics.

Nasal Obstruction

Postoperative nasal obstruction can be particularly disturbing, as it may render an otherwise excellent rhinoplasty a failure. Causes include inadequate management of a deviated septum or enlarged inferior turbinates, synechiae, or nasal valve collapse. Nasal valve collapse may occur if the ULC attachments to the dorsal septum, the cephalic edge of the lateral crus or the undersurface of the caudal nasal bones are compromised during dorsal reduction or when nasal mucosa in this area is violated. Repair may require spreader, lateral crural strut or batten grafts or intranasal Z-plasty.

Saddle Nose

A saddle nose deformity describes a nasal deformity when the dorsum falls below a straight line in running from the radix to the supratip, and can occur after over resection of the bony or cartilaginous dorsum or loss of middle vault support from extensive resection or mobilization of the quadrangular cartilage. Minor saddle nose deformities can be corrected with autologous cartilage grafts, while major saddle nose deformities require larger grafts of calvarial bone or costal cartilage.

Bossa

A bossa, or point, may develop in the nasal tip postoperatively and cause tip asymmetry. Maintaining sufficient integrity of the LLCs will reduce the chance of a postoperative bossa, as the risk of unplanned contracture of the cartilage, especially in the area of the domes, is reduced. Management may require camouflage grafts, resection of cartilage or contouring of the contralateral cartilage to increase symmetry.

Polybeak Deformity

Polybeak is a descriptive term that refers to noses with an inversion of the desired nasal contour. The lower third of the nose becomes dominant compared to the upper third, due to (1) over resection of the bony dorsum; (2) under resection of the cartilaginous dorsum; (3) soft tissue excess; (4) excess length of the lateral crura, and/or insufficient length or strength of the medial crura. Appropriate treatment may include serial injections of triamcinolone acetate (1-10 mg/cc) or revision surgery.

AFTERCARE

The nasal cast and tape, as well as transcolumellar sutures, are removed 5-7 days after surgery. The nose is retaped for an additional 5-7 days. The patient is counseled to avoid any nasal trauma for the first weeks after surgery, and more rapid resolution of nasal obstruction may require endoscopic nasal debridement in the office.

BIBLIOGRAPHY

1. Gunter JP, Landecker A, Cochran CS. Frequently used grafts in rhinoplasty: nomenclature and analysis. Plast Reconstr Surg. 2006;118(1):14e-29e.
2. Rohrich RJ, Ahmad J. Rhnoplasty. Plast Reconstr Surg. 2011;128(2):49e-73e.
3. Tebbetts JB. Primary rhinoplasty: redefining the logic and techniques. Mosby: St. Louis; 2008.
4. Toriumi DM, Josen J, Weinberger M, et al. Use of alar batten grafts for correction of nasal valve collapse. Arch Otolaryngol Head Neck Surg. 1997;123(8):802-8.
5. Toriumi DM. New concepts in nasal tip contouring. Arch Facial Plast Surg. 2006;8(3):156-85.

CHAPTER

10

Cervical Liposuction

Anthony P Sclafani

OVERVIEW

Removal of subcutaneous fat can aid in improving the contour of the neck. Open lipectomy can remove similar or greater amounts of tissue, but unless a large incision is already planned for another purpose, entails additional morbidity. Cervical liposuction of large volumes is rarely necessary in the face, but liposuction can be useful in subtly contouring the gentle curves of the neck.

SPECIAL CONSIDERATIONS

Multiple factors may contribute to a heavy neck with an oblique cervicomental angle: these include lax skin, submental fat accumulation (subcutaneous or subplatysmal), hypertonic platysmal muscle contraction, submandibular gland ptosis, microgenia and a low hyoid (Figs 10.1A to F). A careful preoperative analysis is essential, and often multiple procedures are necessary to maximally improve the appearance of the neck.

ALTERNATIVES TO PROCEDURE

Alternatives to submental liposuction include open lipectomy (which requires a larger submental incision but may be more appropriate), radio frequency-induced tightening of skin, platysmaplasty, chin augmentation of a formal face and neck lift.

TECHNIQUES

Incision Placement

A stab incision is made in the midline in the first submental skin crease to gain access to the central neck. In patients without an obvious skin crease, the incision is made posterior to the posterior border of the mandible. Additional incisions are often, but not always, made just behind the earlobes to provide enhanced access to the neck below the lateral mandible and to allow a cross-hatching pattern (Fig. 10.2). Each incision is made only sufficiently large enough to allow passage of the liposuction cannula.

Anesthetic Infiltration

Anesthetic infiltration is an important part of the dissection, as the tumescent solution distends local tissue septae and facilitates passage of the cannula. A thin, blunt tipped needle with multiple circumferential ports is smoothly passed in a radial fashion, injecting tumescent solution slowly until the treatment area is both distended and anesthetized by the solution. The author's preferred solution is 25 cc of 1% lidocaine with 1:100,000 epinephrine mixed freshly with 250 cc of normal saline, yielding a final concentration of approximately 0.1% lidocaine with 1:1,000,000 epinephrine, which provides sufficient anesthesia and vasoconstriction for the duration of the procedure; typically 150–200 cc is injected into the subcutaneous plane.

Extent of Undermining/Dissection

The passage of the infiltration cannula begins the process of creating discrete tunnels through which the liposuction cannulae will be passed (Fig. 10.3). The small tunnels are progressively enlarged by passing increasingly larger cannulae without any suction applied.

Tissue Modifications

Excision

Once the single port cannula of choice can be passed with ease, it is passed (without suction) through the incision with the port pointed toward the deep tissue and away from the dermis. Once the tip is beneath the skin, suction is applied. Once one atmosphere of vacuum

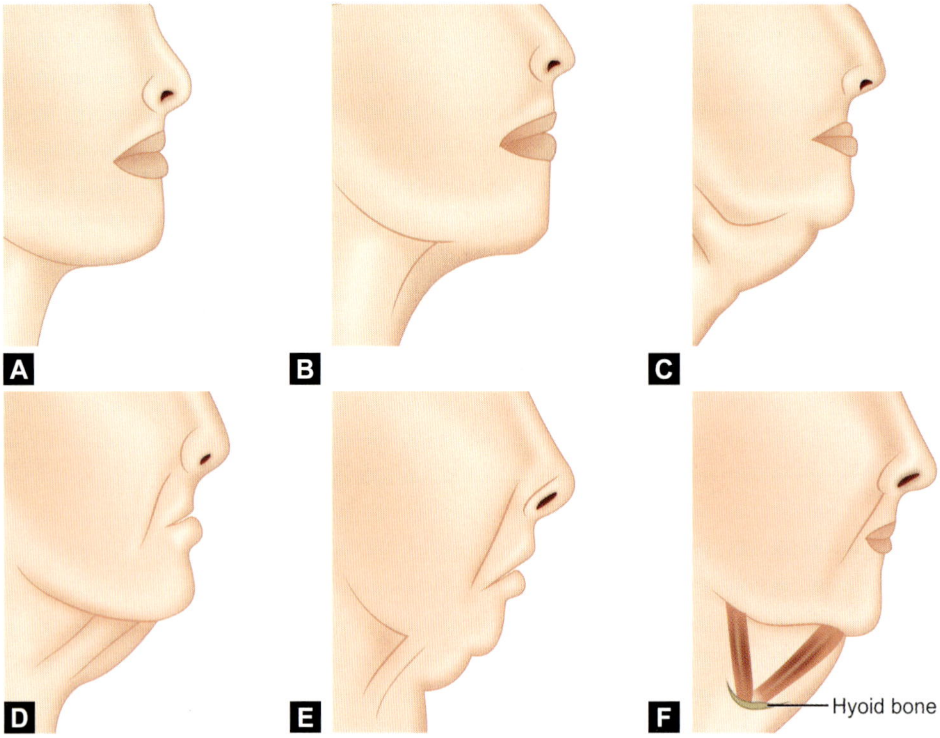

Figs 10.1A to F: Different etiologies of neck deformity: (A) Minimal deformity; (B) Cervical skin laxity; (C) Submental fat accumulation; (D) Platysmal muscle "banding"; (E) Retrogenia and (F) Low position of hyoid bone

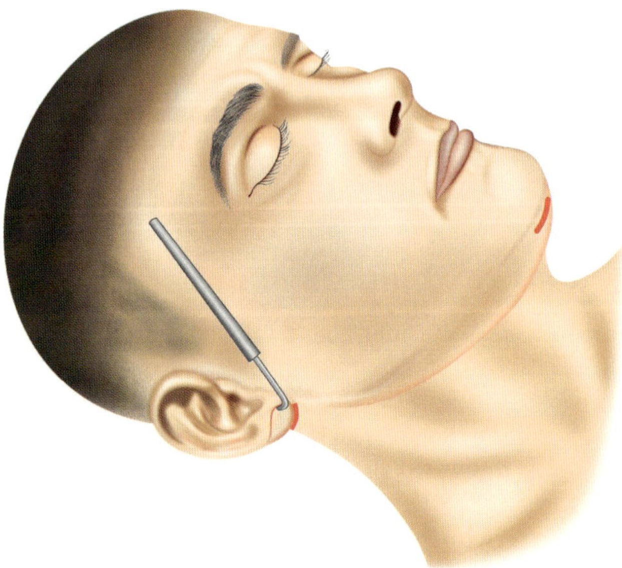

Fig. 10.2: Liposuction incisions are easily hidden in the midline of the first submental crease and just behind the earlobe. Incisions are generally no larger than "stab" incisions with a #15 scalpel

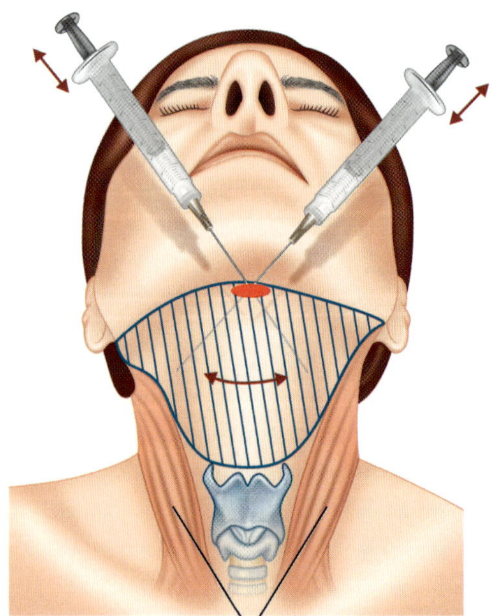

Fig. 10.3: Tumescent anesthetic solution is infiltrated with a narrow infiltration cannula in a fan-like pattern in an area below the mandible, above the thyroid notch and in between the sternocleidomastoid muscles. By passing the cannula in and out and sweeping it in a fan-like pattern, a series of discrete tunnels are created between the dermis and the underlying muscle, bounded by fibrous bands traversing the fat

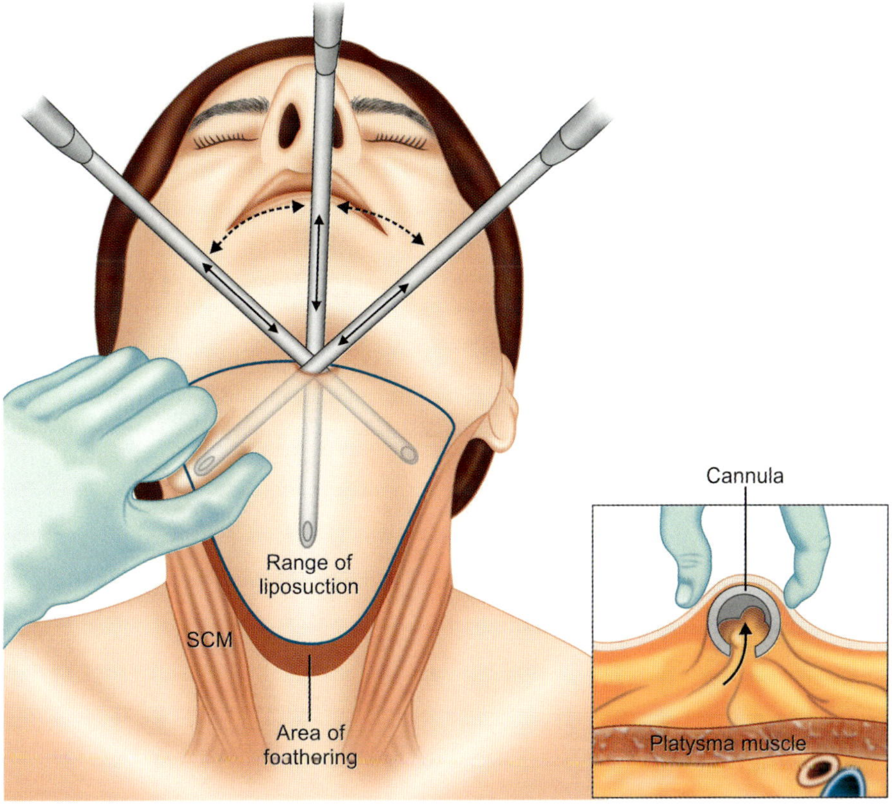

Fig. 10.4: Progressively larger single port suction cannulae are passed in and out, in a fan-like pattern, in the area of liposuction. The port of the cannula is always kept facing away from the dermis. The surgeon manipulates the skin externally by pinching a segment of skin and fat, making passage of the cannula more effective in suctioning the fat. An area beyond the target area is also suctioned, albeit it less aggressively, to feather the effects of the suctioning

is reached, the cannula is advanced in long, steady strokes through the subcutaneous fat by following the previously created tunnels. The dominant hand grasps and compresses a roll of skin and soft tissue while the non-dominant hand passes the cannula back and forth through the encompassed subcutaneous fat. As each area is treated sufficiently, the cannula is moved in a fan pattern (Fig. 10.4). Care is taken to ensure that an even, thin layer of subcutaneous fat remains under the dermis. A cross-hatching pattern of suction tunnels is created using multiple incisions, and is used to facilitate a smooth contour.

Closure

- *Sutures*: Simple skin closure is performed with 5-0 chromic sutures.
- *Dressings*: An elastic band compressive dressing should be applied below the chin and over the head in the operating room.

POTENTIAL COMPLICATIONS

Skin Necrosis

It is essential to maintain the open liposuction port away from the dermis and pointed into deep tissue. Trauma to the dermis from suction may lead to vascular injury to the skin and ultimately cause skin necrosis.

Ridges and Irregularities

Nodules, lumps and ridges may develop postoperatively if care is not taken to ensure smooth and even liposuction.

Marginal Mandibular Nerve Injury

A full assessment of the function of the marginal mandibular nerve function should be performed after the effect of the local anesthetic has worn off. Asymmetry of lower lip eversion (as opposed to lip depression, a function of depressor labii inferioris) indicates injury to the marginal mandibular nerve. Since only blunt-tipped cannulae should be used, these nerve injuries are neuropractic and should be expected to recover.

Cobra-Neck Deformity

This deformity occurs when subplatysmal fat is removed. Dehiscences in the normal midline interdigitations between the left and right sides of the platysmal muscle allow easy access to the subplatysmal fat. Postoperatively, an excessive concavity in the midline submental area may develop.

AFTERCARE

It is important to acknowledge that some of the improvement seen after liposuction is due to postoperative fibrosis and contraction. Patients may remove the elastic support on the morning following surgery and are instructed to remove the additional fluff gauze under the elastic. Patients are told they may shower, but should replace the compressive elastic wrap snugly immediately afterward, and should wear this wrap continuously for the first 7 days afterward. From weeks 2 through 4, patients are expected to wear the garment while sleeping only.

BIBLIOGRAPHY

1. Haack J, Friedman O. Facial liposculpture. Facial Plast Surg. 2006;22:147-53.
2. Klein JA. Tumescent Technique: Tumescent Anesthesia and Microcannular Liposuction. St. Louis: Mosby; 2000.
3. Roland B. Safety of liposuction of the neck using tumescent local anesthesia: experience in 320 cases. Derm Surg. 2012;38:1812-5.
4. Zoumalan RA, Larrabee WF. Anatomic considerations in the aging face. Facial Plast Surg. 2011;27:16-22.

CHAPTER 11

Buccal Fat Pad

Anthony P Sclafani

OVERVIEW

Removal of fat from the inframalar area can recontour the midface and highlight the cheekbones. An intraoral approach to the buccal fat pad of Bichat allows rapid and simple fat removal.

SPECIAL CONSIDERATIONS

The buccal fat pad is a component of the deep temporal fat pad. The buccal fat is contiguous with the deep temporal fat pad superiorly and below the zygomatic arch, as well as the pterygoid extension posteriorly. Stenson's duct runs in proximity to the fat pad, as do small buccal branches of the facial nerve (Fig. 11.1).

ALTERNATIVES TO PROCEDURE

The malar arch can be highlighted by augmentation with a solid implant; alternatively, autologous fat or injectable soft tissue fillers can be injected to augment the soft tissues overlying the malar arch. Finally, a midface lift can be performed, which accentuates the midfacial contours by elevating soft tissues from the submalar area back over the malar eminence.

TECHNIQUES

Incision Placement

A small incision is made approximately 1 cm above the gingivobuccal sulcus opposite the first and second maxillary molar (Figs 11.2A and B)

Tissue Modifications

- *Incision*: The buccinator muscle and buccopharyngeal membrane are then bluntly pierced with a fine hemostat.
- *Excision*: When the clamp is then gently spread (Fig. 11.3), buccal fat is identified and teased out of

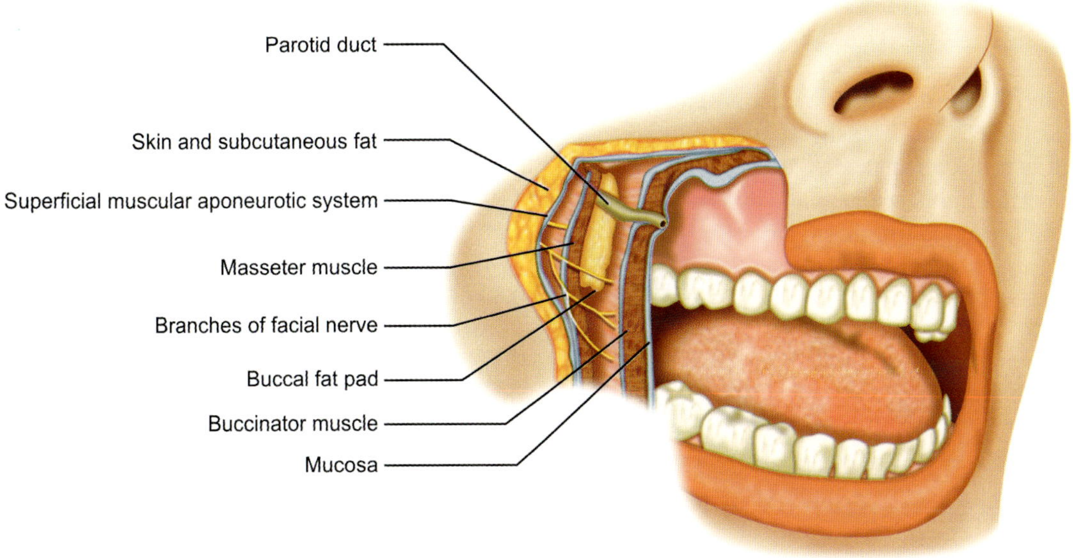

Fig. 11.1: Relevant anatomy in buccal fat pad excision

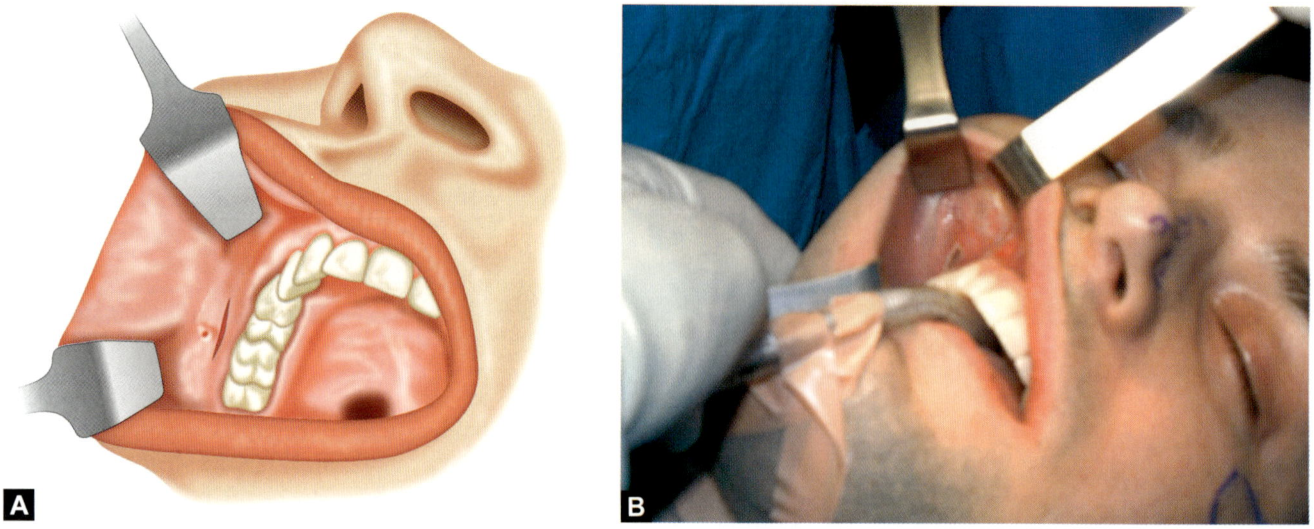

Figs 11.2A and B: An incision is made in the upper gingivobuccal mucosa opposite the first and second molars, carefully avoiding Stenson's duct orifice

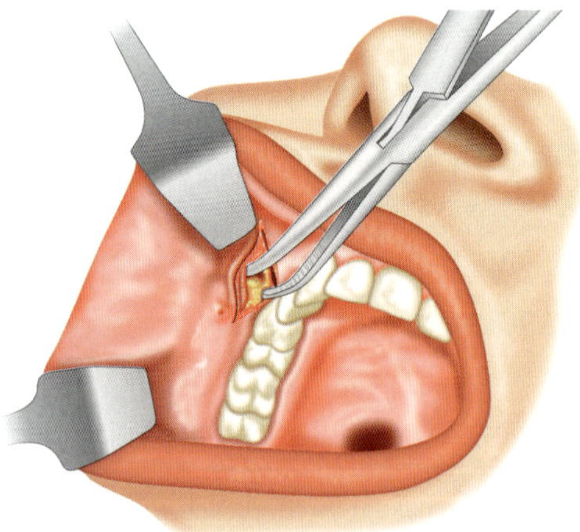

Fig. 11.3: A pointed clamp is used to pierce the buccopharyngeal fascia and is spread to identify the buccal fat pad

the incision (Figs 11.4A and B). External pressure can be applied to facilitate fat delivery. Once a sufficient amount of fat is delivered through the incision, the fat is cauterized with a bipolar cautery and excised. Generally 3–5 cc of fat is excised from each side (Fig. 11.5).

Closure

- *Sutures*: Each incision is closed with interrupted 3-0 chromic sutures
- *Dressings*: No dressings are necessary.

POTENTIAL COMPLICATIONS

Asymmetric Fat Removal

Care should be taken to remove symmetrical amounts of fat. Because of edema, the final result of fat removal is not fully evident for several weeks, and intraoperative fat removal should be guided by volume removed.

Buccal Nerve Weakness

Clamps should be spread parallel to the anticipated course of the buccal branches of the facial nerve to avoid stretch injury.

Stenson's Duct Injury

Stenson's duct runs through the buccal fat pad, with the transverse facial artery running above it and buccal branches of the facial nerve above and below it. Bipolar cautery only should be used, and only when these structures have been excluded.

AFTERCARE

There is no significant aftercare needed. Early mouth opening is recommended, as there will be some trismus secondary to muscular inflammation.

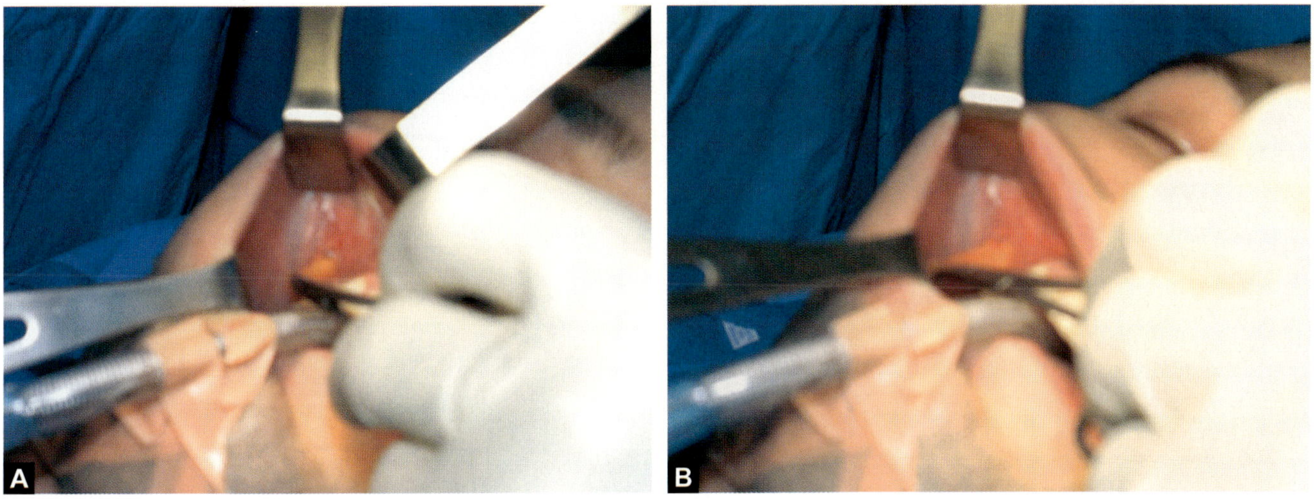

Figs 11.4A and B: Once the fat is identified, it is teased out

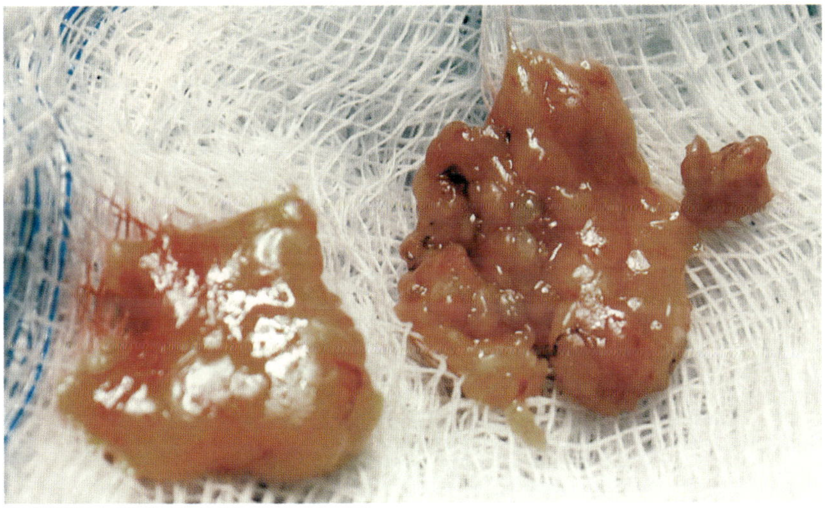

Fig. 11.5: Bilateral fat specimen after excision

BIBLIOGRAPHY

1. Dubin B, Jackson IT, Halim A, et al. Anatomy of the buccal fat pad and its clinical significance. Plast Reconstr Surg. 1989;83:257-62.
2. Jackson IT. Anatomy of the buccal fat pad and its clinical significance. Plast Reconstr Surg. 1999;103:2059-60.
3. Matarasso A. Managing the buccal fat pad. Aesth Surg J. 2006;26:330-6.

CHAPTER

12

Cheek and Chin Implants

Anthony P Sclafani

OVERVIEW

Synthetic implants have been used for several decades to alter the facial contour. In general, these implants are placed over bony surfaces to augment facial volume in focused areas, and in the past, these materials were also used to complement facial soft tissue volume. However, with the increasing emphasis on restoration of facial volume with autologous or exogenous injectable fillers, facial implants have been more appropriately used to augment bony facial deficiencies. The most appropriate and commonly addressed areas are the chin and the cheeks. In the past, a variety of materials have been used for this purpose, but currently the most common materials are silicone, expanded-polytetrafluoroethylene (e-PTFE) and porous high density polyethylene (PHDPE). All of these materials are well-tolerated and can produce long-lasting aesthetic results.

SPECIAL CONSIDERATIONS

The facial implants currently available are preformed into specific shapes and sizes which must be selected based on the individual patient's requirements, and each can be tailored intraoperatively. Silicone implants are solid surfaced, while e-PTFE and PHDPE are microporous, allowing tissue ingrowth into the implant surface. This difference makes porous implants more susceptible to early infection (prior to soft tissue ingrowth) while more resistant to infection later. Soft tissue ingrowth also provides stability for e-PTFE and PHDPE implants, while silicone implants rely on a precise pocket and subsequent capsule to maintain the implant in the correct position. All synthetic implants are much more rigid than normal soft tissue, so placement of these in areas of thin skin and soft tissue coverage potentially may lead to implant visibility and/or extrusion; these implants should be placed anatomically as deep as possible.

Regardless of where the implant is to be placed, it should be soaked for at least 15 minutes in an antibacterial saline bath immediately prior to use. If a microporous implant is being used, the plunger of a 20 cc syringe is removed and the implant placed in the syringe barrel; the plunger is then replaced and the syringe filled with the antibacterial solution. Once all air has been expressed from the syringe, a gloved finger is placed over the tip of the syringe and the plunger pulled back: the vacuum produced will evacuate air from the pores in the material, with the antibacterial solution replacing the air. As this happens, bubbles will be seen emerging from the implant surface. The plunger is released and the air again expressed from the syringe; this process is repeated until bubbles are no longer seen escaping from the implant surface, indicating that the interior pores of the implant have been saturated with antibacterial solution.

ALTERNATIVES TO PROCEDURE

Bony malar deficiency can be treated with soft tissue augmentation using autologous fat or injectable fillers. If significant soft tissue volume is present, a midface lift can restore some volume over key areas such as the malar eminence and infraorbital rim, while resected or mobilized SMAS can be sutured to the medial zygomatic arch for enhanced volume. Soft tissue fillers or fat can be injected over the mentum to enhance the anterior projection of the chin pad. Additionally, a sliding genioplasty can be performed, in which the lower border of the mentum is cut horizontally; the free piece is slid forward to advance it anteriorly and secured to the main body of the mentum in place with titanium plates.

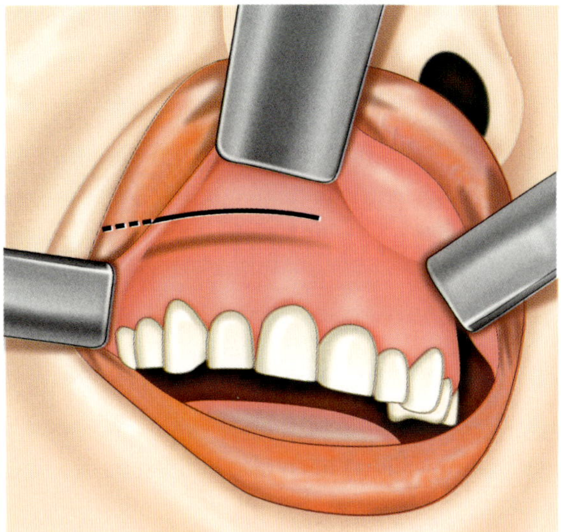

Fig. 12.1: An incision is made 1 cm above the gingivobuccal sulcus from the midline to the first molar and dissection carried down to bone

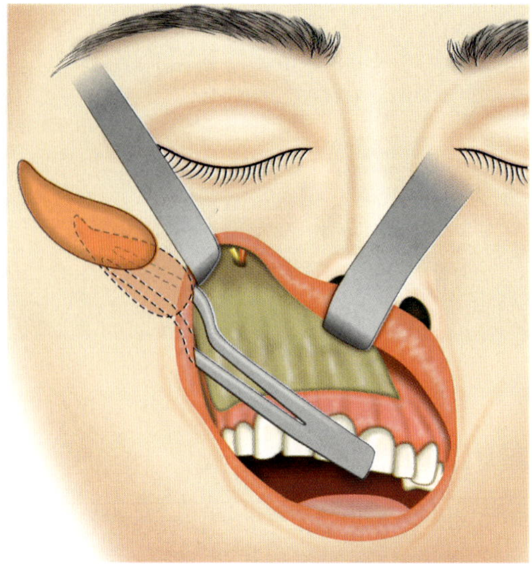

Fig. 12.2: The implant is introduced once a subperiosteal pocket has been dissected directly below the chosen location for the implant (as marked preoperatively on the skin). It is important to ensure that the implant lies flat against the bone without buckling

TECHNIQUES

Cheek Implants

Cheek implants can augment one or more areas, based on the design shape of the implant. Malar arch, malar eminence, subzygomatic hollow, infraorbital rim and tear trough augmentation are possible, so the surgeon must be familiar with the different design shapes and the specific locations of their placement.

Incision Placement

Cheek implants can be placed either through a transpalpebral or sublabial approach. As cheek implants have become larger and more complex in shape, the transpalpebral approach has become less useful, and most of these implants are placed using a sublabial approach. An incision is made through the mucosa of the upper gingivobuccal sulcus between the first molar and the midline, carefully preserving a 1 cm cuff of mucosa on the gingival side (Fig. 12.1). The cautery is then used to dissect down to the maxilla. The periosteum is incised with a #15 blade, and the maxillary periosteum is elevated with a Freer elevator.

Extent of Undermining/Dissection

Prior to beginning dissection, the implant is placed on the skin in the desired location and orientation, and the outline is circumscribed on the skin with a sterile surgical marker. This is used as a guide to elevate periosteum sufficiently, without creating too large a dissection pocket. Care is taken to avoid injury to the infraorbital neurovascular bundle, typically found below the medial limbus of the eye just below the orbital rim (less distinct in women). The pocket created should be only large enough to allow placement of the implant. Implants with orbital rim and tear trough portions will require dissection on both sides of the infraorbital rim. Implants with significant zygomatic arch portions will require dissection of the arch, and it is essential to maintain a subperiosteal dissection plane. PHDPE implants require larger pockets than silicone or e-PTFE implants, as soft tissue tends to adhere to the implant edges and prevents proper implant positioning unless a generous pocket is created (Fig. 12.2).

Tissue Modifications

Suturing: e-PTFE and PHDPE implants are stable if the pocket created is not excessively large and they are in direct contact with bone. Silicone implants, even one with a textured base, may be prone to movement in a larger-than-needed pocket. A 2-0 permanent monofilament suture can be passed through a dental roll bolster and then transcutaneously, recovering the needle in the implant pocket. The needle is then passed through the implant and then returned through it again to the implant's superficial surface. The needle is regrasped and then driven transcutaneously through the bolster and lightly tied. Additionally, some surgeons prefer to drill a

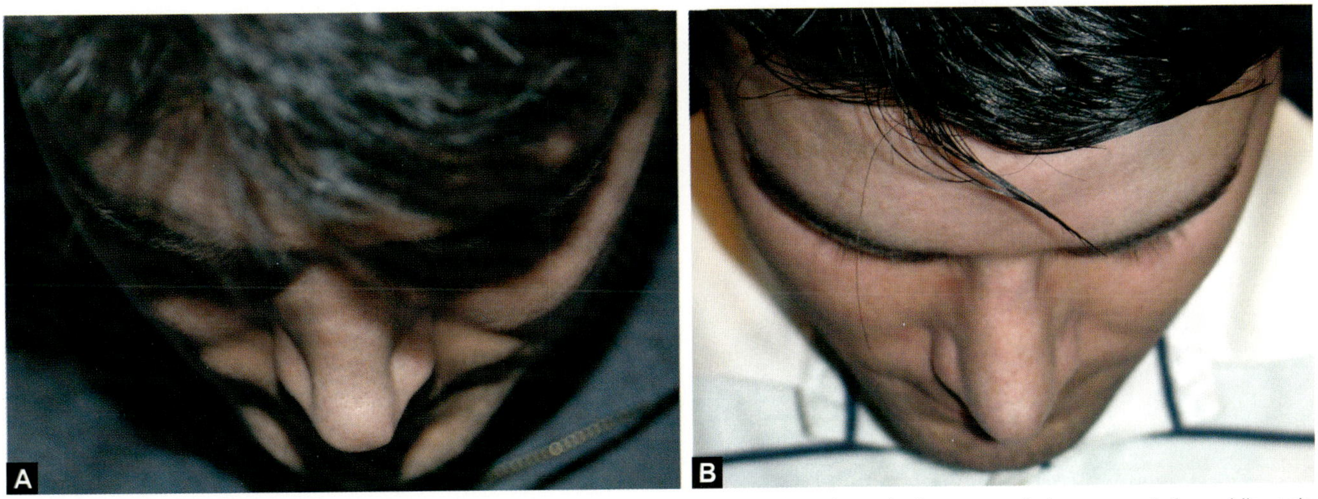

Figs 12.3A and B: (A) Before and (B) after cheek augmentation. In general, female patients desire more anterior augmentation, while male patients seek to highlight the malar arch; however, the specific implant shape and position should be tailored to the individual

hole through PHDPE implants and the underlying bone and secure the implant in place with a titanium screw. It should be noted, however, that the heat generated from drilling will fuse some implant pores closed and prevent tissue ingrowth, and the screw serves as additional foreign material in the wound. In general, this technique should only be used when the PHDPE implant cannot be held securely in position by surrounding soft tissue.

Closure

- *Layers/Sutures*: Whenever possible, soft tissue from the cheek flap should be sutured with a 3-0 or 4-0 braided absorbable suture such as polyglactin 910 (Vicryl, Ethicon, Inc., Somerville, New Jersey) to remaining soft tissue surrounding the implant in order to most effectively isolate the implant from the external environment. The gingivobuccal sulcus incision is closed with a water-tight, running, locking 3-0 Vicryl suture, started 5–8 mm distal to the distal end of the incision and running mesially to a point 5–8 mm medial to the proximal end of the incision (Figs 12.3A and B).

Dressings

No dressings are applied. Antibacterial ointment is applied to the bolsters if used.

Chin Implants

Chin implants are more uniform in size and shape than cheek implants, varying mostly in terms of anterior projection, height and the degree of extension laterally beyond the mentum. Chin implants commonly used are also made of silicone, e-PTFE coated silicone and PHDPE. Anatomic implants typically do not extend beyond the mentum, while extended implants will have longer, more gradually tapering arms which continue laterally to blend with the mandibular ramus.

Incision Placement

Chin implants can be placed through either an intraoral or external (submental) approach. Reported infection rates are roughly equivalent for these two approaches. However, the intraoral approach necessarily transects the mentalis muscle; incomplete or inadequate healing of this muscle will lead to a dimpled and distorted chin pad. While the external approach leaves a visible scar, it is well-hidden if properly placed.

- *Intraoral approach*: The lower lip is appropriately anesthetized with a 1% xylocaine with 1:100,000 epinephrine solution by blocking both mental nerves and by direct infiltration of the gingivolabial sulcus. Cutting cautery is used to incise the mucosa approximately 1 cm on the labial side of the sulcus (Fig. 12.4). The cautery is then used to divide the mentalis muscle, carefully preserving a stump of muscle attached to the mentum. Once this is done, the periosteum has been exposed and is incised. Using a Freer elevator, the periosteum is elevated down to the lower border of the mandible, and then laterally along the lower mandibular border.
- *External approach*: The first submental skin crease is identified and marked, marking the midline as well (Fig. 12.5). In a patient with a severely hypoplastic mentum, the appropriate position of the incision can

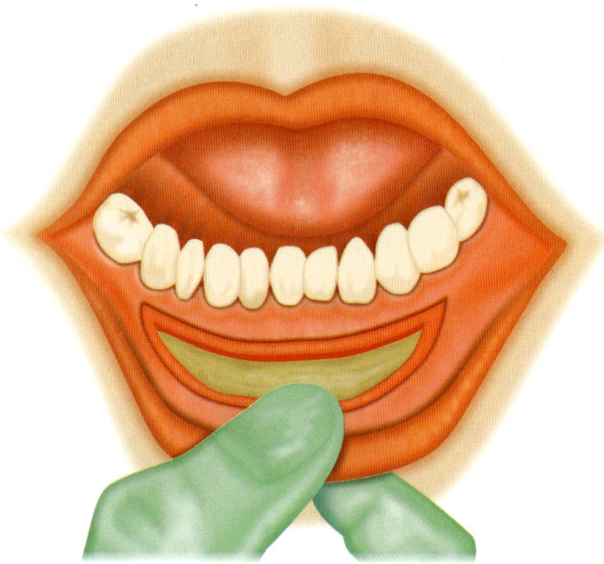

Fig. 12.4: Chin implants can be placed transorally by incision near the apex of the gingivolabial sulcus, leaving a cuff of mucosa for later closure and requiring sectioning of the mentalis muscle

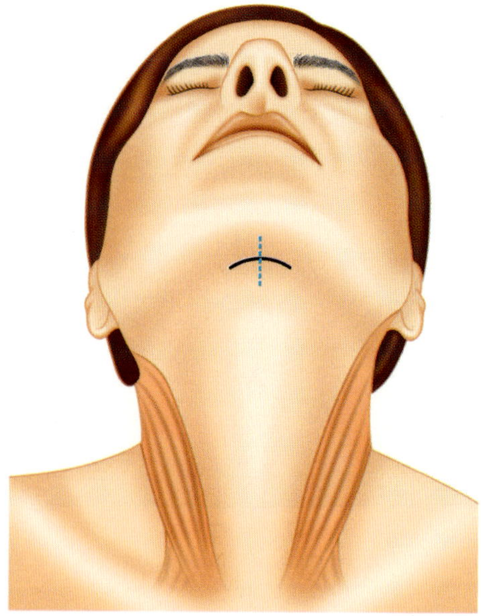

Fig. 12.5: A submental incision centered over the midline and placed just behind the chin fat pad allowed placement of chin implants transcutaneously

be planned by locating it at the posterior edge of the chin fat pad; once the implant is place, this incision will be hidden on the undersurface of the chin. The incision is no more than 3 cm in length, unless a PHDPE implant is used, which necessitates a larger incision. The skin incision is made with a #15 blade after the chin has been anesthetized with mental nerve blocks and local infiltration. The platysma muscle is exposed and carefully transected with cautery. Soft tissue can be swept aside until the periosteum of the midline lower mandibular border is seen. A Freer or Obwegeser elevator is then used to sweep the soft tissues overlying the mental periosteum upward until the mental crease is exposed. A 1–1.5 cm strip of periosteum in the midline is left intact, and vertical incisions through the periosteum are made on either side of this strip from the lower mandibular border to the mental crease (Fig. 12.6). The periosteum can be elevated laterally along the lower mandibular border through these periosteal incisions, while an intact strip of periosteum in the midline is maintained (Fig. 12.7).

Extent of Undermining/Dissection

Even more so than with cheek implants, proper placement and secure stabilization is essential for the success of chin implants. Overly large implant pockets will allow movement of the implant. As with cheek implants, prior to incision, the implant is placed externally on the skin in the desired location and outlined on the skin with a sterile surgical marker (Figs 12.8A and B). The dissection pocket is just slightly larger than the marking, unless a PHDPE implant is being used, in which case the pocket needs to be considerably larger, as the implant must be placed directly in position and cannot be slid into the appropriate location. Care is taken to dissect along the lower mandibular border and superiorly only as much as necessary to accommodate the implant.

Implant Placement

As with cheek implants, chin implants should be soaked in an antibiotic solution and handled as little as possible (see above discussion for proper preparation of implants). Silicone and hybrid e-PTFE implants are placed into the dissection pocket one limb at a time. Once the surgeon has slid one side of the implant into the pocket on one side and is satisfied with positioning, the implant is bent at its midpoint and the remaining limb is slid into the contralateral pocket (Fig. 12.9). Prior to implant placement, the midline of the implant is marked on the exterior surface of the implant; after the implant has been placed, symmetric placement of the implant is checked using the marking at the implant midline. Minor adjustments in position are possible without fully removing the implant, but the soft tissues overlying the implant must be elevated to move the implant; significant deviations from correct placement symmetrically over the mentum and along the lower mandibular border generally require removal of the implant, confirmation of the symmetry of the dissection pockets and implant replacement.

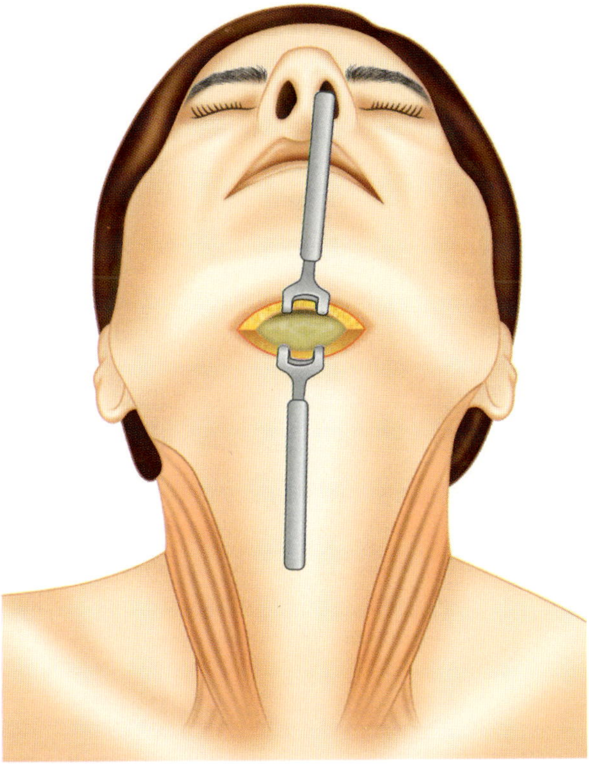

Fig. 12.6: After the fat and platysma muscle are divided and retracted, the periosteum of the lower mandible is exposed. Two paramedian vertical incisions are made, leaving a bridge of intact periosteum in the midline

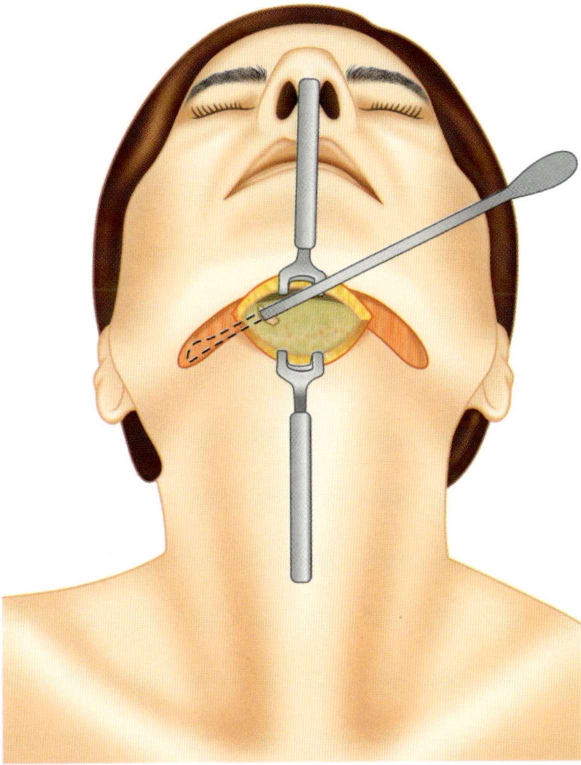

Fig. 12.7: Using a Freer elevator, a subperiosteal pocket is dissected under the marked area of planned implant placement. It is important to hug the lower mandibular border during this dissection

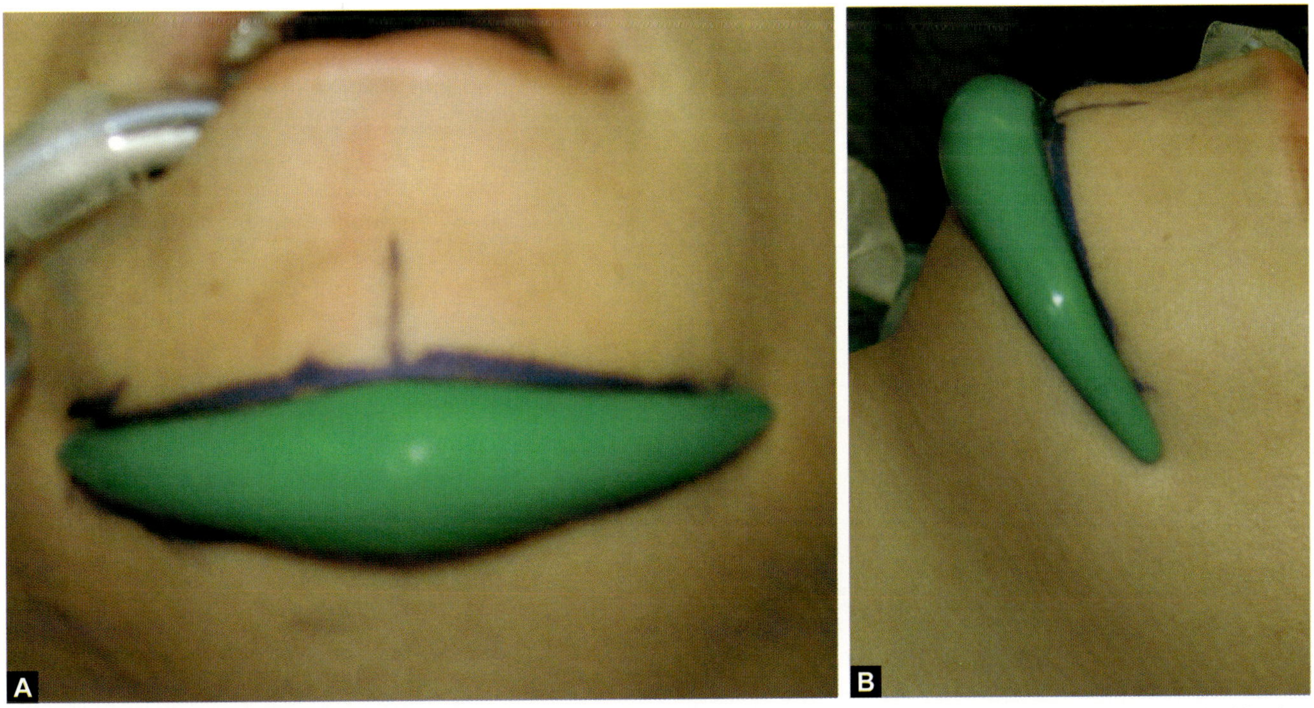

Figs 12.8A and B: Proper placement of the chin implant is facilitated with the use of nonsterile "sizer" implants to mark the desired implant location on the skin preoperatively

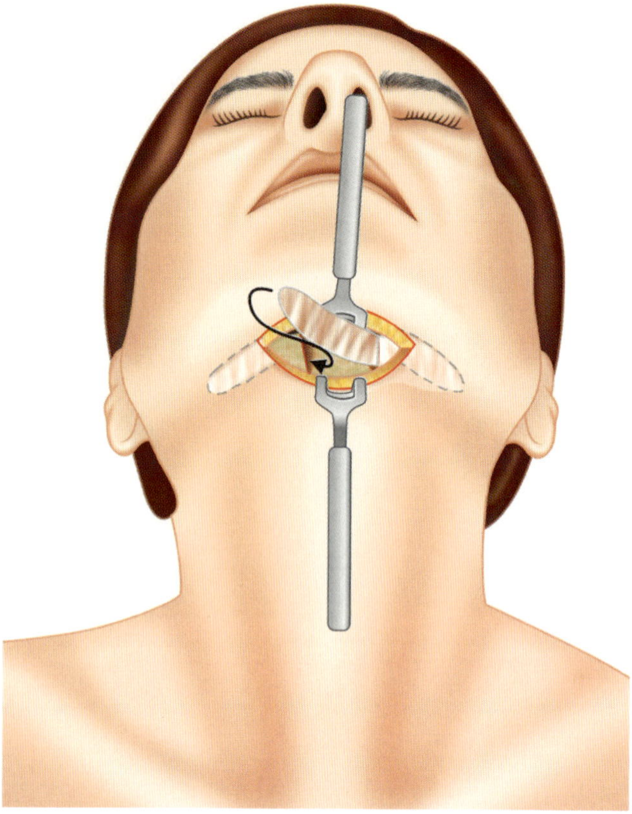

Fig. 12.9: Once one half of the implant is place, it is bent and inserted into the contralateral subperiosteal pocket. Symmetry is checked by aligning the midline of the implant (marked preoperatively) with the midline as marked on the skin

Closure

Layers/Sutures

- *Intraoral approach*: It is essential to re-establish the proper continuity and orientation of the mentalis muscle, which should be reapproximated with 3-0 polyglactin 910 sutures. The mucosa should then be closed with the same suture, placed in a running locking fashion to ensure a water-tight closure.
- *External approach*: The platysma muscle fibers are closed with 3-0 polyglactin 910 sutures, while the dermis is closed with 4-0 sutures. The epidermis can be closed with either interrupted 6-0 polypropylene sutures or liquid skin closure (2-octyl-cyanoacrylate, Dermabond, Ethicon, Somerville, New Jersey) (Figs 12.10A and B).

Dressings

An elastic tape is applied over the chin to secure the implant in position after covering any external wound with a nonadhesive pad.

POTENTIAL COMPLICATIONS

Extrusion and Infection

Implant extrusion is rare if the above techniques are followed, and generally follows bacterial colonization and infection of the implant. Infection rates are not significantly different between the intraoral and external approach, and should be between 1–3%. Early infection of microporous implants, and infection of solid implants at any time, generally leads to formation of a bacterial biofilm on the implant, a mucopolysaccharide covering which makes treatment much more difficult. Antibiotic treatment should be instituted as soon as an infection is suspected, with broad spectrum antibiotics and continued for at least 6–8 weeks if treatment appears to be successful, while if no improvement is noted after a few days, the implant should be removed, the cavity rinsed with antibiotic solution and the wound allowed to heal before a new implant is placed.

Implant Movement/Asymmetry

Issues of asymmetry, if the above techniques are followed, are typically rare if the implant was seated correctly initially. Overly ample dissection pockets facilitate implant movement and these should only be large enough to allow for implant placement. Likewise, it is essential that the pocket be shaped to the exact specifications of the implant. Softer implants such as silicone may bend into the appropriate position in a poorly created pocket temporarily, but postoperatively will seem to "rotate" as the bent portion of the implant flattens into an undesirable position. Additionally, in the chin, placement of a portion of the implant subperiosteally and the center preperitoneally creates a plane transition at two points which helps "lock" the implant in this position.

Bony Erosion

Bone erosion has been shown to occur with hard silicone implants placed direct on the bone of the mentum. Maintenance of a periosteal bridge over the bone preserves osteoblasts over the bone to prevent excessive remodeling.

Nerve Injury

The infraorbital nerve is generally at risk for injury during placement of cheek implants, and great care in dissection around the foramen is necessary. Any bleeding from the

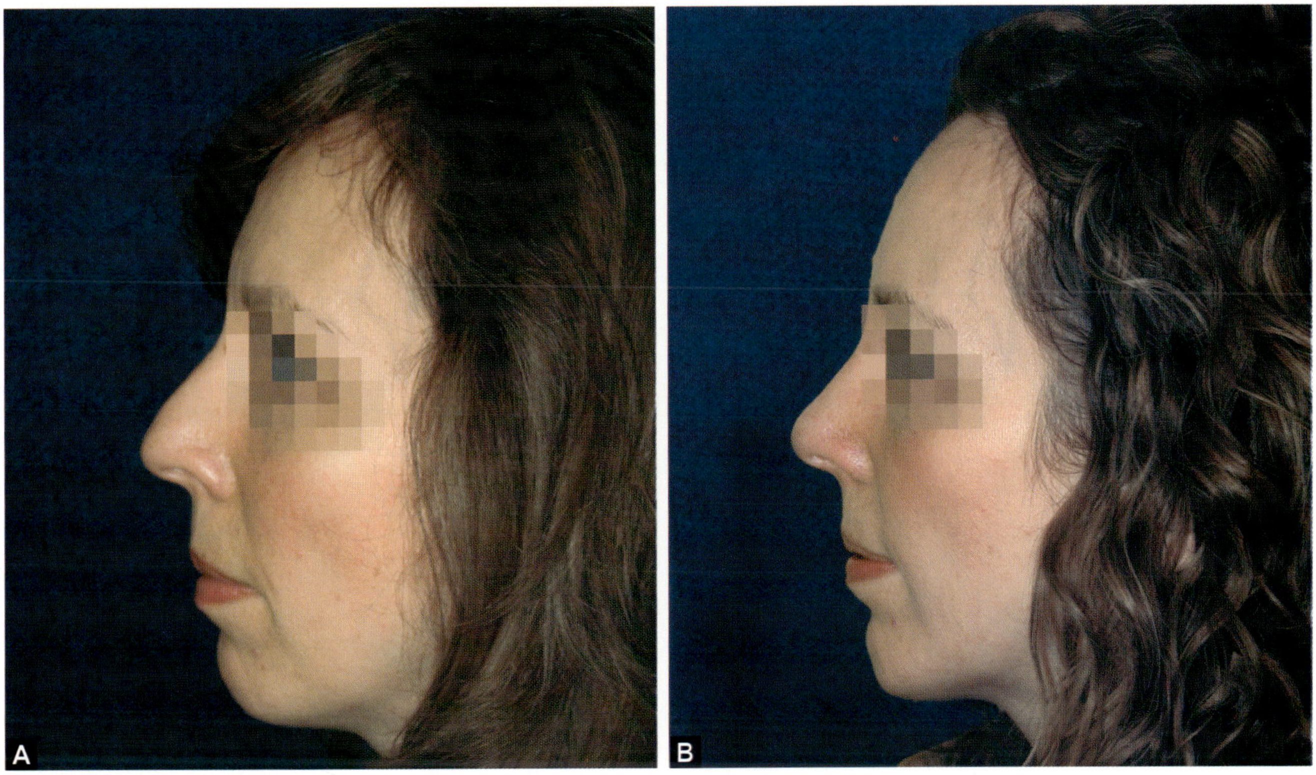

Figs 12.10A and B: (A) Before and (B) after chin augmentation and rhinoplasty

infraorbital neurovascular pedicle should be managed with bipolar cautery only, if necessary. Extensive dissection over the superior aspect of the malar eminence places the zygomaticofacial nerve at risk. Extensive traction on the facial flap may cause temporary anesthesia or dysesthesia of the cheek. During dissection for a chin implant, the mental nerves are placed at risk, and dissection should extend superiorly from the lower mandibular border only as much as needed.

AFTERCARE

Postoperative care is fairly simple. Patients are instructed to rinse their mouths gently with a warm salt water solution 3–4 times per day and brush their teeth gently. They are asked not to lean on their cheeks or chin for at least 3 weeks.

BIBLIOGRAPHY

1. Choe KS, Stucki-McCormick SU. Chin augmentation. Facial Plast Surg. 2000;16:45-54.
2. Mladick RA. Alloplastic cheek augmentation. Clin Plast Surg. 1991;18:29-38.
3. Warren SM, Spector JA, Zide BM. Chin surgery VII: the textured secured implant—a recipe for success. Plast Reconstr Surg. 2007;120:1378-85.
4. Yaremchuk MJ. Atlas of Facial Implants. Philadelphia: Saunders/Elsevier; 2006.

CHAPTER 13

Otoplasty

Anthony P Sclafani

OVERVIEW

Congenital auricular prominence may be associated with other congenital syndromes, but most often is found in isolation. While correcting this deformity addresses the patient's physical appearance, it is performed to restore a normal appearance of the ears and is rightly classified as reconstructive surgery. While this procedure can be performed at any age, correction of ear deformities is best done in childhood, before the patient has suffered psychologically from social stigmatization and prior to developing a sense of physical "self". Approximately 5% of Caucasians in the United States have protruding ears. The 2008 American Society for Aesthetic Plastic Surgery (ASAPS) survey estimated just slightly less than 25,000 "cosmetic" ear surgeries were performed; 59% of patients with prominent ears have a family history, and transmission is thought to be autosomal dominant with variable penetrance.

SPECIAL CONSIDERATIONS

A variety of common names have been used to phenotypically describe the prominent auricle, such as lop ear, bat ear, Satyr's ear, shell ear and cup ear, among others. It is more valuable to identify the specific defects of the malformed ear, as these features will directly be addressed during otoplasty.

The auricle will grow after birth and will attain approximately 85% its adult size by 5–6 years of age. Prominent ears do not progress or cause a physical debility. However, the social stigma of deformed ears can cause significant emotional distress. Children rarely suffer from teasing by peers before the age of 6, and surgery can be delayed until that time, allowing for surgery with a more mature and cooperative patient.

The helical rim should have a gentle furl and graceful arch and should evenly protrude 1–2 mm more than the antihelix. There should be a defined antihelix forming a 90 degree angle between the scaphoid fossa and conchal wall, with similarly defined superior and inferior crura enclosing a fossa triangularis (Fig. 13.1). The conchal bowl should rise away from the mastoid cortex (conchomastoid angle) at a roughly 90 degree angle and should not extend excessively laterally. The lobule should continue smoothly from the inferior extent of the helix, and the ear should angle away from the scalp at an angle (auriculocephalic angle) no greater than 25 degrees. Overall, the height and width of the auricle should be 5–6 cm and 2.5–3.5 cm respectively. The ear should protrude no more than 10–12 mm superiorly, 16–18 mm in the midpoint of the helical rim and 20–22 mm at the lobule from the head (Fig. 13.2).

ALTERNATIVES TO PROCEDURE

Minor auricular deformities can sometimes be partially or fully corrected noninvasively. Especially within the first year of life, the auricular cartilage is quite soft and pliable. Taping and splinting of prominent or folded auricles during the first several months of life can aid in correcting, or at least improving, the contour of the auricle. Otherwise, hairstyling remains the only way to camouflage auricular prominence.

TECHNIQUES

Modern otoplasty maneuvers fall into two distinct categories: (1) cartilage cutting and (2) cartilage sparing techniques. Cartilage cutting techniques are powerful steps which can significantly remodel and reposition the auricle; however, these techniques can lead to unnatural, sharp edges when cuts through firm cartilage are seen through thin auricular skin. Cartilage sparing techniques avoid sharp angles by relying mainly on sutures and postoperative fibrosis to bend, fold and maintain the corrected shape

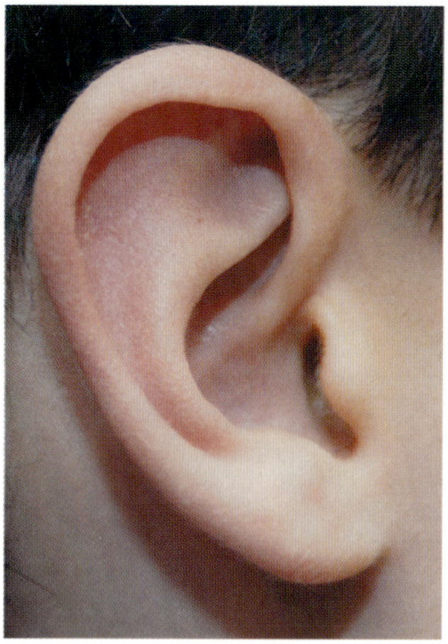

Fig. 13.1: The aesthetic ear has a smooth helical rim, a well-formed antihelix and a defined conchal bowl

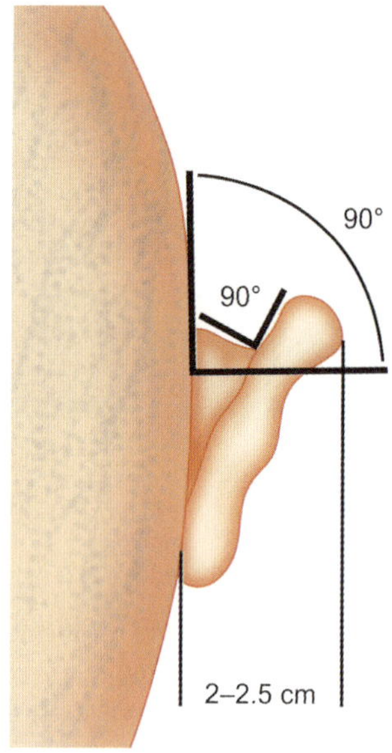

Fig. 13.2: The normal ear with lateral ear projection of no more than 20–22 mm. Both the conchomastoid angle and the conchohelical angle are each approximately 90°, and the auriculocephalic angle should be about 25°

and position of the auricular cartilage. The utility of this approach can be limited in adult patients, whose cartilage is stiffer and less pliable than pediatric patients.

Incision Placement

A postauricular approach is generally used for otoplasty. An ellipse of skin is based over the postauricular crease and excised down to the auricular perichondrium (Fig. 13.3).

Extent of Undermining or Dissection

A pre-perichondrial plane is dissected radially to the helical rim along the length of the incision, while the dissection proceeds posteriorly to expose the entire conchal bowl cartilage and the mastoid periosteum (Fig. 13.4).

Tissue Modifications

The ear should be evaluated at the superior pole, level of the external auditory meatus, antitragus and lobule, and specific needs at each point addressed. Common deformities, seen either together or in isolation, include incomplete antihelical folding, excess depth of the conchal bowl, lateral-inferior furling of the superior pole, lateralization of the lobule and lobule excess. Depending on the specific findings of each ear and the resilience or stiffness of the auricular cartilage, particular techniques can be chosen to best accomplish surgical goals.

Cartilage Excision

Cartilage is rarely excised except for conchal bowl excess, in which a crescent of the conchal bowl wall can be excised to medialize the position of the antihelix (Figs 13.5A and B). By excising the cartilage at the junction of the cartilage with the conchal bowl floor, the lateral extent of the conchal bowl wall is reduced as the cartilage is then sutured medially to the mastoid periosteum. Alternatively, an excessively convex conchal bowl base may make medializing sutures difficult; in such cases, the conchal bowl base can be excised to allow medialization without excessive suture tension.

Cartilage Incision

The anterior scoring approach attempts to take advantage of cartilage's tendency to warp. Either through a posterior incision or a small anterior one, a wire brush or other scoring device is advanced along the subperichondrial plane at the apex of the antihelix (Fig. 13.6). The cartilage is then scored with partial thickness cuts parallel to and along the length of the antihelix. The cartilage can then be more easily folded and braced in position with the postoperative dressing (Fig. 13.7).

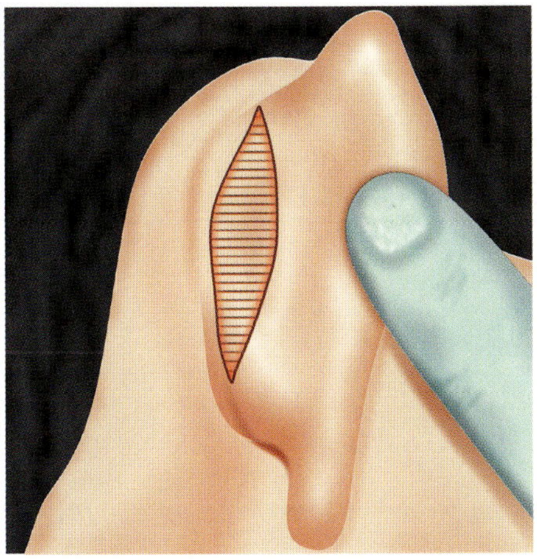

Fig. 13.3: The postauricular incision appears to be centered over the medial concha when the ear is retracted forward, but falls into the crease when the ear is released

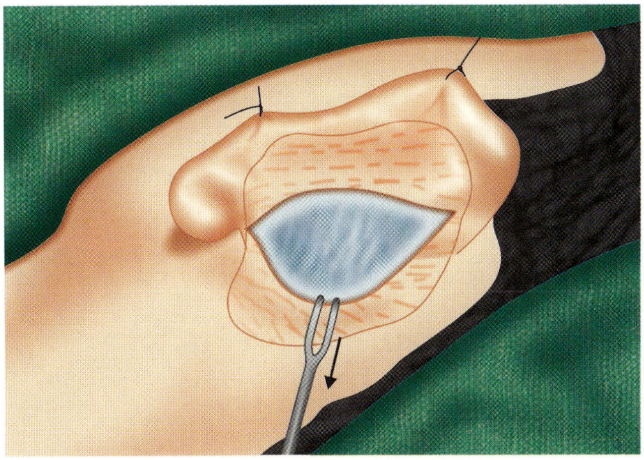

Fig. 13.4: Through the postauricular incision, skin is undermined just above the perichondrium to the edge of the helical rim laterally and posteriorly to expose 2–3 cm of mastoid periosteum. This typically requires cauterization and transection of the posterior auricular muscle

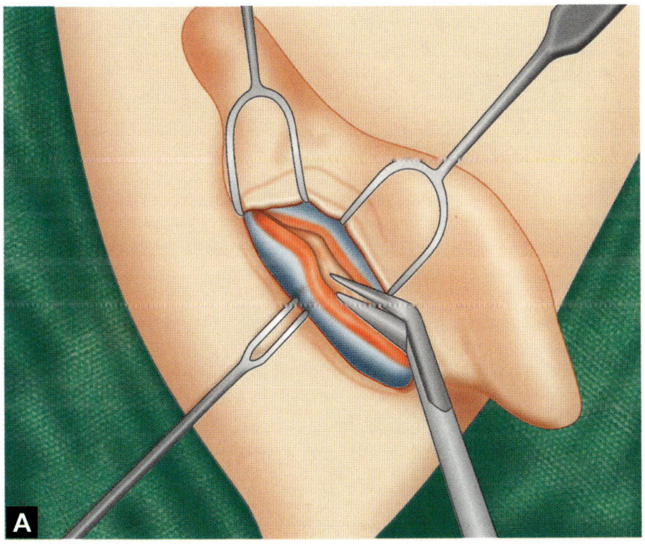

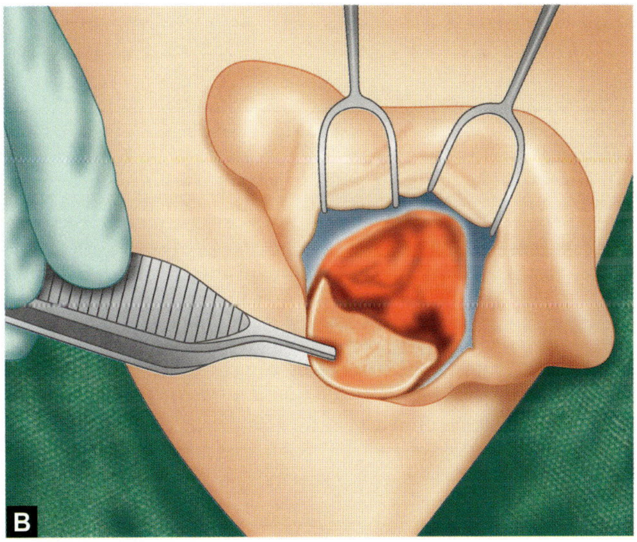

Figs 13.5A and B: If excessive lateral wall of the concha causes a protruding ear, the cartilage can be incised at the point where the lateral conchal wall meets the mastoid periosteum, and an ellipse of cartilage lateral to this incision is excised

Other cartilage cutting techniques utilize full-thickness cuts in the cartilage to break the natural spring of the cartilage and allow repositioning of the cartilage segments with sutures. Because of the thinness of the skin and the rigid nature of the cartilage, care must be taken to camouflage the edges of these cartilage segments. The sites of these cuts should allow undisturbed, natural curvatures of the auricular cartilage to cover or telescope over the cut edges. This can be particularly useful in treating auricular cartilage with limited flexibility in the conchal bowl and particularly in the antihelix. To correct a poorly formed antihelix, parallel incisions on either side of the apex of the antihelical curve can be made, followed by sutures placed between the two larger segments to allow the strip of antihelical apex to ride over the sutured cartilage segments and camouflage the sharp angle formed by the junction of the two larger cartilage segments (Figs 13.8A and B).

Suturing

Cartilage sparing procedures can be used to form a more defined antihelix, medialize the conchal bowl, correct prominence of the superior pole of the auricle and correct earlobe prominence. Mustardé mattress sutures

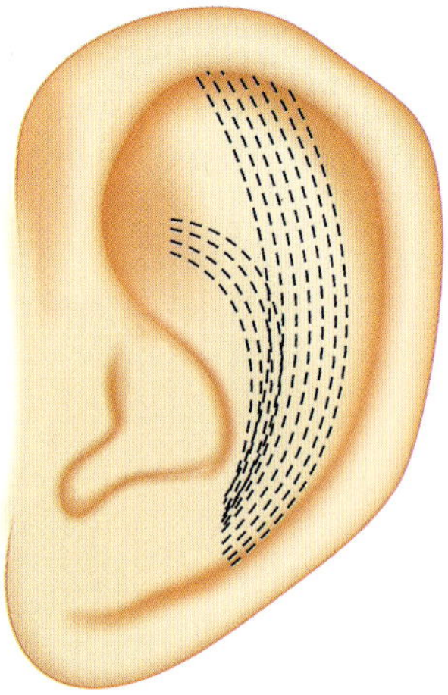

Fig. 13.6: Anterior scoring of the cartilage with a wire brush will allow folding of the cartilage and healing in this position

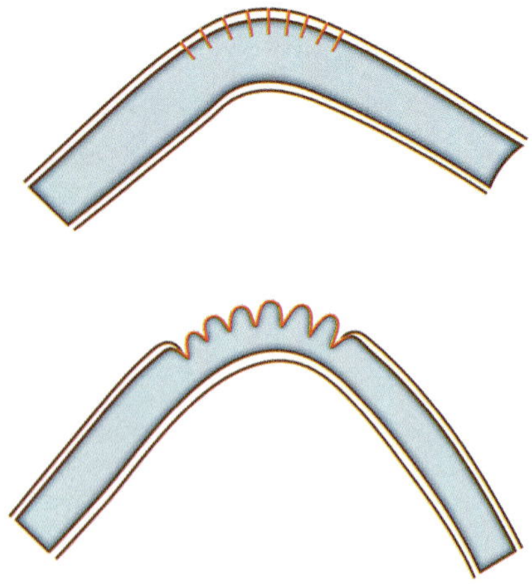

Fig. 13.7: Partially incised cartilage will allow folding to the contralateral side

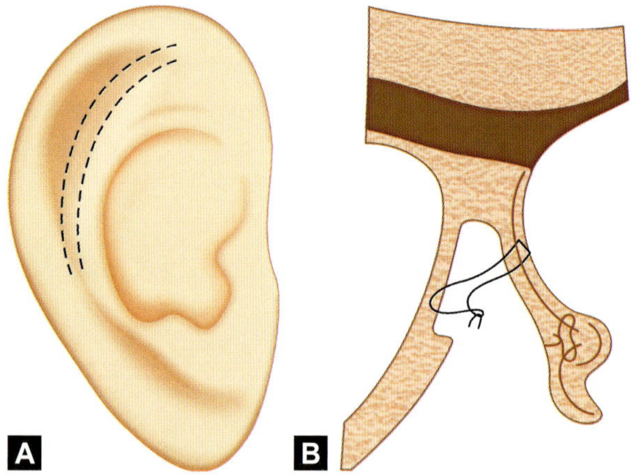

Figs 13.8A and B: (A) Incisions are made through the cartilage on either side of the planned antihelix; (B) The medial and lateral cartilaginous segments are then sutured together to form a more acute antihelical fold, while the intervening cartilage strip "floats" above to blunt the sharp cartilage edges

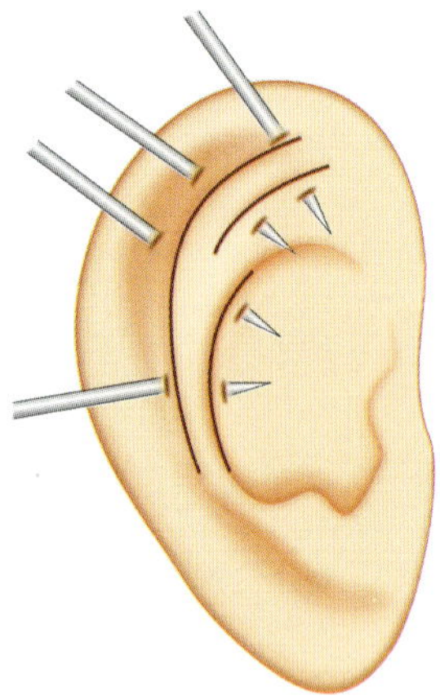

Fig. 13.9: The antihelix is manually folded and Keith needles are passed through the planned antihelix. When the ear is folded forward, the sites where needles are seen entering and exiting the cartilage are marked for placement of Mustardé sutures

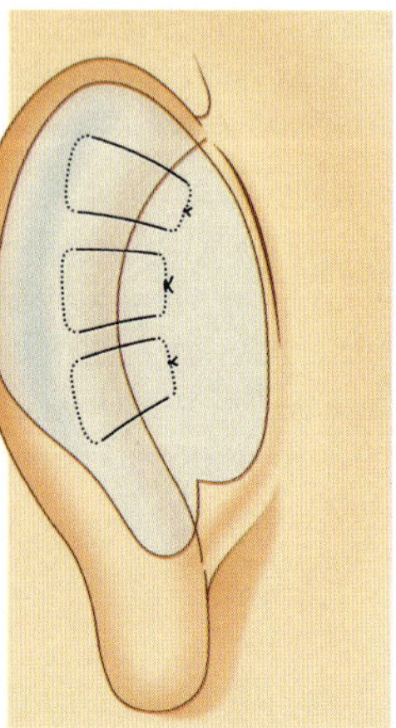

Fig. 13.10: Mustardé mattress sutures span across the medial surface of the antihelix and increasingly define it as the sutures are tightened and tied

are placed between the sides of the antihelical fold and tied sufficiently tightly to better define the antihelix. The antihelix should be manually folded by the surgeon and a Keith needle can be passed through the cartilage and across the antihelix about 1 cm below its apex and the entry and exit sites on the medial side of the cartilage marked as placement sites for mattress sutures (Fig. 13.9). Horizontal mattress sutures of a 3-0 or 4-0 braided, nonabsorbable suture material such as Mersilene are placed at these sites and tied while an assistant folds the antihelix appropriately. Three to five sutures are placed along the length of the common and superior crura of the antihelix (Fig. 13.10). Suture bites should be about 1 cm wide, purchasing cartilage and lateral perichondrium but not skin, to allow for a gentle rolling antihelical curve; however, sutures should not be placed too superiorly

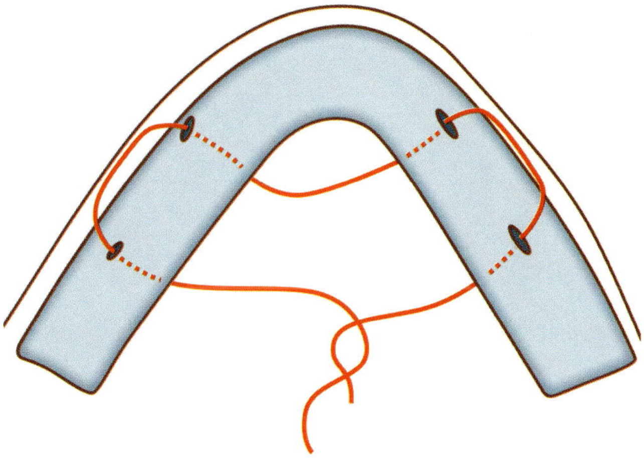

Fig. 13.11: Mattress sutures include a full thickness portion of cartilage but should not penetrate the lateral perichondrium. Postoperative fibrosis between the two sides of cartilage ultimately aid in maintaining cartilage position

along the superior crus to avoid a "tentpole" deformity, where the superior crus of the antihelix is well-defined across the scaphoid fossa and up to the helix (Fig. 13.11).

The conchal bowl can be sutured more medially to reduce its lateral extension in cases of prominence. Partial thickness cartilage excision is performed to "flatten" this surface of the cartilage if the medial surface of the conchal bowl is excessively convex. Horizontal mattress sutures are placed through the portion of the conchal cartilage extending laterally away from the mastoid and tied to a suture bite of mastoid periosteum (Figs 13.12A and B). It is important that the suture pulls the conchal bowl posteriorly as well as medially; mastoid sutures placed too anteriorly will cause the anterior lip of the conchal bowl cartilage to roll anteriorly and constrict the external auditory meatus (Fig. 13.13).

Further contouring of the auricular position and shape can be performed with directed sutures for specific purposes. If the superior pole of the auricle remains prominent, a 3-0 Mersilene mattress suture is passed between the cartilage of the fossa triangularis and the temporalis fascia after the superior skin is further elevated and fascia clearly exposed (Fig. 13.14). Also, inferior pole prominence can be a result of excessive soft tissue on the medial aspect of the earlobe (best treated by conservative skin excision from the medial surface of the earlobe, in continuity with the postauricular incision) or by a prominent or laterally oriented cauda helicis. This can be treated either by conservative cartilage excision of the cauda helicis after further peripheral undermining of the auricular skin or an additional 3-0 Mersilene mattress suture tied between the cauda helicis and conchal bowl.

Closure

During wound closure, it is important that the repositioned and reformed cartilage should not be stretched or pulled, but instead gently manipulated and sutures supported, as excessive tension may break the sutures or cause them to pull through the cartilage.

Layers or Sutures

The skin is closed in a single layer with a running 4-0 chromic suture.

Skin Excision or Burow's Triangles

Prior to wound closure, the auricle should be repositioned, the postauricular skin redraped and any excess skin is conservatively excised.

Drains

A small, rubber band drain is often placed and brought out through the inferior portion of the incision, if necessary.

Dressings

A form-fitting, lightly compressive dressing is made from cotton soaked in mineral oil, packed lightly to fill the newly created concavities, and then covered with a mastoid dressing.

POTENTIAL COMPLICATIONS

In general, complications of otoplasty are fairly uncommon, and most are technique related: telephone ear or reverse telephone ear, recurrence. Cellulitis can occur, and is generally caused by typical skin flora. Chondritis classically presents as deep ear pain with swelling and erythema developing 3–5 days after surgery. Drainage, culture and antibiotics (including coverage of Pseudomonas in cases of suspected chondritis) should be instituted as soon as the diagnosis is suspected. Suture failure may occur and lead to recurrence of some of or all of the preoperative deformity. Causes include inadequate number or caliber of suture material, failure to properly address the resilience of the auricular cartilage, poor purchase of cartilage by the suture or auricular manipulation or trauma in the early postoperative period. Within several weeks, sufficient fibrosis develops around the newly shaped auricular cartilage to maintain its shape and position without the sutures. Recurrence of auricular deformity is uncommon (approximately 2%) and is generally a result of suture failure. Suture granulomas can develop, and are characterized by a tender focal swelling generally along the scar; these may develop months after

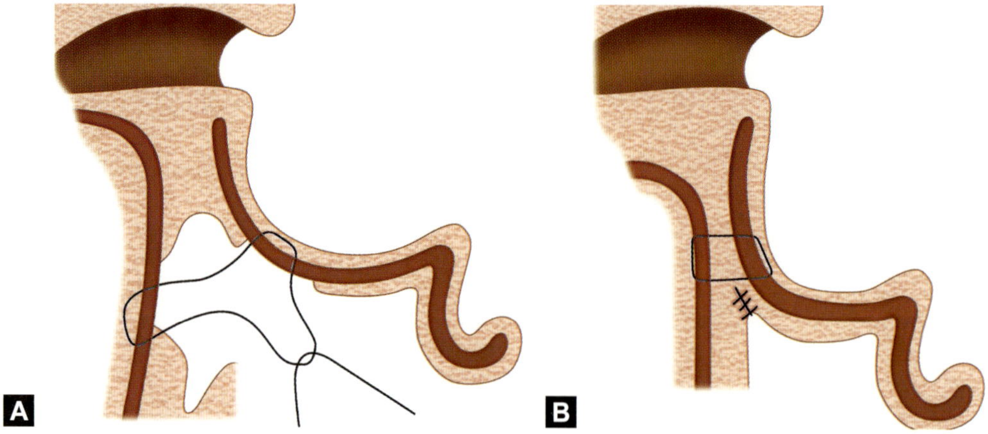

Figs 13.12A and B: Conchal setback sutures from conchal to mastoid periosteum medialize the conchal bowl

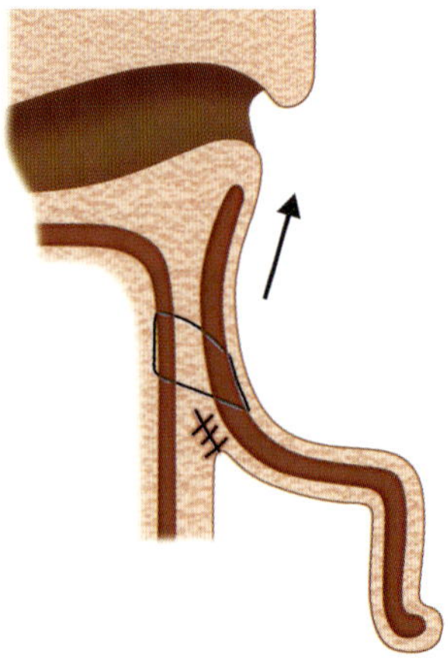

Fig. 13.13: It is important to avoid placing the periosteal suture too anteriorly, or the curved conchal bowl will be pulled forward and advanced to compromise the external auditory meatus

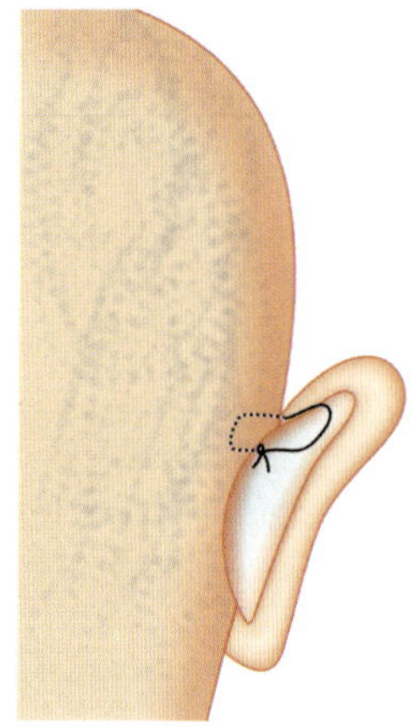

Fig. 13.14: For the persistently lateralized superior auricular pole, a suture can be placed between the medial surface of the fossa triangularis and the temporalis fascia for discrete superior auricular medialization

the surgery. Topical and oral antibiotics may help to reduce inflammation, but the wound may require exploration and suture removal, preferably after development of postoperative fibrosis. Suture bridging is generally the result of excessive skin resection, as the span of sutures across the postauricular crease become visible in relief below the skin. Excessive skin closure tension may predispose to the development of hypertrophic or keloid scars; however, these may develop even in the absence of excessive wound closure tension, and a patient and family history of poor healing should be evaluated preoperatively. Uneven reduction of auricular prominence can cause a "telephone ear" deformity, in which the superior and inferior poles project further from the head than the midportion of the auricle (or a "reverse telephone ear" deformity, with the superior and inferior poles more medialized than the midportion); careful inspection of the intraoperative result should identify this unwanted result prior to wound closure, and sutures revised.

AFTERCARE

The dressing and drain are removed on postoperative day one, and an elastic athletic headband is worn over both ears constantly; after the first week, this is worn at nighttime only for the next 3 weeks.

BIBLIOGRAPHY

1. Furnas DW. Correction of prominent ears with multiple sutures. Clin Plast Surg. 1978;5:491-5.
2. Janis JE, Rohrich RJ, Gutowski KA. Otoplasty. Plast Reconstr Surg. 2005;115:60e-72e.
3. Mustardé JC. The correction of prominent ears using simple mattress sutures. Br J Plast Surg. 1963;16:170-8.
4. Porter CJW, Tan ST. Congenital auricular anomalies: topographic anatomy, embryology, classification, and treatment strategies. Plast Reconstr Surg. 2005;115:1701-12.

CHAPTER 14

Hair Transplantation

Anthony P Sclafani

OVERVIEW

Hair restoration initially developed as a mass manipulation of skin, whether by transposing hair-bearing skin to a desired area or by excising bald scalp. The introduction of hair transplantation has revolutionized hair restoration treatments by introducing the capacity to more closely simulate a natural hair pattern. Topical (minoxidil) and oral (finasteride) medications have aided the hair loss patient by stimulating the regrowth of hair, especially in the crown, but have not replaced hair replacement surgery.

SPECIAL CONSIDERATIONS

Since the description of the concept of "donor dominance" by Orentreich, physicians have understood the underpinnings of hair transfer technique. Simply put, hair follicles are genetically preprogrammed to stop producing hairs at a certain point, regardless of location. Hence, occipital and temporal hair follicles, which in most patients continue to produce hairs throughout the patient's lifetime, can be transferred to bald scalp and will continue to behave as occipital hair follicles and produce hair. The determination of optimal donor areas depends upon the anticipated ultimate hair loss in a particular patient. This will affect not only the donor site but also the amount of hair harvested, as sufficient hair should remain to camouflage the scars from graft harvesting as well as produce an aesthetic appearance. Conversely, the number, density and location of grafts placed is determined also by the anticipated hair loss; for example, a 40-year-old man, distressed by a mild receding hairline should not be densely grafted at the former location of his hairline if significant frontal crown and temporal hair loss is anticipated (based on his family history), as there will be insufficient donor follicles remaining for these other areas.

ALTERNATIVES TO PROCEDURE

In addition to medical treatment of hair loss, scar flaps or scalp excision can be used. A temporal (Juri) flap can be raised from the temporal area after two delay procedures to increase vascularity of the flap. Based anteriorly, the flap is cut with an irregular border in an attempt to recreate the irregular anterior hairline, and then transposed to the desired position of the frontal hairline to replace a segment of excised scalp skin. Bilateral flaps can be used to increase the coverage of the scalp. A patient with a reasonable frontal hairline but significant crown baldness can be treated with a scalp excision. An ellipse of skin is excised in a sagittal fashion, the temporal skin is undermined and the hair-bearing temporal skin is advanced medially to close the wound.

TECHNIQUES

Harvesting

Incision Placement

The typical occipital harvesting incision is placed across the occipital scalp at least 3 cm above the occipital hairline. For ease, a multiblade scalpel with 2–4 mm spacers can be used to harvest multiple parallel strips of skin (Fig. 14.1A). The incision is carried down through the dermis, and a #15 blade is used to divide the deep attachments and to remove the individual strips of skin (Fig. 14.1B).

Extent of Undermining/Dissection

Generally, the skin edges are quite mobile and easy to advance together.

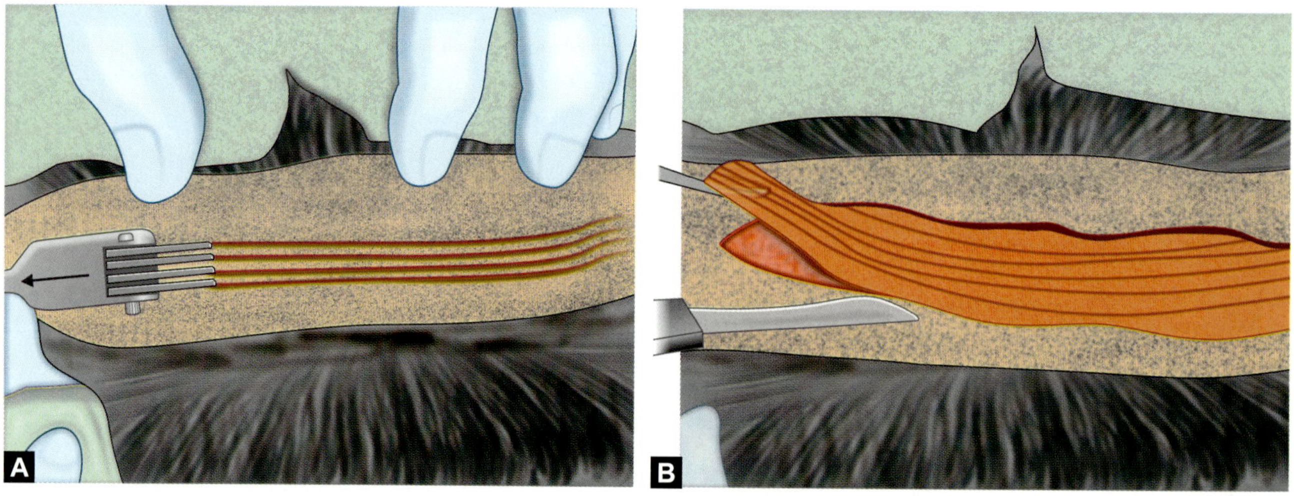

Figs 14.1A and B: (A) A multi-bladed knife is used to excise parallel strips of hair-bearing skin of a specified width; (B) The strips are excised sharply just below the level of the follicles

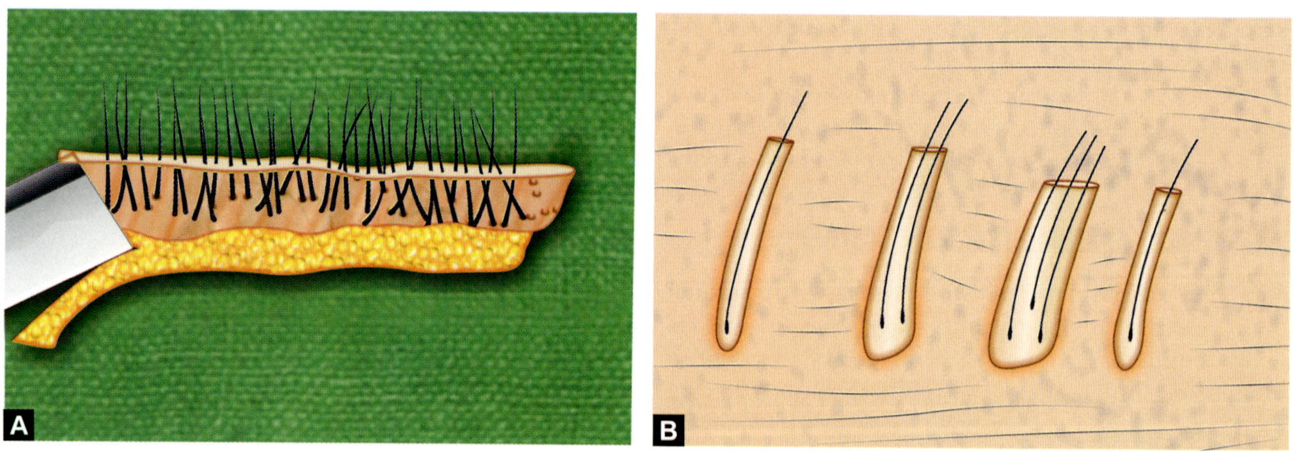

Figs 14.2A and B: (A) Each strip of skin is reviewed and subdermal fat removed just below the follicles; (B) Follicular units of 1–3 follicles are isolated from the strip

Closure

- *Layers/sutures*: Deep dermal sutures of 3-0 polyglactin 910 are used to reapproximate the skin edges, which are then closed with skin staples.

Graft Preparation

Extent of Dissection

Grafts are kept moist with sterile saline during preparation. The strips of skin are laid on edge on a sterile tongue depressor, and with gentle pressure the attached subdermal fat is exposed and removed with a sharp blade (Fig. 14.2A). Under loupe or microscope magnification, the strips are sectioned to precise follicular units, groupings of 1–4 follicles that occur naturally (Fig. 14.2B). Care should be taken to cut these units parallel to the hair shafts to avoid damaging the follicles. The follicular units are trimmed to remove any non-hair bearing skin, and then grouped into similar sized units.

Tissue Modifications

- *Incision/excision*: The recipient areas are carefully marked. If the frontal hairline is being treated, it is important to graft no less than 7–8 cm from the brows, unless one is certain that there will be sufficient donor hair to ensure good scalp coverage posterior to the hairline when maximal hair loss has occurred. It is

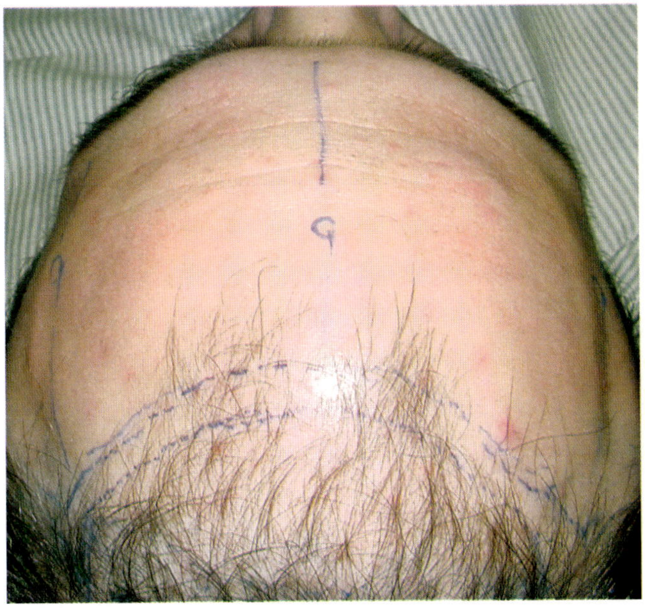

Fig. 14.3: Especially in patients with advanced or early-onset alopecia, a conservative hairline should be created to ensure sufficient follicles for coverage. The frontal hairline is feathered with single hair grafts in a random pattern

important to establish a seemingly irregular frontal hairline that is feathered, with scattered single hair grafts as a fringe anteriorly, blending into a more dense hairline with 1–4 hairs per graft posteriorly (Fig. 14.3). Single follicle grafts can be placed in slits, while larger grafts require removal of bald skin to accommodate the graft using hollow punches ranging in size from 1 mm to 3 mm in inner diameter. Donor sites are prepared by first injecting a dilute anesthetic to anesthetize the scalp as well as increase the tissue turgor of the scalp. With the scalp more rigid, the specific calibrated dagger-shaped scalpel blades are pierced through the skin in a random pattern to accommodate single hair grafts at the frontal fringe (Fig. 14.4A). More posteriorly, punches are pushed with a twisting motion to remove a core of skin; slotted punches allow the excised skin to be pushed out of the slot for greater speed (Fig. 14.4B). Light pressure with a sterile cotton tip applicator is generally all that is needed to achieve hemostasis.

Graft Placement

The appropriate graft is then grasped with a Jeweler's forceps and placed into the slit incision (Figs 14.5A and B). A cotton applicator is applied to the graft for a moment to ensure the graft skin sits level with the surrounding skin. Punch sites often will ooze blood, which may push the graft upward; in these cases, the cotton applicator is held for a few additional seconds over the graft. Speed of placement is essential, as grafting sessions may place between 300 hairs and 2,000 hairs; prolonged sessions will require additional analgesia, and edema of the scalp may make placement and retention of grafts difficult.

Dressings

Grafted areas should be treated gently to avoid disturbing the grafts (Fig. 14.6). A Telfa pad (Covidien, Mansfield, Massachusetts, US) is placed over the grafts and the scalp dressed with Kerlix gauze (Covidien, Mansfield, Massachusetts, US). If needed, patients may wear a winter cap over the dressing.

Potential Complications

Hair Loss

Some loss of hair may be seen, as the follicles respond to the grafting nearby by entering telogen phase. These hair shafts fall out as the follicles enter the resting phase; this is much more common in the grafted follicles (Figs 14.7A to C). Typically, these follicles exit the telogen phase in 3–4 months and resume producing hair.

Graft Loss

Most grafts survive and heal into surrounding skin. However, it is expected that some grafts will fall out initially, and patients should be advised to expect to see some follicles rinse out of their hair along with shampoo during their first shower. However, beyond this early period, graft loss is uncommon, and as long as follicles were harvested from skin genetically programmed for persistent hair.

Halo Deformity

It is essential to account for the possibility of further hair loss when planning hair graft recipient areas. Aggressive vertex grafting, followed by additional progression of loss of the lateral vertex hair will leave a halo deformity, densely grafted vertex hair surrounded by a ring of bald scalp. This can subsequently be grafted, but only if sufficient donor hair remains.

Doll's Hair

Transplantation of hair in a routine pattern will immediately be identified as unnatural, and rows must be avoided. Grafts should be placed in a deliberately random pattern, including a thin fringe in front of the frontal hairline to appear natural.

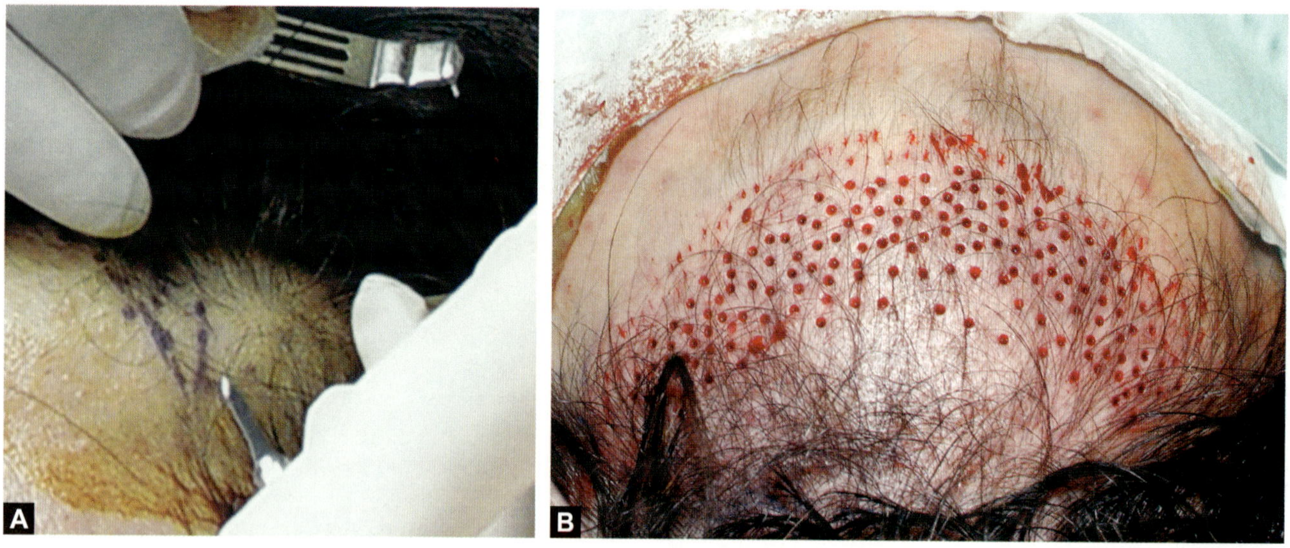

Figs 14.4A and B: (A) Stab incisions are made to accommodate single hair grafts; (B) Larger grafts are placed posterior to the zone of feathering for greater coverage

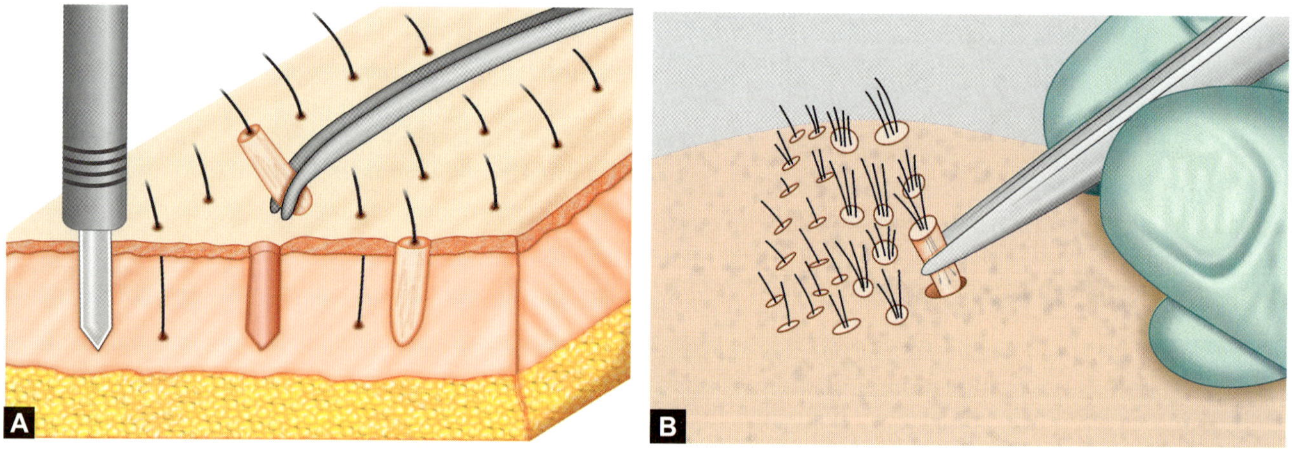

Figs 14.5A and B: (A) Single grafts are placed into the slits prepared in the recipient sites; (B) Skin removal is required to accommodate larger grafts

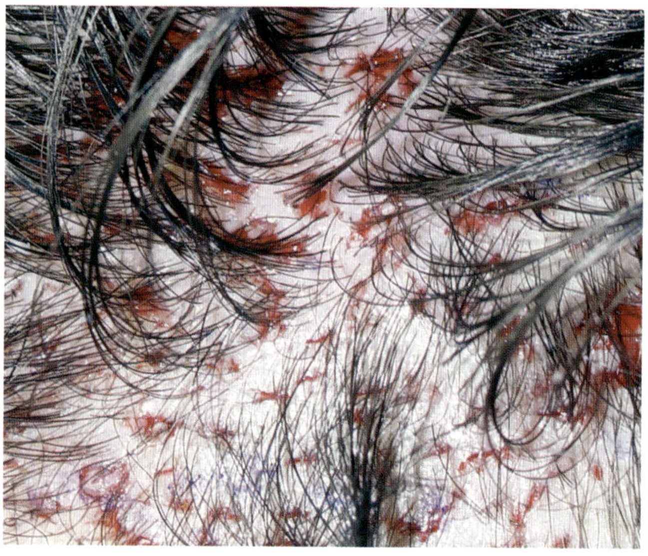

Fig. 14.6: Once placed, grafts are treated gently to avoid disturbing placement

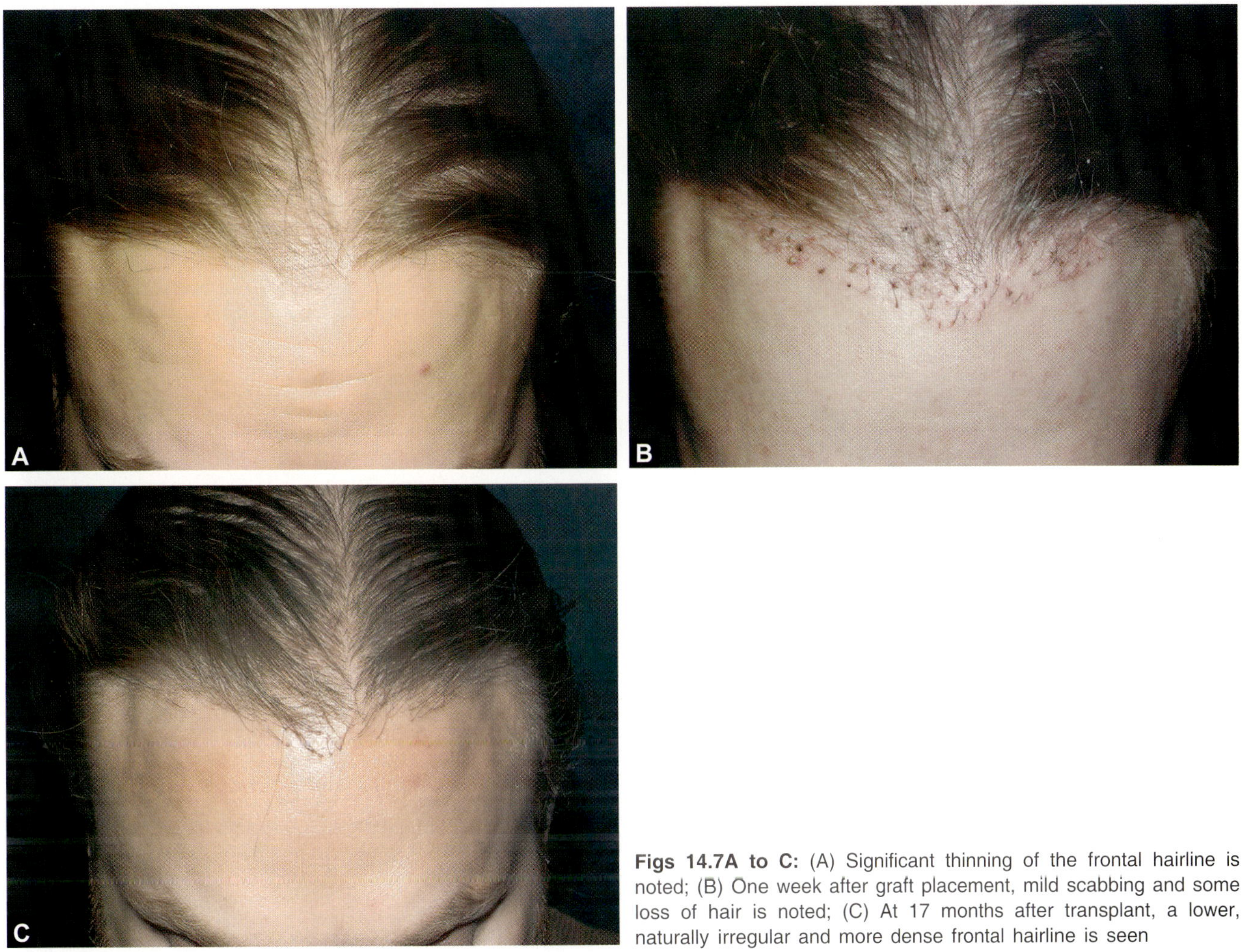

Figs 14.7A to C: (A) Significant thinning of the frontal hairline is noted; (B) One week after graft placement, mild scabbing and some loss of hair is noted; (C) At 17 months after transplant, a lower, naturally irregular and more dense frontal hairline is seen

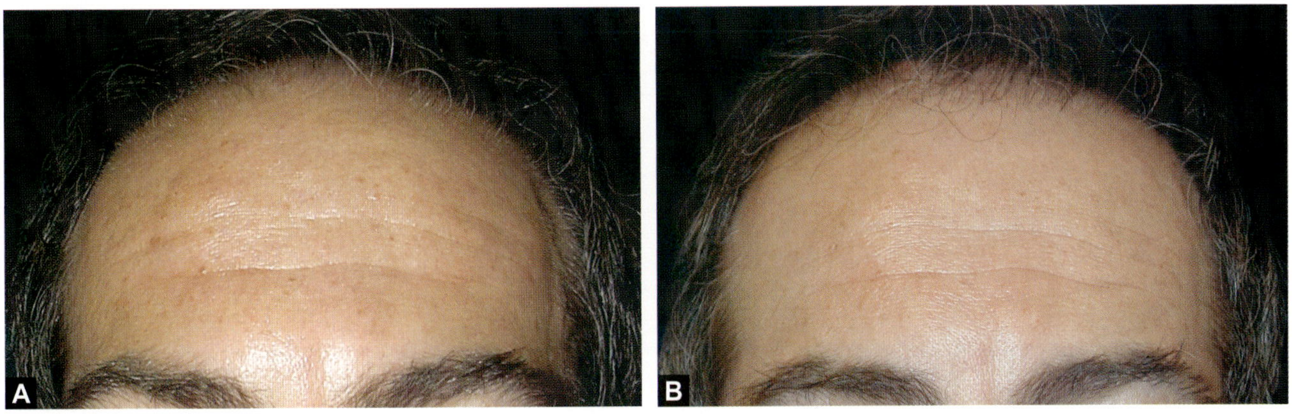

Figs 14.8A and B

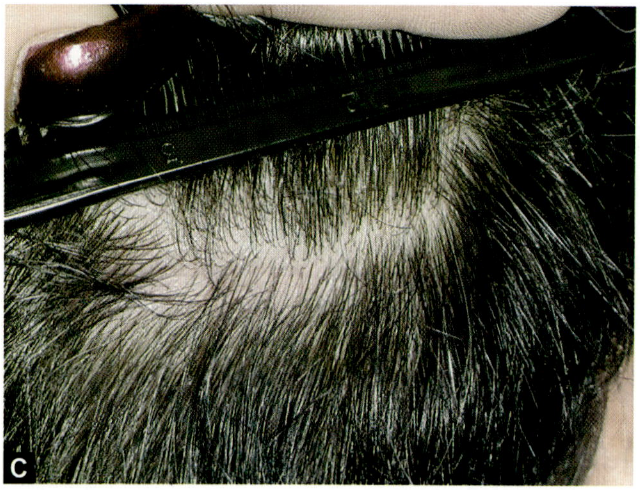

Figs 14.8A to C: (A) Before and (B) After transplants to the frontal hairline; (C) Donor site scar generally heals well if appropriately closed

Scarring

Hypertrophic scars are rare but possible, and grafting in patients with a history of poor wound healing or keloid formation should be avoided if possible. The donor site scar generally heals well (Figs 14.8A to C) but will widen if not properly closed.

Follicular Cyst

Occasionally, hair may become ingrown as the local tissue is somewhat compressed by the additional tissue of the grafts. These are generally self-limited.

AFTERCARE

If not done in the office by staff, patients are instructed to wash their hair gently on the day after transplantation by pouring warm soapy water over the hair and similarly rinsing with warm water until clear. Strenuous activity should be avoided for 7 days, and patients are generally advised to take 3–4 days off from work.

BIBLIOGRAPHY

1. Avram M, Rogers N. Contemporary hair transplantation. Dermatol Surg. 2009;35(11):1705-19.
2. Orentreich N. Hair transplants. Long-term results and new advances. Arch Otolaryngol. 1970;92(6):576-7.
3. Stough DB, Berger RA, Orentreich N. Surgical improvement of cicatricial alopecia of diverse etiology. Arch Dermatol. 1968;97(3):331-4.
4. Unger W. Defining the frontal area in hair restoration surgery. Dermatol Surg. 2010;36(12):2085-6.

CHAPTER 15

Introduction to Reconstructive Facial Plastic Surgery

Thomas C Spalla

BACKGROUND

Reconstructive surgery of the head and neck is an immense field which overlaps with numerous care providers playing a role in the evaluation, management, and long term care of these patients. The gamut of problems faced ranges from something as straightforward as a laceration to as complex as facial transplantation. When faced with a complex problem, the primary surgeon would be remiss to not involve other colleagues. This is by no means a shortcoming and it should not be perceived as weakness or lack of ability, but these consultations serve to deliver the best care available for patients presenting with complex defects. The following providers should be kept in mind as they may serve a unique purpose in the patient's recovery: otolaryngology, oral and maxillofacial surgery, plastic surgery, neurosurgery, trauma surgery and dentistry. Enlist the help of medical colleagues, as many of these patients have several comorbidities which should be maximally medically managed to optimize care. Do not forget that ancillary services, such as physical and occupational therapy, speech pathology, home care nurses and social work play a tremendous role in the long-term success and satisfaction with the reconstructive intervention.

A career in facial reconstructive surgery will certainly keep the surgeon busy and continually challenged as the variety of conditions seen is so diverse and the field itself evolves with new technologies and paradigms.

CONSULTATION

Consultation for elective reconstructive surgery does not differ greatly from a purely aesthetic evaluation. During the reconstructive consultation, the patient and surgeon must identify the defects and/or loss of function and seek goals to remedy these issues. The surgeon must come up with plans of action, as there is often more than one, and present them to the patient for a discussion of the options and allow the patient come to a solution which is acceptable. Often the patient leaves it up to the surgeon to decide, but this should not dissuade the surgeon from discussing all reasonable options with their associated risks and benefits, for this constitutes a necessary portion of the informed consent process. When the surgeon is presented with an elective reconstruction, the opportunity allows for a complete evaluation of not just the injury but the patient as well. Motivations, expectations and fears are able to be discussed as would be done during an aesthetic evaluation. Once informed consent is obtained, reconstructive efforts and rehabilitation may begin.

In emergent reconstructive surgery, the consultation process may be abbreviated. Emergency department consultation and rapid intervention is often required. In situations of airway instability or severe hemorrhage, time must not be spent taking a history. Obtaining and maintaining the airway and control of life-threatening vascular injury is of paramount importance and trumps any other issue the facial reconstructive surgeon must deal with at that moment. Barring these extreme circumstances, a history and physical examination is permissible even in the emergency setting. Taking an AMPLE (Allergies, Medicines, Past medical/surgical history, Last known menstrual period, Extenuating circumstances) history is necessary for best care of the trauma patient. If the patient is not obtunded from injury or intoxicating substances, the surgeon should take the time to proceed as above with the elective consultation.

EVALUATION

Evaluating the patient needing facial reconstructive surgery should be broken down into two broad categories: (1) those whose reconstructions are elective and (2) those whose injuries are emergent.

Photodocumentation of injuries can be invaluable for the surgeon as well as the patient. For the surgeon, photographs can help to provide a record of injuries and subsequent outcome. This helps in the lifelong learning of the surgeon and can also be an effective teaching tool for other surgeons, residents and medical students. These photographs may become a crucial part of the patient's record in cases brought before legal counsel. Additionally, as in aesthetic surgery, preoperative photographs provide an important part of the record in cases brought against the surgeon. This documentation (e.g. of a facial paralysis) may save the surgeon from a potential lawsuit.

In the elective situation, reconstructive surgical evaluation should be undertaken in a stepwise and systematic fashion comfortable to the head and neck surgeon. It is recommended that the surgeon proceed with his or her standard head and neck examination prior to examining the defect/deficit at hand. This serves several purposes. First, it serves to ensure a complete and thorough examination which may lead to the discovery of other issues unknown by the patient or undetected by the initial examination, by the emergency department or trauma team. Second, a complete examination provides documentation of the complete preoperative status of the patient which may serve as an important record should deficits or defects present postoperatively. Finally, the complete examination lets the patient know that the surgeon is not only cognizant of the presented problem but is interested in the patient as a whole. This helps to build trust and understanding between the patient and the surgeon.

Emergency Considerations

As briefly mentioned above, the facial reconstructive surgeon will be presented with situations which require immediate attention. The reconstructive surgeon trained in otolaryngology should be amply prepared for any airway emergency. It is doubtful that any other member of the evaluating team will be better prepared to manage the airway than this surgeon, and he or she must take the leadership role in establishing a safe and secure airway. Emergent airway management is beyond the scope of this chapter, and the reader is encouraged to develop a firm understanding of this prior to engaging in the management of these situations. Once the airway is secured, evaluation of other life-threatening injuries may begin. Except in cases of airway compromise or significant head and neck hemorrhage, the head and neck surgeon can generally defer to the trauma surgeon and emergency room physicians for evaluation and management of the trauma patient in the early, life-threatening stages. However, the head and neck surgeon should stay close by in case the airway becomes unstable, head and neck hemorrhage occurs, or to simply assist with the resuscitative efforts as an active team member.

CONSENT

In elective reconstructive situations, standard informed consent must be obtained with the patient or patient's surrogate. Risks, benefits, alternatives and proposed outcomes must be discussed in detail. In certain traumatic situations, these discussions are often brief due to lack of acceptable alternatives. However, this should not deter the surgeon from fulfilling his or her duties to explain the procedure(s) in detail and reiterate potential risks. By explaining the procedure, the surgeon can often help to alleviate the patient's anxiety and fears. The patient may have a completely distorted perception of facial reconstructive surgery, and this affords the surgeon the opportunity for patient education and connection. Even though defects, malformations and deficits may be present preoperatively, the surgeon should teach the patient about what is present preoperatively and explain the goals and anticipated outcomes. Despite the surgeon's best efforts, problems and complications may arise, and it behooves the surgeon to discuss potential adverse outcomes. It is also important that the surgeon explain the complications that may arise from the initial insult or injury so that the patient understands that this is part of the disease process and not the reconstruction. If not explained preoperatively, the patient may blame the surgical efforts when in fact the outcomes were expected sequelae.

In cases of an incapacitated trauma patient, all attempts for informed consent should be made with the appropriate family member or patient representative providing this does not delay care and impair outcomes. By doing so, the surgeon has the opportunity to meet and discuss the patient's status with the caregivers, which may help to alleviate anxiety and fear. In situations where consent cannot be obtained, the surgeon may proceed with interventions he or she perceives that are in the patient's best interest as long as the patient is medically stable for said interventions such as the closure of open wounds. Facial reconstruction is generally nonemergent and going through the proper chain of consent is in the surgeon's best interest. Even in large defects, heroic reconstructive efforts with the potential for significant risk or donor site morbidity are usually best reserved for situations in which informed consent can be obtained. If the opportunity for informed consent does not arise in a timely fashion, the window of time during which the surgeon feels affords the best possible outcome, the surgeon may desire an interdisciplinary meeting with the other medical and surgical teams providing care to the patient, creation of a legal decision maker, and a consultation to the ethics board is not unreasonable.

BEFORE AND AFTERCARE

The care provided to patients before and after reconstructive surgery can be just as important as the surgery itself. Undergoing any surgery can be particularly trying for patients and their caregivers, and since the postoperative care is so crucial with facial plastic surgery, the instructions must be clearly stated.

If a patient has significant medical comorbidities and is at high risk for surgery and postoperative complications, the surgeon must carefully weigh the pros and cons prior to the commencement of any intervention. Additionally, there can be significant psychosocial issues with the reconstructive patient that needs to be addressed before and after surgery. For example, a head and neck cancer patient may have limited social support when he or she returns home and activities of daily living may become impossible, or, take for instance, the assault victim who is suffering from post-traumatic stress disorder whose psychological well-being is suffering despite a good surgical outcome.

Prior to the procedure, part of the patient selection and consent process should be to review the required postoperative care. If the patient is unable or unwilling to follow the directions, then alternatives should be considered. If no alternatives exist or are distinctly not in the patient's best interest, ancillary support such as a skilled nursing facility or homecare nurse should be considered. It is beneficial to provide the patient with clearly written instructions regarding postoperative care. This allows them to understand the process better and also avoids them scrambling for any necessary supplies (e.g. bandages, saline) after the surgery. Each encounter the physician and physician's staff have with the patient affords the opportunity for continued education, discussion and reassurance.

Close follow-up allows for the detection and management of any untoward issues. It also helps to set the patient's mind at ease that he or she is being cared for. This bond can be especially meaningful for both the patient and the physician. An additional benefit for the surgeon is the lifelong learning and education provided by managing a variety of complex head and neck reconstructions.

CHAPTER

16

Healing, Soft Tissue Trauma and Wound Care

Thomas C Spalla

HEALING

A brief overview of the healing process is worthwhile, because by developing an understanding of it the surgeon is better equipped to understand the visible changes occurring and how to affect them, if necessary, for an optimal outcome. Also, as new medicines and technologies for wound healing come along, developing knowledge in the basic science of wound healing allows the surgeon to understand these new developments and their applications. The three basic phases through which healing progresses are the: inflammatory phase, proliferative phase, and remodeling phase.[1]

Inflammatory Phase

This phase begins immediately with the disruption of blood vessels and the subsequent influx of blood products, proteins, collagen and clotting factors (Fig. 16.1). These mediators promote cell migration through the vessel walls into the wound bed to initiate the healing process. Within hours, neutrophils are present and begin to destroy bacteria. Monocytes begin accumulating which assist in fighting bacteria, but they also aid in debridement and the release of growth factors which incite granulation tissue.[1] Fibronectin begins to cross-link with collagen and cell surfaces to cause clot formation.[2]

Proliferative Phase

This phase begins 3–4 days after injury and is heralded by fibroblast proliferation. Cell mitoses increase and subsequently, epithelialization does as well. Along with these processes, angiogenesis also begins to occur more rapidly and is promulgated by various chemotactic factors.[2] Collagen synthesis increases and strength is enhanced by the joining of collagen bundles in the midportion of the wound within the edges.[3]

Remodeling Phase

Wound vascularity, fibroblasts and macrophages begin to decrease and type I collagen dominates initially. Type III collagen forms later and a cell, the myofibroblast, is responsible for wound contraction. This phase may take up to 18 months.[2]

Types of Healing

Primary intention healing is the process by which wound edges are reapproximated shortly after injury.

- *Delayed primary closure*: It refers to surgical closure of the wound after a period of time has elapsed. This may be utilized in contaminated wounds.
- *Secondary intention healing*: It refers to the situation by which healing occurs without closure. This may be a prolonged process which involves the formation of granulation tissue and can result in contracture.

EVALUATION

This chapter focuses solely on the evaluation and management of soft tissue injuries of the head and neck. The reader is directed to the chapter on reconstructive surgery for information regarding the work-up and management of the trauma patient.

After an appropriate history and complete head and neck examination, determining the extent of soft tissue trauma can be undertaken. The surgeon should note, to the best of his or her abilities, when and how the injury occurred. This helps to better estimate the possibility and type of foreign material which may be present, and may also make the surgeon expect a higher chance of infection if the time to wound closure is significantly delayed (usually greater than 24 hours). At first glance, even minor injuries can appear quite impressive due to the propensity for

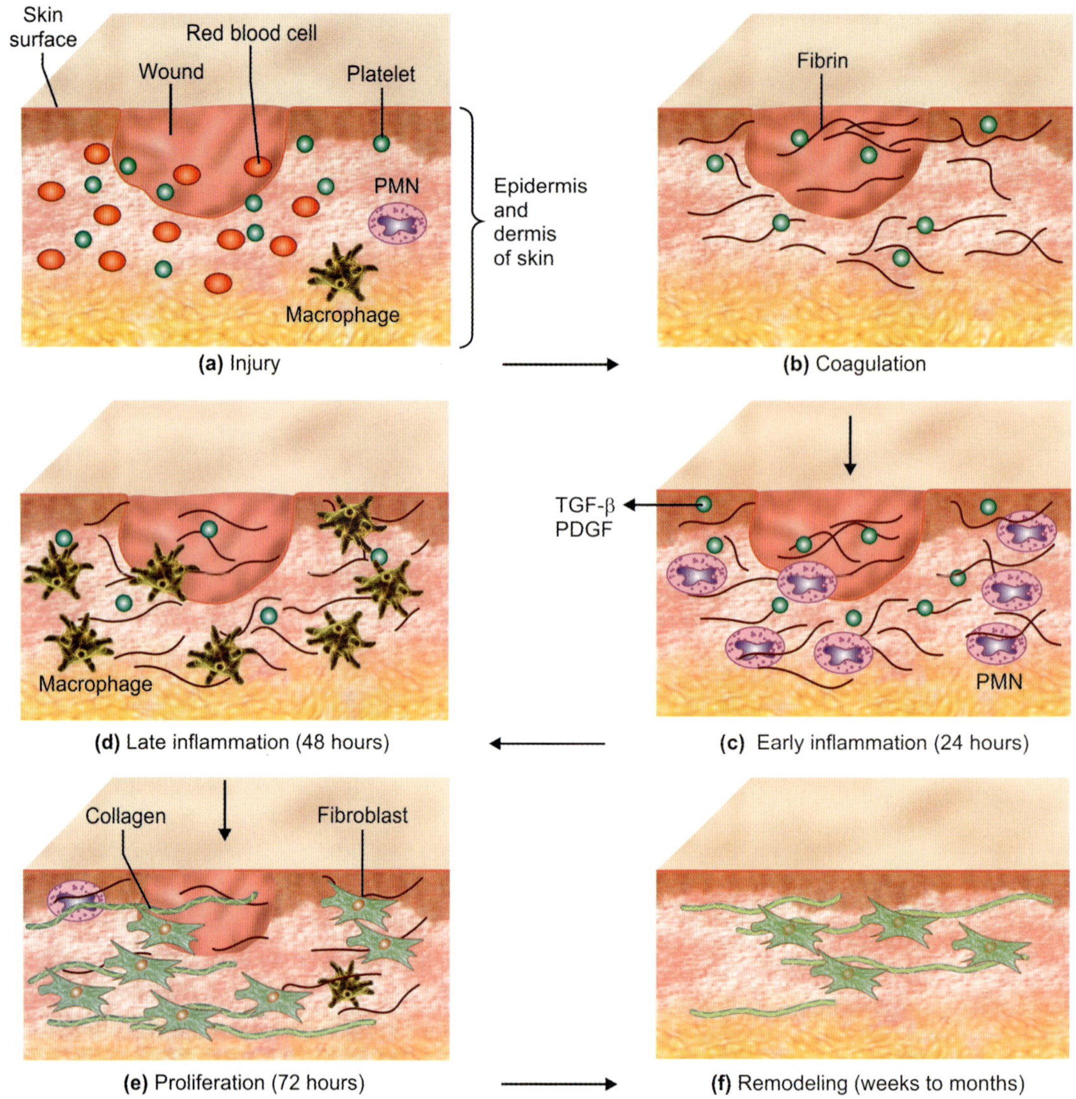

Fig. 16.1: The process of wound healing
(PMN: Polymorphonuclear leukocytes; TGF-β: Transforming growth factor; PDGF: Platelet-derived growth factor)
Source: Expert Reviews in Molecular Medicine. Cambridge University Press; 2003

significant blood loss from the extremely well-vascularized head and neck. It is helpful to clean the patient of blood and foreign materials to best assess the extent of injuries.

When cleaning the patient, it is helpful to have an assistant available to manipulate the patient's head and pass materials to the surgeon to expedite this process. Ensure that the entire head and neck has been evaluated. It is not uncommon to find significant injuries that were initially missed due to dried blood, debris, and obstructing cervical collars.

When the cervical collar prohibits complete examination, the surgeon requires assistance in these situations. If the patient is combative, and removing the cervical collar places the patient at risk for spinal injury, the examination may be deferred until the earliest safe possibility Document this limitation in the chart and coordinate this examination in the near future with the other physicians involved in the patient's care. When the patient is alert and following commands, instruct the patient that you will need to remove the collar momentarily to perform an examination. Instruct them to lie perfectly still and allow the surgical team to log roll them, while maintaining cervical spine stability, for assessing the occiput and nape of the neck. As soon as the examination is complete, the cervical collar must be replaced until the patient meets criteria for cervical spine clearance.

When initially cleaning the patient, use sterile saline to do so. Resist the urge to use antiseptics at this time. Work far away from the wounds initially. This allows for examination of these more remote sites that may be overlooked. It also allows the patient to acclimate to the cleaning and examination which may be anxiety-provoking as most patients are expecting pain at the moment the wound is touched.

When it comes to cleansing of the open wounds themselves, local anesthesia may be extremely helpful. However, perform a detailed neurologic examination prior to the use of local anesthetics and document any sensory or motor deficits. For most situations, 1% lidocaine is sufficient. The addition of epinephrine is beneficial for decreasing bleeding, increasing the duration of the anesthetic and decreasing the chance for systemic toxicity. However, ensure that the use of epinephrine is not contraindicated with the patient's medical history or current condition. The anesthetic solution may be buffered with bicarbonate to decrease some of the pain associated with injection. Also, consider the addition of a long-acting local anesthetic such as bupivacaine in situations where long-term (6–8 hours) pain control would be beneficial. Always follow guidelines regarding combining local anesthetics, the amounts given (based on the patient's weight), and always avoid intravascular injection.

Once the patient is comfortable, copious use of sterile saline is used to cleanse the wound(s). Ample lighting and magnification is mandatory to help ensure no foreign materials are left behind. Gentle debridement with sterile gauze can be helpful. Do not get too aggressive with the debridement in the emergency room setting if great amounts of foreign material are present. These situations are best managed in the operating room setting for optimal patient comfort, surgical instrumentation, control of exacerbated hemorrhage and assistance.

Even when in the emergency room setting, the surgeon must be prepared for bleeding which may be provoked by accidentally traumatizing a vessel, removal of a protecting clot or exposing a vessel which is no longer under vasospasm. Therefore, a basic set of sterile instruments (forceps, hemostats and retractors), cautery, and potentially, suction equipment should be on hand for the rapid control of such situations.

If, after the wound(s) are thoroughly cleaned, there remains the suspicion for foreign material, a soft tissue X-ray may be helpful. Ultrasound can also be useful in the hands of a skilled operator in locating foreign material. Once this is ruled out, detailed survey of the injury can take place.

In characterizing the injury, the surgeon should note: the location (in detailed anatomic terms), the length of the lacerations, the character (linear, jagged, stellate, etc.), the depth, the tissues involved, the amount and type of tissues lost, presence and type of foreign bodies, and associated neurologic deficits. Once this inventory is taken, repair may commence. Figure 16.2A shows a patient presenting after a motor vehicle accident with numerous lacerations secondary to the windshield and Figure 16.2B shows the same patient after cleaning and primary repair of the wounds.

WOUND CARE

If the patient is admitted to the hospital, regular follow-up by the surgeon and his or her team is necessary. Wound checks serve several purposes. They allow for the early identification and intervention of any issues with healing. Additionally, these visits strengthen the bond between the patient and surgeon, and afford the patient and caregivers the opportunity to have their questions answered regarding the injury, wound care and expected outcomes.

Closed Wounds

Just because a wound has been closed, this does not imply that wound care is unnecessary. Wounds that have been sutured generally require less effort than wounds allowed to heal by secondary attention, but they still require regular attention.

Keep the incision free of crusts by gently wiping with a cotton-tipped applicator soaked in saline. If this fails to remove the crust, peroxide may be substituted for the saline. If this still fails, simply apply a thin layer of antibiotic and repeat the cleaning again later. Patient often asks how often they need to clean the area or apply ointment. The author recommends cleaning at least three times daily but also stresses that any crusts that develop in the interim should be removed. The incision should be kept moist with a thin layer of antibiotic ointment. The author generally avoids the use of ointments containing neomycin due to the propensity for dermatitis associated with this agent. The application of a non-stick dressing after applying ointment is helpful in preventing the ointment from rubbing off onto clothing or bedding.

Sutures may be removed between 5 days and 7 days after repair. Just prior to removal, the incision line should be cleaned and the surrounding skin degreased of antibiotic ointment. Performing this prior to suture removal lessens the chance for any incisional trauma or microdehiscence. Atraumatically remove the sutures; use magnification if sutures are difficult to see or manipulate. The patient has generally been examining the incision

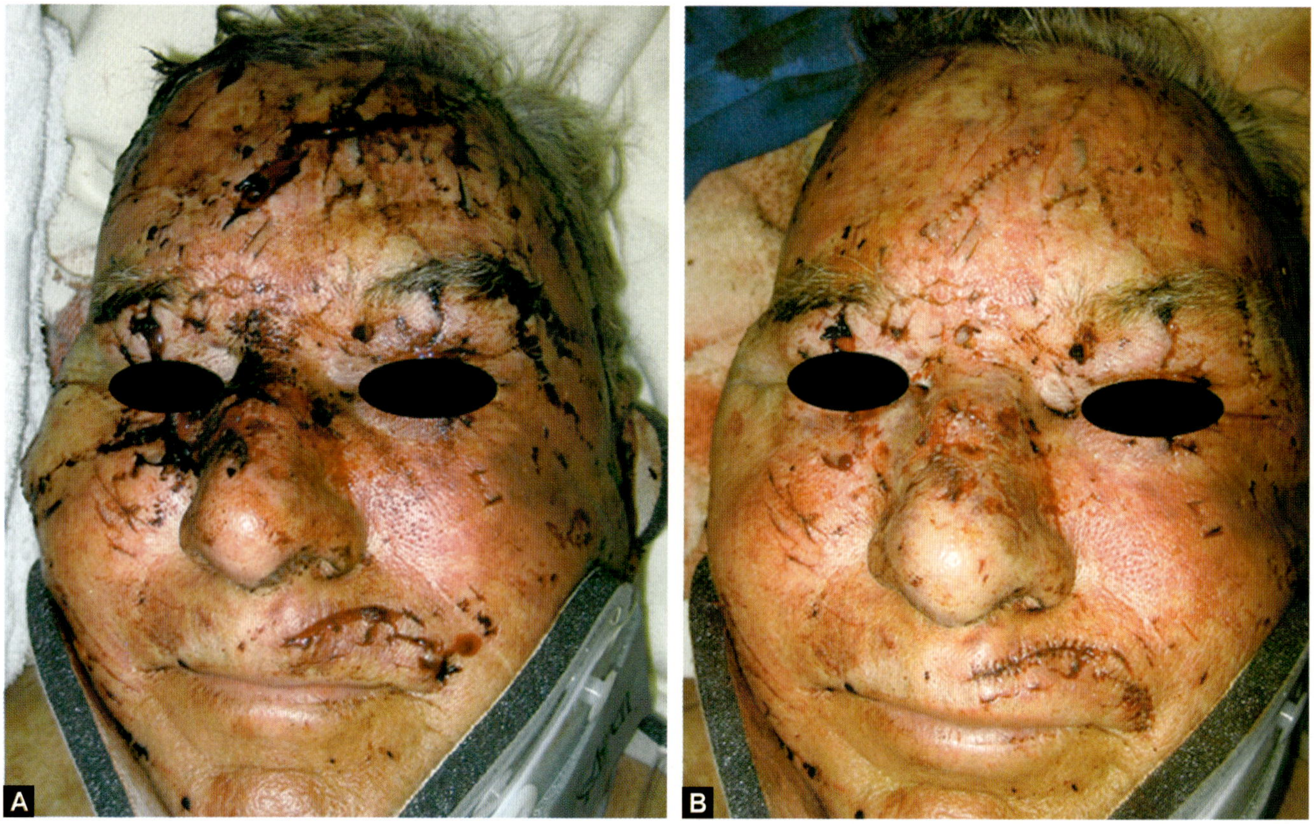

Figs 16.2A and B: (A) Patient presenting with extensive facial lacerations after a motor vehicle accident; (B) Same patient as in Figure 2A after repair in the emergency department
Source: Nadir Ahmad, MD FACS

line during the past week, so it is appreciated to let the patient see his or her incision now unobstructed by sutures. Reassure the patient that it is very early in the healing process and that the final outcome will not be apparent for several weeks to months in most cases.

At this time, supporting the wound with tapes placed perpendicularly across the incision helps to lessen tension on the wound now that the sutures are removed. Doing so should help to prevent widening of the scar by keeping tension of the incision. Additionally, the tapes help to prevent accidental pull across the incision by creating mass movement of the area which limits the force from being applied across the weakest point, the incision.

A follow-up visit in 7 more days is helpful. Photographs are taken at this point. The tapes may be removed with the aid of adhesive remover and the wound examined. It is the author's preference to continue taping for the next 4–5 weeks if the patient allows. Simply teach the patients how to apply the tapes so that weekly visits are not necessary. Some patients develop a mild contact dermatitis from the adhesive or inflammation from having the skin occluded. If this develops, a rest period of a few days should be instituted and consideration for a low potency steroid cream should be given.

If no further surgical revisions are anticipated, at 6 weeks from the initial repair, dermabrasion may be undertaken to improve the final result of the scar. The reader is directed to the chapter in this book regarding dermabrasion for full details of this technique.

Avoidance of UV light is extremely important to prevent permanent dyschromias. Application of sunblock or sunscreen with SPF 30 or greater is recommended, and it must be stressed that reapplication during sun exposure is mandatory. This should continue for at least 6 months, and ideally this should become a part of the patient's daily routine for any exposed skin to minimize additional solar damage.

Open Wounds

Healing by secondary intention can be a viable solution in several situations. Areas which are concave (e.g. the temple) may heal with excellent aesthetic results if meticulous wound care is continued though the healing

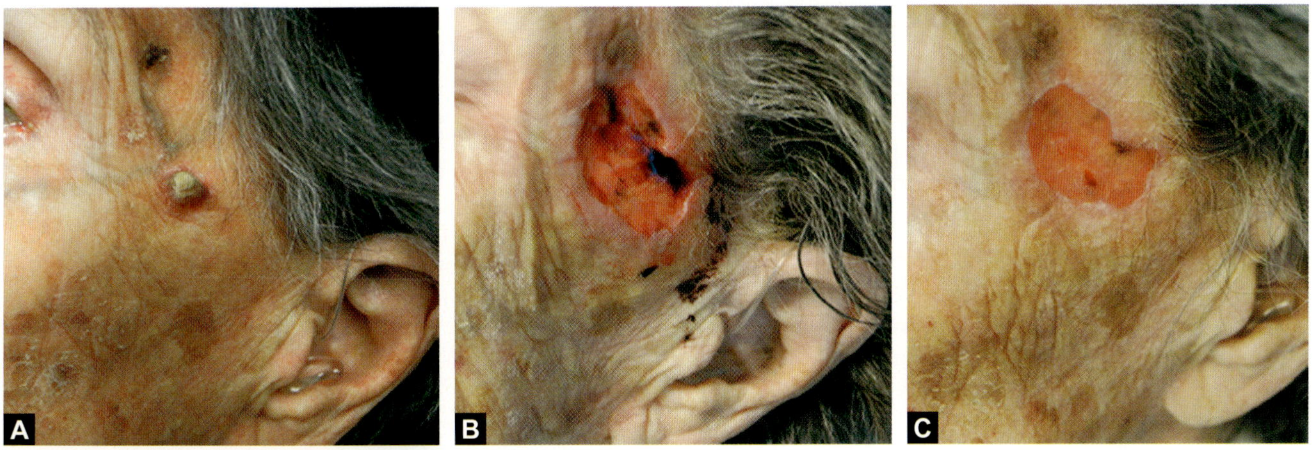

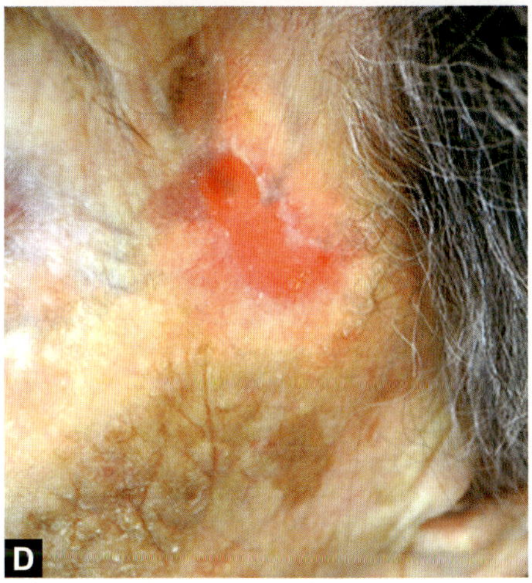

Figs 16.3A to D: Elderly female with squamous cell carcinoma in situ and actinic keratosis with cutaneous horn; (B) Same patient as in Figure 16.3B after Mohs surgery; (C) After 2 weeks of local wound care consisting of washing three times daily and keeping a thin layer of antibiotic ointment on the wound; (D) Secondary intention healing 6 weeks after Mohs surgery

process. Another great example of this is in the midline of the forehead. This can come in handy when the donor site from a paramedian forehead flap cannot be closed without undo wound tension or the use of advancement flaps.

Also, when dealing with an aggressive cutaneous malignancy (e.g. squamous cell carcinoma, melanoma, Merkel cell carcinoma), closure with a local or distant flap may prohibit cancer surveillance. Some of these situations are best managed by secondary intention healing. However, if wound contraction is felt to significant distort form of function, then a skin graft can be an alternative in these situations since skin grafts will decrease, but not eliminate, the degree of contracture that would be present if the wound was left to heal via secondary intention.

It must be emphasized to the patient and caregivers that healing via secondary intention can be more labor intensive than a closed wound. Open wounds should be cleansed with gentle soap and warm water several times daily followed by the application of a layer of antibiotic ointment. Close follow-up with the surgeon is helpful, because this allows the surgeon to perform gentle debridements of any significant crusts which may develop. The patient must be made aware that it may take several weeks before the wound is healed to the point that it does not require cleaning.

The end result can be expected to be smooth, shiny, hairless, flatter than the surrounding tissue, and slightly hypochromic. Teaching the patient this at the outset is part of the consent process in choosing this healing pathway. As with any healing tissue, avoidance of UV light for months helps to improve the final outcome.

Figure 16.3A shows a patient who presented to the author's clinic for hearing-related complaints. However, upon inspection of the face, a cutaneous horn was seen. She was sent for Mohs surgery and the pathology revealed squamous cell carcinoma in situ. Due to the location of the wound and tissue frailty (it tore when forceps were applied), secondary intention wound healing was chosen. With the aid of her caregivers, the results were obtained 6 weeks later (Figs 16.3B to D)

CONCLUSION

As with all surgical interventions, being available for the patient throughout this process will not only alleviate his or her anxiety but will also allow the surgeon the advantage of early detection of any healing issues that will undoubtedly occur at some point in the surgeon's career. Soft tissue trauma can be a complex, yet extremely rewarding experience for the facial reconstructive surgeon. Patients are generally injured both physically and emotionally by the experience, and the surgeon is in a unique position to aid in healing both of these aspects of the patient's life.

REFERENCES

1. Koopmann CF. Wound healing: A review of factors affecting wound repair. Otolaryngology. In: English G (Ed). Philadelphia: JB Lippincott; 1991.
2. Koopmann CF. Cutaneous wound healing. An overview. Otolaryngol Clin North Am. 1995;28(5):835-45.
3. Wheeland RG. The newer surgical dressings and wound healing. Dermatol Clin. 1987:5(2);393-407.

CHAPTER

17

Soft Tissue Reconstruction

Thomas C Spalla

BACKGROUND

Reconstructing skin and associated soft tissues occurs to some degree in most aspects of facial plastic surgery. Therefore, a profound understanding of methods of repair and the associated rationale for such repairs is crucial. Reconstruction can be for traumatic and nontraumatic causes. Soft tissue trauma will be encountered by every facial plastic surgeon at some point and injuries range in severity from the mildest of abrasions to devastating tissue loss. Nontraumatic causes of soft tissue reconstruction can encompass such etiologies as acne scarring and Mohs surgery repair. Regardless of the etiology, the basic tenets of repair are the same and illustrated herein.

LACERATION REPAIR

As with any surgical procedure, consent should be obtained, if possible. While the patient's options are relatively limited in these situations, and he or she understandably just wants to return to their preinjury status, it is worthwhile to spend a few minutes explaining the injury, how the repair will benefit them and the potential outcomes. It is beneficial to tell the patient that a scar will be present (if dermal or greater injury has occurred), but that all means to minimize this possibility are going to be undertaken. This is the first step in the creation of a realistic understanding of the situation as well as the limitations of any intervention. Also, emphasize that he or she must be active in the healing process, and compliance with postoperative instructions will help the final outcome. Finally, it helps to educate the patient that additional procedures may be required for the best results, and reassure the patient that he or she will not be abandoned, or lost to follow-up, throughout the healing process.

Injury Limited to the Epidermis

Few wounds brought to the attention of the head and neck surgeon meet this criterion. Due to the lack of dermal involvement, scarring is not expected. Basic wound care such as washing with mild soap and water and the application of an antibiotic ointment is all that is required. If there is some wound edge separation, simply applying tapes across the wound to approximate the tissues may be all that is required. If this fails to address the situation, consideration for a single-layered closure would be appropriate.

Injury Limited to the Epidermis and Dermis

A number of head and neck lacerations meet these criteria (i.e. no underlying structures are transected). When dermal injury is present, layered wound closure is mandatory. By closing the deep dermal layer, the surgeon is able to reapproximate the wound edges and keep any wound tension in this deep layer away from the upper dermis and epidermis which would tend to cause widening of the scar. The epidermis can then be closed with proper wound eversion (Figs 17.1A to D).

The surgeon has numerous options in terms of suture material for wound closure. With regards to the most superficial layer, the choice must be made whether to use a dissolvable or nondissolvable suture. Dissolvable sutures have the drawback of inducing erythema at the incisional site while being resorbed. However, their use is particularly tempting in the noncompliant trauma population who has a low propensity (at least in the author's experience) of routine follow-up. When using permanent sutures, which mandate removal (usually 5–7 days later) to prevent a "railroad track" appearance,

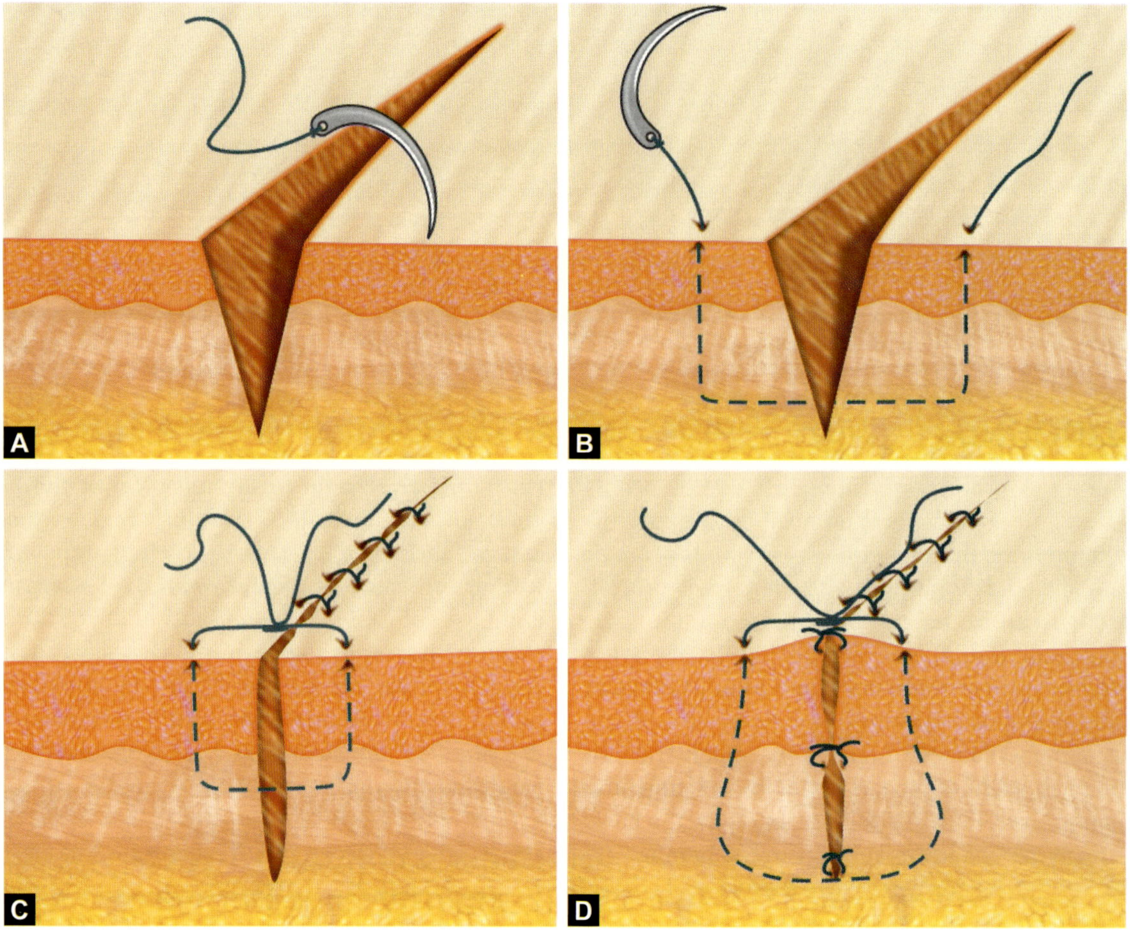

Figs 17.1A to D: Layered (dermal and epidermal) wound closure

the surgeon depends on the patient to return for suture removal or else the work is compromised. If any question about compliance and reliability exist, the use of dissolvable sutures is preferred to prevent these untoward results.

When closing the dermis, a dissolvable suture is typically used. However, some dissolvable sutures may induce inflammation in the dermis and may lead to sterile stitch abscesses which may lead to scarring. If this history exists in the patient, or in the surgeon's prior experience, consideration should be given for a very slowly dissolving or even a permanent suture. In the author's experience, the use of such sutures can lead to the sutures slowly "spitting" or becoming palpable and slowly extruding through the skin. However, these are easily trimmed and do not lead to an inflammatory reaction and these pinpoint areas heal inconspicuously.

The surgeon has many options when closing the epidermis. The key to repair is performing meticulous atraumatic technique and careful alignment of equal tissue layers while providing wound eversion. A mistake often observed early in training programs is the urge to make the incision appear flat and even with the surrounding tissue. However, wounds invariably contract, thus an everted wound will gradually flatten with time. If a wound starts flat, it will contract and become inverted. If an untoward aesthetic results, inverted scars can be difficult to revise.

Muscle

Muscle should be realigned and repaired with a dissolvable suture to minimize scarring in this region, to decrease the chances of bleeding from the raw ends, and to close the dead space created from the separation. Healing of the apposed muscle bellies also increases the chance for return of function.

Nerve

Thorough examination of the head and neck seeks to find any neurologic injury, and a strong foundation in neuroanatomy provides the surgeon with the ability to "see" the wound in three dimensions and suspect a neurologic injury when a neurologic examination cannot be performed. Neurorrhaphy (nerve repair) should occur as soon as feasible. Performing proper nerve anastomosis is almost impossible in the emergency room, and therefore a planned trip to the operating room with microsurgical instrumentation, microscopic evaluation and repair can be undertaken. If during wound examination the severed nerve is seen and repair cannot be undertaken at that moment, the surgeon should identify the ends of the nerve and tag them with a permanent, colored suture for later reidentification because the ability to electrically stimulate the nerve disappears in approximately 3 days.

If possible, at the time of initial wound repair, neurorrhaphy should be undertaken with primary anastomosis being the first choice. If primary anastomosis cannot be undertaken due to tissue loss or the repair is under *any* tension, an interposition nerve graft is required. The reader is directed to the chapter regarding facial paralysis management for details of neurorrhaphy.

TECHNIQUE FOR SOFT TISSUE REPAIR

Prophylactic antibiotics for skin flora coverage are recommended due to the contaminated means by which the trauma took place. Broaden coverage if gross contamination is present or there is aerodigestive tract communication. Check the tetanus immunization history and administer a booster if one is indicated. Once the patient is adequately cleaned and local anesthesia has taken effect, the repair may begin. Additional injuries may be noted that were not as readily apparent during the cleansing, and these should be noted. Debride any obviously nonviable tissue. Tissue of questionable viability should be left in place. The head and neck's vascularity is robust and even tenuously vascularized tissue may survive. Bring like tissues together to the preinjury alignment as best as possible. In cases of tissue loss, undermining may be required to prevent tension across the healing incision. As with any plastic repair, avoid any undue tissue trauma, particularly of the epidermis and dermis as unsightly scarring may result. When closing the skin, utilize skin hooks to avoid superficial trauma. If skin hooks are not available, use forceps, but do not crush the tissue between the forceps' teeth.

Any bleeding encountered should be addressed to prevent postoperative hematoma formation which could lead to compromised vascularity, tissue loss, infection and scar. The offending vessel(s) should be isolated and cautery sparingly used so that additional trauma is minimized. Care must be taken when using the cautery near the dermis of hair-bearing skin, because this may result in the permanent alopecia. Vessels may be isolated and tied off or addressed with a figure-8 suture technique.

The author (TCS) reserves the use of tissue adhesives for specific populations in whom suture removal may not be possible without the use of anesthesia such as children and the mentally impaired. Tissue glues are also useful in patients in whom follow-up or wound care (cleaning sutures, applying an ointment, etc.) is very questionable such as in the indigent population. Otherwise, the author avoids the use of these agents, because optimal wound eversion is impaired, and these glues limit local wound care. Additionally, the cost of these agents should be considered as they are generally more expensive than several packs of suture. Since the wound requires layered closure, one additional suture is more cost-effective than opening a new tissue adhesive. Figure 17.2A illustrates a partial avulsion of the scalp after a motor vehicle accident. Primary repair was achieved and a jackson-Pratt drain was used due to the large amount of dead-space created by the injury (Figs 17.2A to C).

Avoid the temptation to perform a complicated repair, such as a transposition flap, during this initial intervention. Understandably, certain situations mandate local tissue flaps due to paucity of local tissues, but these measures should be reserved for these situations. By performing such measures in less extreme circumstances, the ability to utilize these flaps for secondary repair, should infection or ongoing tissue injury result (e.g. in ballistic injuries), is lost.

After the repair is complete, cover the wound in a thin layer of antibiotic ointment. A nonstick dressing is helpful to prevent the ointment from rubbing off onto clothing or bedding. However, closure with sutures mandates local wound care, and the use of dressings does not mean this does not need to take place.

The incision should be gently cleaned regularly with a mild soap and warm water several times daily, and the ointment reapplied. If difficult to remove crusts develop, they should be soaked with peroxide to gently soften and atraumatically remove them. Resist the temptation to pull off any scabs. Softening them with peroxide and antibiotic ointment will allow them to slowly resolve. By tearing them off, healing must begin anew at any newly traumatized sites which will only further delay the process.

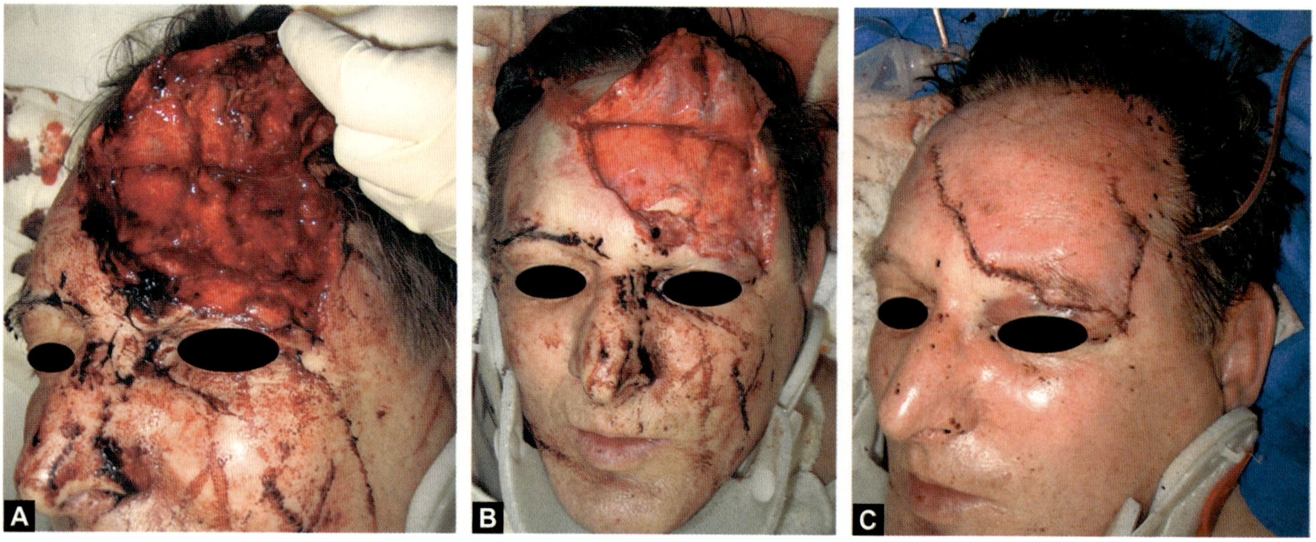

Figs 17.2A to C: (A) Patient brought in after a motor vehicle accident with a partial scalp avulsion; (B) The same patient as in Figure 17.2A after cleaning the wound; (C) After wound closure. A drain was placed due to the large dead space
Source: Nadir Ahmad, MD FACS

AVULSED TISSUE

Avulsed tissue can be difficult to manage, because its survival is highly dependent on its blood supply as well as the patient's general medical status. After cleansing, suturing the avulsed tissue back into its alignment may be successful. However, the patient and surgeon must understand that partial or complete loss of this tissue is a strong possibility. This could necessitate further surgery to improve the result. Figure 17.3A demonstrates a patient with a partial avulsion of the auricle. The auricle was still attached the enough of a degree that the vascular supply was felt to be adequate (Figs 17.3A and B).

BITE WOUNDS

Bite wounds may be of human or animal origin. All bite wounds are, by definition, contaminated and need to be managed as such. A tetanus booster should be given if the patient is due and broad-spectrum antibiotics (e.g. amoxicillin with clavulanate) should be initiated. Strong consideration for photographs should be given since many of these cases, particularly human bites, may proceed to litigation. Thorough cleansing of the wound with copious amounts of normal saline should occur and local anesthesia administered for patient comfort. Do not hesitate to get soft tissue X-rays to help rule out the presence of foreign material such as a tooth fragment. Ultrasound may also be ordered if suspicion exists and the X-ray is negative. Undetected foreign material could lead to suppuration and failure of the reconstructive effort.

Puncture Wounds

If the wound consists of deep punctures, secondary intention healing should be allowed to proceed. During this time, local wound care should be undertaken and oral antibiotics given. Future scar revision can always be considered.

Lacerating Bite Wounds

Repair may be considered in a primary or delayed fashion. If primary repair is used, then meticulous cleansing and antibiotic usage should be utilized. Additionally, by loosely approximating the tissues, this will allow for the egress of edematous fluid. Many surgeons prefer to close these in a delayed fashion after allowing for the initial contamination to resolve through local wound care and antibiotics.

Bites Resulting in Loss of Tissue

In some cases, the tissue is completely detached from the patient. Resist the urge to replace these tissues. They have been significantly contaminated, devascularized for some time and handled traumatically both at the time of injury and likely afterwards as well. It is highly

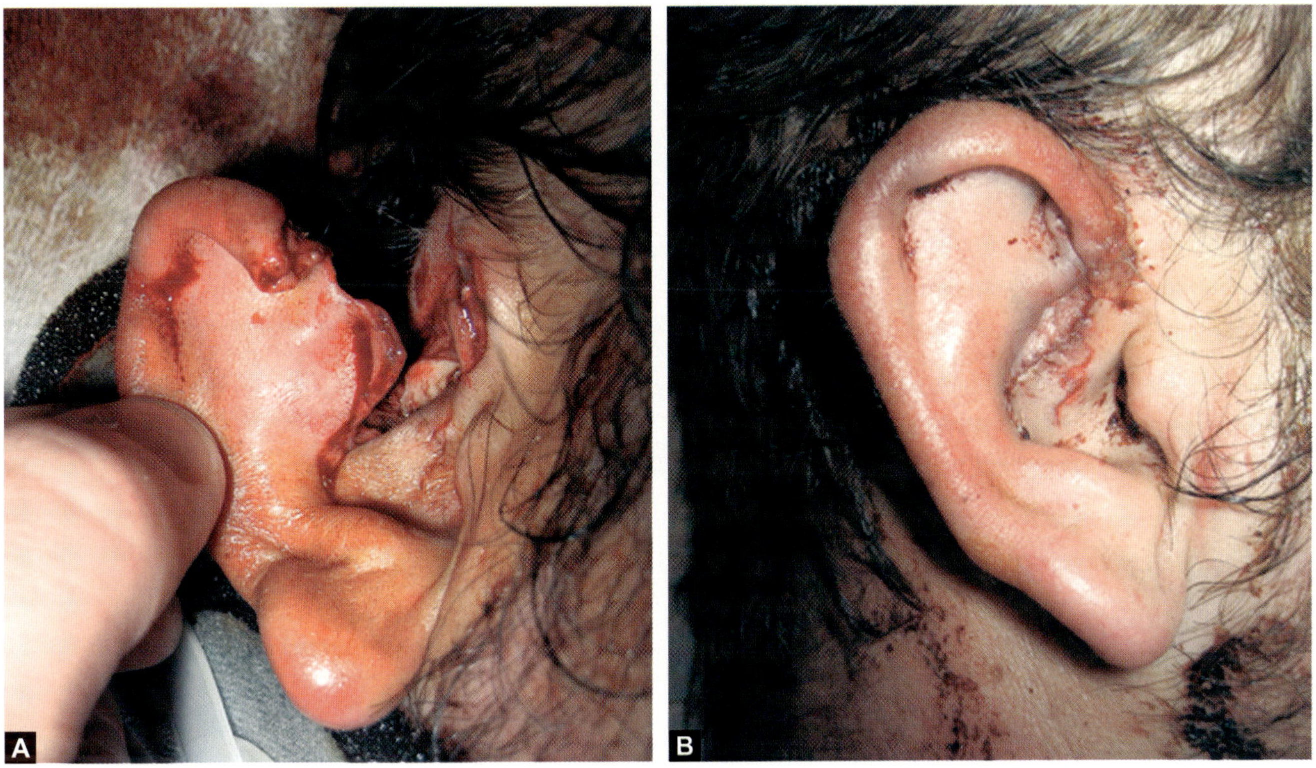

Figs 17.3A and B: (A) Partial auricular avulsion; (B) After repair in the emergency department. No healing issues were present long-term
Source: Nadir Ahmad, MD FACS

unlikely that significant vasculature is present and in a good state to justify a microvascular anastomosis. The surgeon is safest in treating this patient like a patient who has undergone a skin cancer excision and employ these forms of reconstructions once the wound is clean.

Follow-up

Close follow-up to examine for signs of infection is warranted. Make sure that wound care is appropriate and that all questions are answered. Perform serial photographs of the healing wounds for education purposes and also to serve as a record should the patient seek legal counsel.

If scarring is present, secondary scar revision may be considered in the future, but allow adequate time to pass. If the patient will allow, permit several months to a year to pass, assuming that doing so will not compromise function or significantly psychologically harm the patient, as this will allow the scars to mature, and a more predictable result is possible. Also, the patient may be satisfied with the result which may, or may not, be improved by further intervention. An additional benefit of allowing time to pass is that it allows for a psychological adjustment period where the patient begins to acclimate to the appearance of the injury which may permit the "new wounds" of reconstructive efforts to be better accepted. No matter what efforts are taken (resurfacing, scar revision, tissue replacement), informed consent and preoperatively photography is mandatory.

BURNS

After emergent and systemic management of the burn patient, attention may be then turned to the head and neck involvement. First, a thorough assessment of the extent of burn injury and the method of thermal injury is necessary. Once, this is done, coverage with an antibiotic ointment (e.g. silver sulfadiazine cream) followed by nonadherent dressings may be applied. Obvious nonviable skin and tissues may be sharply debrided away so that they do not act as a growth medium for bacteria. However, any questionable tissue should be left alone to demarcate if it is nonviable.

When considering soft tissue reconstruction in the burn patient, several issues must be kept in mind. Several reconstructions may be necessary over the patient's life, and therefore donor site morbidity becomes a strong consideration when regional or distant tissues are utilized in the repair. Additionally, scar contractures cannot only result in significant disfigurement, but they can result in crippling disability and loss of function such as neck immobility, ectropion and microstomia. Therefore, functional preservation and restoration are of paramount importance. Compression garments and splints (e.g. an oral appliance) may be helpful in decreasing these issues and should be considered early in the management.

Due to the complexity that arises in these patients, a multidisciplinary team is the best way to manage the reconstructive, rehabilitative and psychosocial needs of the burn patient. Efforts are underway in the development of skin substitutes and hopefully these advancements will allow for early intervention, avoidance or donor site morbidity, and better long-term outcomes.

FOLLOW-UP AFTER REPAIR

If the patient is admitted to the hospital, regular follow-up by the surgeon and his or her team is necessary. Wound checks serve several purposes. They allow for the early identification and intervention of any issues with healing. Additionally, these visits strengthen the bond between the patient and surgeon and afford the patient and caregivers the opportunity to have their questions answered regarding the injury and expected outcomes.

In general, sutures may be removed between 5 days and 7 days after repair. However, consider leaving sutures in longer in previously irradiated patients as the vascular supply, and thus healing, is compromised. Just prior to removal, the incision line should be cleaned and the surrounding skin degreased of antibiotic ointment. Performing this prior to suture removal lessens the chance for any incisional trauma or microdehiscence. Atraumatically remove the sutures; use magnification if sutures are difficult to see or manipulate. Reassure the patient that it is very early in the healing process and that the final outcome will not be apparent for several weeks to months in most cases.

At this time, supporting the wound with tapes placed perpendicularly across the incision helps to lesson tension on the wound now that the sutures are removed. Doing so should help to prevent widening of the scar by keeping tension off the incision. Additionally, the tapes help to prevent accidental pull across the incision by creating mass movement of the area which limits the force from being applied across the weakest point: the incision. If any areas have been left to heal secondarily, these areas should not be taped and local wound care should continue.

A follow-up visit in 7 more days is helpful. Photographs are taken at this point. The tapes may be removed with the aid of adhesive remover and the wound examined. It is the author's preference to continue taping for the next 4–5 weeks if the patient allows. Simply teach the patients how to apply the tapes so that weekly visits are not necessary. Some patients develop a mild contact dermatitis from the adhesive or inflammation from having the skin occluded. If this develops, a rest period of a few days should be instituted and consideration for a low potency steroid cream given.

If no further surgical revisions are anticipated, at 6 weeks from the initial repair, dermabrasion may be undertaken to improve the final result of the scar. The reader is directed to the chapter on dermabrasion for full details of this technique. Predermabrasion and postdermabrasion photography should be taken.

As with all surgical interventions, being available for the patient throughout this process with not only alleviate his or her anxiety but will also allow the surgeon the advantage of early detection of any healing issues that will undoubtedly occur at some point in the surgeon's career.

CHAPTER

18

Scar Revision

Thomas C Spalla

INTRODUCTION

Whether from trauma, cancer, surgery, radiation, or other means, scarring can be extremely upsetting for both the patient and the surgeon. Scarring can lead to loss of both form and function. For the patient, this could mean the inability to close the eye or mouth, the loss of hearing associated with an external auditory canal stenosis, or even neck immobility. Also, from the patient's perspective, this can be psychologically devastating. He or she may spend a significant portion of the day worrying about other's perception of the scar. As these thoughts progress, he or she may not wish to be seen in public or by loved ones. This could lead to loss of employment and relationships, and may even lead to severe depression and suicide. Thankfully, these extremes do not apply to the majority of patients. However, the surgeon would be remiss to not strongly consider the psychosocial effects scarring may have on the patient. Despite the tenacity the scar process presents to both patient and surgeon, there are numerous methods the surgeon possesses in his or her armamentarium for combating this.

HISTORY

A thorough history is critical. The surgeon should aim to determine the method by which the scar was created, when it occurred, whether anything was unique about this (e.g. postoperative infection), whether the patient has had past attempts at improving it, and the patient's goals, expectation and motivations. Of course, a complete medical and surgical history is obtained, and a family history of problematic scarring can be helpful, but do not be deterred by the patient who tells you that a family member had a "keloid". Oftentimes, a hypertrophic scar is mislabeled as a keloid. This is a good opportunity to ask the patient about his or her history of scarring. Look for other iatrogenic or traumatic scars (e.g. a bicycle mishap as a child) to gauge the patient's previous healing response. If the patient reports a self-history of "keloids", examine this site and determine whether or not a true keloid exists.

TIMING

With some exceptions, scars will generally improve over time. What is meant by improvement is flattening, softening and improved color match with time. Also, as time progresses, most patients become more accepting of, and cope better with, the presence of the scars.

There are some scars that do not improve over time. Some scars hypertrophy and some may even keloid (Figs 18.1A and B). There are histological features which distinguish the two conditions. However, both conditions, particularly the latter, are highly undesirable, and these conditions are the reason that close follow-up is mandatory after surgery to help in the early detection and slowing, and hopefully, halting of these processes.

All scars undergo some degree of contracture. In situations where scars lie close to functional structures, this contracture may lead to functional loss, and therefore early intervention may be necessary to prevent such loss.

REVISABLE SCARS

Before taking the time to determine whether the patient is medically and psychologically fit for scar revision, the surgeon must determine whether or not the scar itself can be improved through intervention.

Scars that are considered unsightly generally have one or more of the following characteristics:

- Excessive in size—width, length or thickness
- Poor color match to surrounding tissues
- Alopecia—in a hair-bearing region

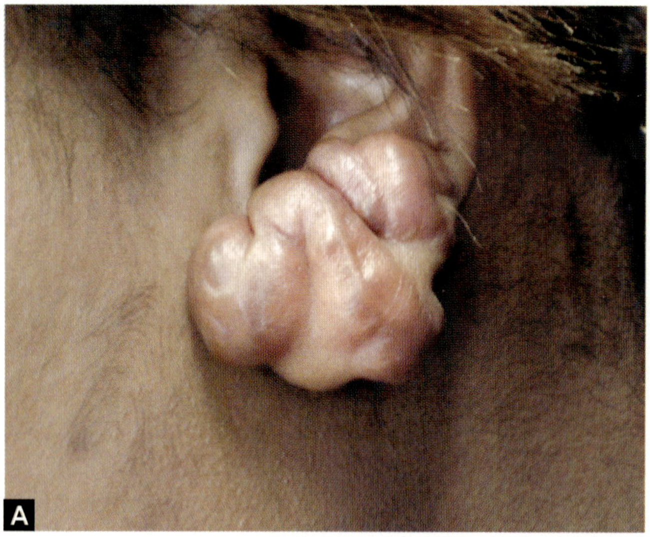

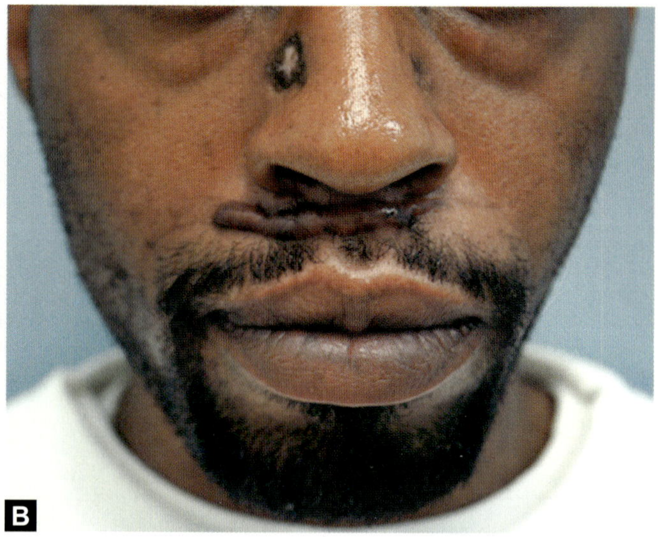

Figs 18.1A and B: (A) Left auricular keloid; (B) Upper lip keloid from endotracheal tube taping

- Crosses anatomic/aesthetic boundaries
- Pulls and distorts a structure causing aesthetic changes and/or functional loss

Scars possessing one or more of these findings may be amenable to revision with the goal being improvement. It is crucial to stress the goal of improvement to the patient. No "magic scar eraser" exists at this time, and despite the surgeon's expertise, any injury to the skin of sufficient depth will result in a scar. The time spent explaining this to the patient and counseling him/her on reasonable expectations cannot be overstated. If the time is not spent, even the best outcome in the surgeon's eye may fall short of the patient's expectations.

Steroid Injections to Treat Scars

Physicians are cognizant of the beneficial anti-inflammatory effects steroids possess, and this property along with collagen synthesis inhibition makes the use of steroid injections into scars, a favorable way of managing thickened and raised scars.

A depot steroid such as triamcinolone can be used and injections are usually repeated on a 3–4 week interval basis. This allows for periodic evaluations of the progress and to detect any untoward side effects which may occur. These visits also allow the patient-physician bond to strengthen and afford the opportunity to discuss future scar revisions which may be desirable.

Care must be taken when using steroid injections. The injection must be delivered within the scar itself and not allowed to diffuse into the surrounding tissues. At times, these injections may be very difficult due to the scar's density. Steroids cause fat necrosis and this could lead to a wasting of the surrounding tissues and a depressed segment of tissue. Additionally, thinning of the skin may result in a shiny, atrophic appearance and the development of telangiectasias may occur. Inform the patient of these potential risks prior to injections.

Relaxed Skin Tension Lines and Facial Subunits

The understanding of relaxed skin tension lines (RSTLs) and facial subunits is at the core of facial scar revision. RSTLs are demonstrated in Figures 18.2A and B. Lines of maximal extensibility (LMEs) lie perpendicular to the RSTLs and represent the direction in which the skin can be stretched with minimal force. Undermining in these directions is necessary when closing wounds within, or parallel to, RSTLs.

Facial subunits are illustrated in Figures 18.3A and B. If possible, designing incisions which lie along these borders will allow for the final scar to be less noticeable. Also, when greater than 50% of the subunit requires excision (e.g. in Mohs surgery), it may be most aesthetically desirable to replace the entire subunit as this tends not to draw as much attention to the area and thus makes it a more aesthetic outcome, as this will allow the new scar to lie on the subunit boundary.

Excision

Excision represents the simplest and most common method of scar revision (Figs 18.4A to C). Scars that are

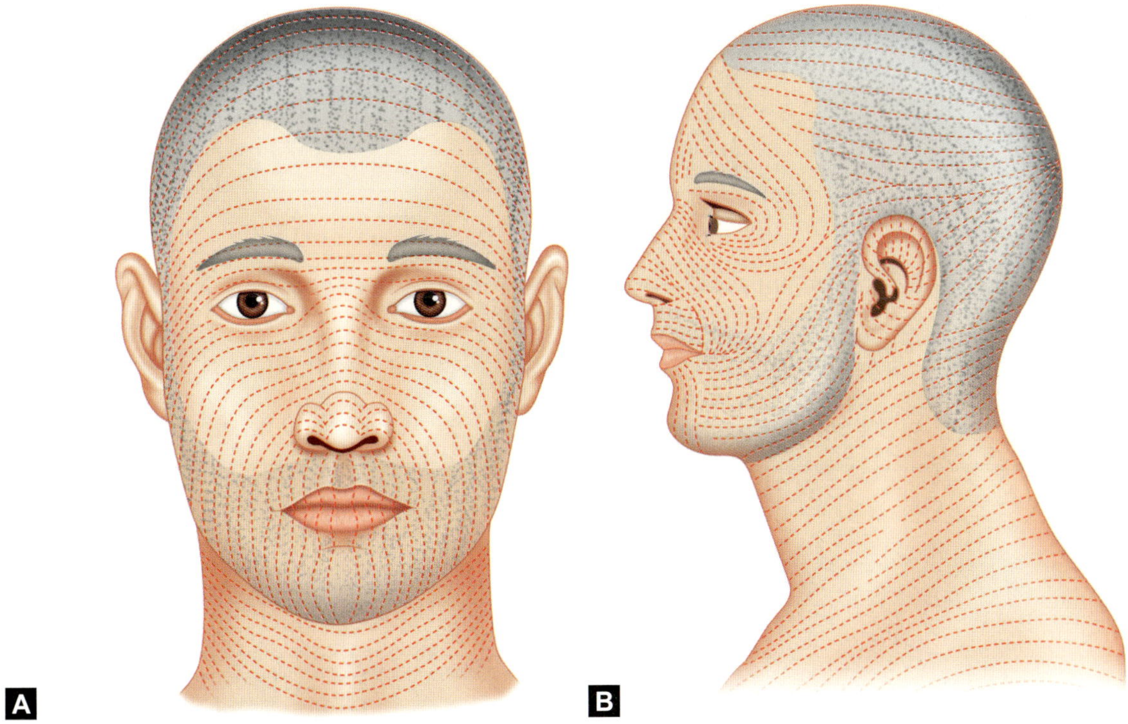

Figs 18.2A and B: Relaxed skin tension lines

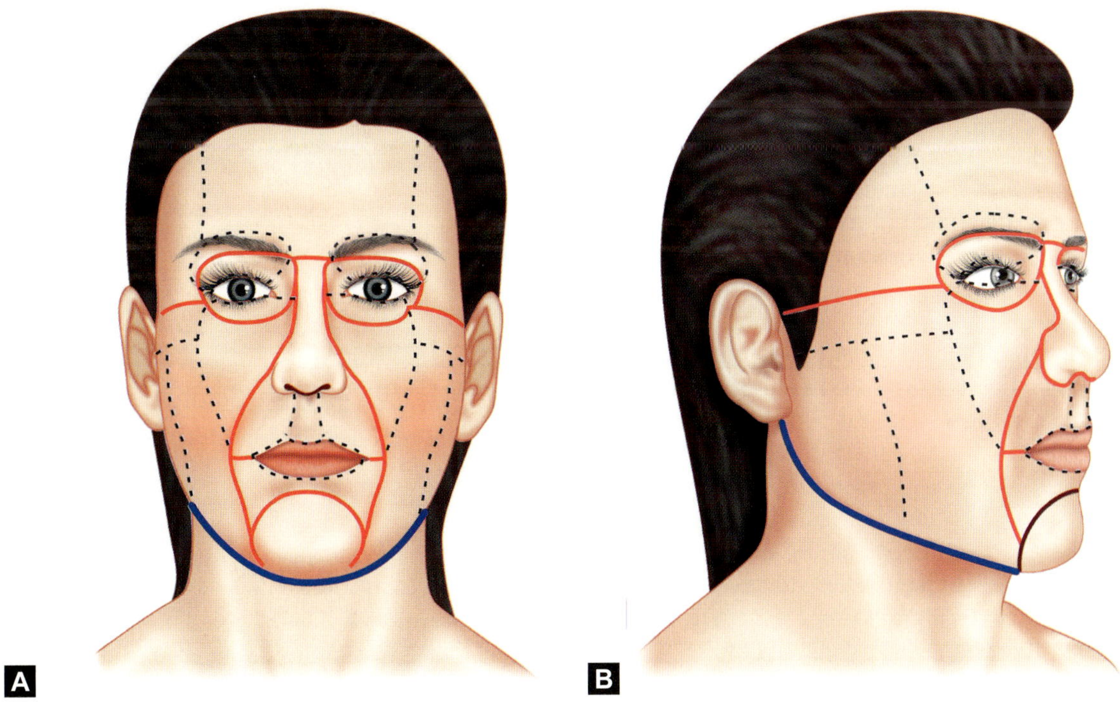

Figs 18.3A and B: Facial subunits

amenable to this form of reconstruction generally run parallel, or close, to RSTLs. If they do not, consider using one of the rearrangement techniques detailed below, or else the incision may end up being excessively long, although oriented with the RSTLs, and may not be the best possible outcome.

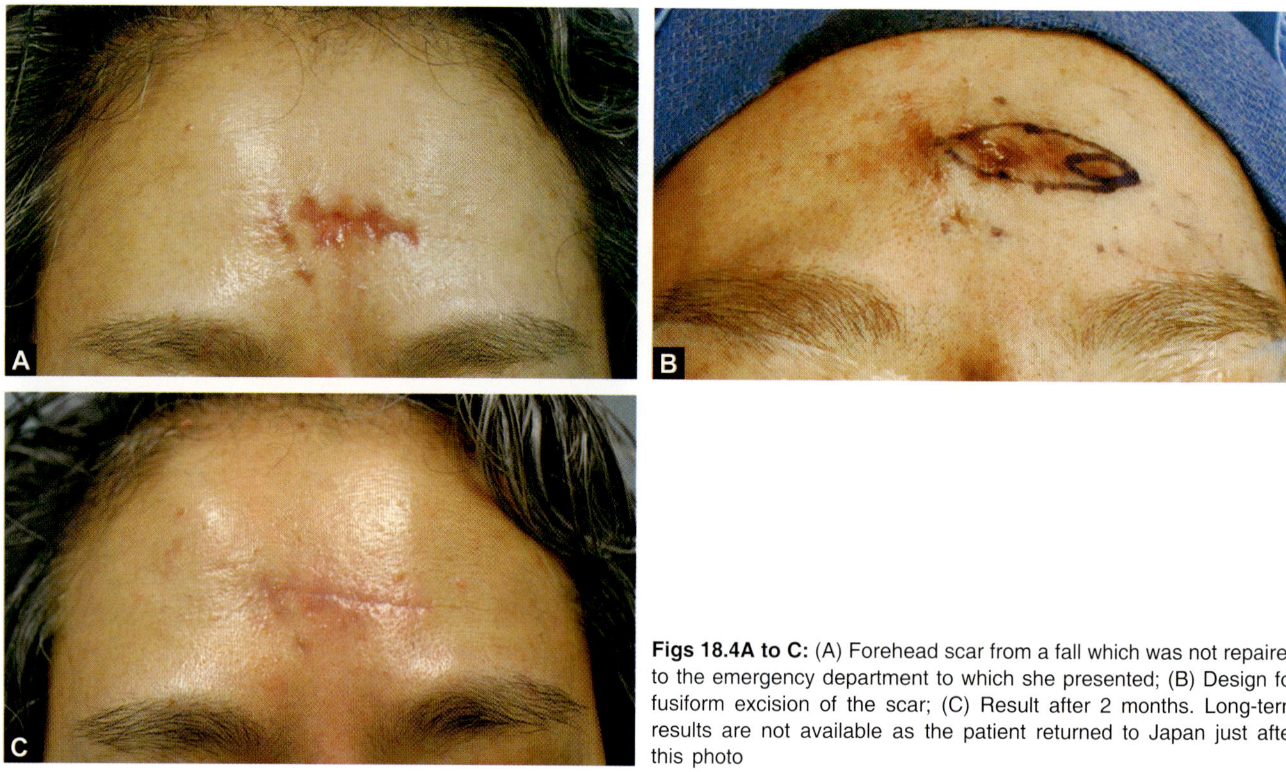

Figs 18.4A to C: (A) Forehead scar from a fall which was not repaired to the emergency department to which she presented; (B) Design for fusiform excision of the scar; (C) Result after 2 months. Long-term results are not available as the patient returned to Japan just after this photo

Technique

To perform this, the surgeon first outlines the scar with a narrow (1-2 mm) margin. The fusiform shape (see Fig. 18.4B) should have a width to length ratio of at least 1:3. The creation of less than this may result in a dog-ear deformity at the ends of the incision. Increasing the ratio lessens this chance at the expense of the creation of a longer incision.

Sharply excise the fusiform shape and slightly beveling the blade away from the incisional site helps to ensure good wound eversion upon closure. Do not hesitate to use forceps on the material to be excised. However, the use of single-pronged hooks during undermining and closure helps to prevent unnecessary tissue trauma. Sharply undermine the tissues in the immediate subdermal plane. Ensure that adequate undermining has occurred by gently reapproximating the tissues with two single-pronged hooks. The edges should come together with little to no tension. If tension exists, widening of the final scar may occur. Excessive undermining (i.e. greater than four times the length of the incision) may be detrimental, however. Close the dermal layers with buried dissolvable sutures in an interrupted fashion.

Superficial closure methods vary between surgeons. Atraumatic, aseptic, and meticulous/atraumatic technique, and proper postoperative wound care matter more than the specific method of epidermal closure. Superficial closure, in scar revision, is generally done with sutures, but tissue glue could be considered in the population in whom suture removal can be difficult or require anesthesia.

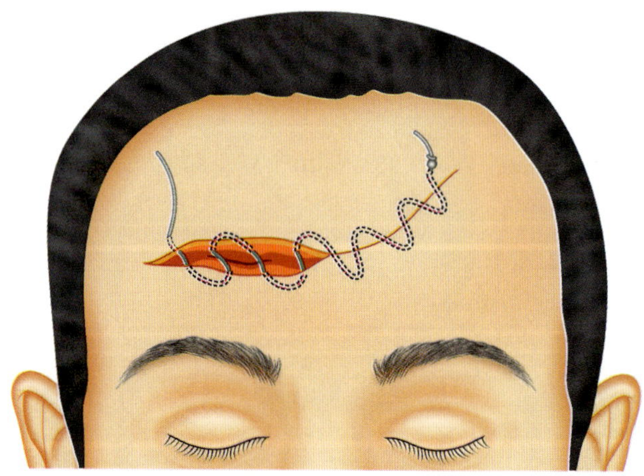

Fig. 18.5: Intracuticular suturing

The intracuticular technique, shown in Figure 18.5, is useful in several situations:

- Patients in whom suture removal may be difficult
- Patients who are apprehensive about seeing sutures (e.g. mental disability)
- Wounds that typically heal extremely well without much eversion (e.g. blepharoplasty).

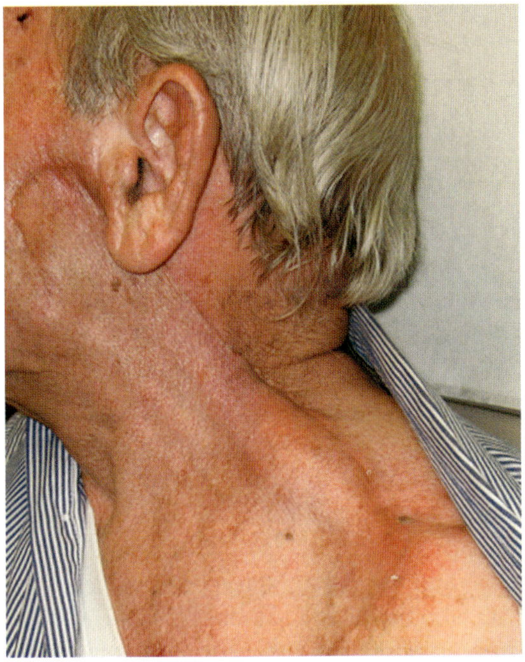

Fig. 18.6: Scar running across relaxed skin tension lines on the neck after a cervicofacial advancement flap. This scar band could be improved through the Z-plasty technique
Source: Nadir Ahmad, MD FACS

Dissolvable sutures are an additional consideration with regards to superficial wound closure. Dissolvable sutures offer the benefit of the lack of suture removal. However, this comes with the cost of increased erythema at the incisional site as the sutures dissolve. They can be useful in the following situations:

- Patients in whom suture removal is difficult
- Patients who are unlikely to follow-up (e.g. trauma patients or patients with poor social support) These patients are not good candidates for elective scar revision due to the lack of necessary postoperative wound care and surveillance.

Typically, sutures may be removed 5–7 days after repair. Suture removal should not simply be designated to the nearest available assistant. This is a process in the scar revision and in the patient's overall experience. Atraumatic technique during removal is necessary, and if this is not done by the surgeon, he or she should ensure that the designated assistant is facile with this. Just prior to removal, the wound can be gently cleaned by the surgeon or assistant and pictures taken, if necessary or desired.

Once the sutures are removed, the wound is now weaker than it was just moments ago and this fact should be stressed to the patient, so he/she is still very delicate in cleaning the area and avoiding trauma.

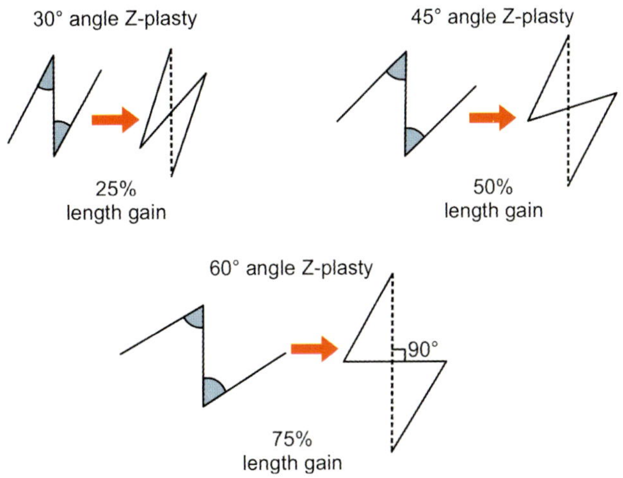

Fig. 18.7: Z-plasty technique demonstrating length changes with increasing angle of rotation

Z-Plasty

Z-plasty is a technique which makes use of additional incisions oriented at various angles to the original scar or proposed incision to allow for several effects. By using it in scar excision and revision, the orientation of the initial axis of the scar will be rotated. This can be useful in reorienting scars which lie perpendicular to RSTLs. Keep in mind, however, that additional incisions will be made and they will not lie parallel to the RSTLs. This is an inherent sacrifice that must be understood prior to undertaking the Z-plasty reconstructive technique. Also, the total length of the incision will increase. Due to the inherent nature of the triangular shape of the Z-plasty limbs, the contracture forces of healing are not simply oriented in such a way to pull and widen the healing incision. This helps to decrease the chance for a wide or hypertrophic scar. The Z-plasty technique is also helpful to break up scars which may distort anatomic structures (e.g. webbing at the medial canthus). Figure 18.6 shows a cervical scar with banding which lends itself well to a Z-plasty technique.

Figure 18.7 illustrates the principles of lengthening and rotation which occur through the use of the Z-plasty technique.

Figures 18.8A to F demonstrate how the axis of the scar may be realigned to lie within a RSTL. Z-plasty's rotational properties may be useful to realign an anatomic structure such as the corner of the mouth. When posed with a long scar that needs to be realigned, the inherent creation of large limbs for the rotation is undesirable and an alterative means such as W-plasty or geometric broken line closure (GBLC) should be considered.

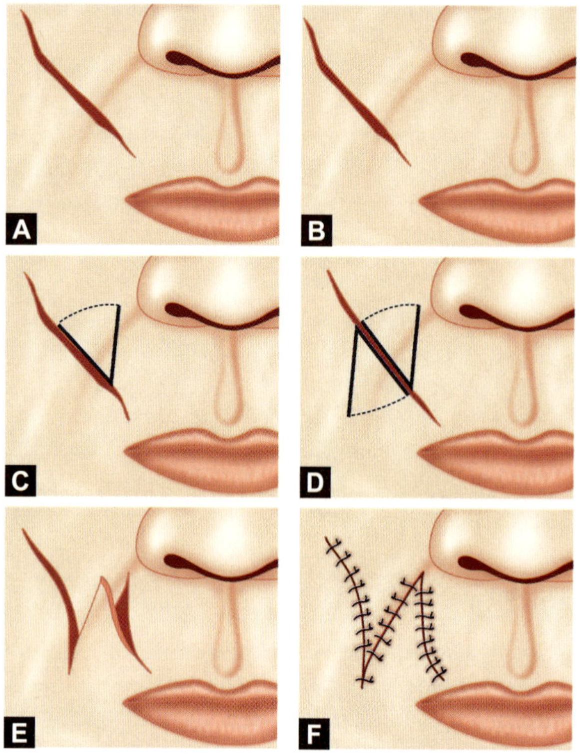

Figs 18.8A to F: Z-plasty technique to realign the axis of a scar

W-Plasty

W-plasty is utilized when presented with a scar which is not oriented parallel to the RSTLs but is too long to utilize a Z-plasty. The limbs of a W-plasty should be limited to 1 cm in length on the face and 1.5 cm on the neck. Figures 18.9A to C demonstrates the way in which a W-plasty is executed.

Geometric Broken Line Closure

When the scar is long and poorly aligned with the RSTLs, or in a scar which is distractingly visible simply due to its length although lying within a RSTL, the GBLC method may be beneficial (Figs 18.10A and B). The GBLC uses various geometric shapes (e.g. triangles, squares and half-circles) to "fool" the observer's eye into not seeing the scar as readily as if it were straight. The shapes break up the observer's line of sight and due to the focusing on various small shapes rather than one long one, the scar becomes less visible. Like the W-plasty, the numerous limbs (5–6 mm in length), help to break up the scar's contractile forces and create a greater surface area for healing thereby reducing the chance of a widened or hypertrophic scar.

Dermabrasion

Dermabrasion has been used for nearly 100 years for the removal of traumatic tattooing during wartime. It has evolved and been refined to manage scarring from nearly any cause. It is particularly useful for acne and traumatic scarring such as may occur after a motor vehicle accident resulting in numerous small lacerations from shattered glass. Dermabrasion consists of removing the epidermis and a varying layer of the dermis mechanically through the use of a handheld device.

The device (Fig. 18.11) consists of a power unit, a handpiece and various tips. The tips come in two basic types: (1) wire brush and (2) diamond fraise. Both types vary in sizes and shapes depending on the site to be dermabraded and surgeon's preference. Like otologic drilling, the larger tips are generally safer, as the risk for creating a single overly deep hole is lessened with this choice. The diamond fraise tips consist of a drum or acorn-shaped head which is coated with industrial grade diamonds. This rough surface spins and gradually removes the skin. Some amount of heat is created with this technique. The wire brush is recommended for more experienced users as it rapidly removes the skin by creating numerous tiny lacerations. It may be that these lacerations, as they heal, have a microscopic Z-plasty-like effect on the healing tissue.

As with iatrogenic scars (e.g. after Mohs reconstruction), dermabrasion is best carried out approximately 6 weeks after the initial injury.

Lasers

Lasers offer a relatively newer way of managing scars. In addition to the resurfacing capabilities that certain ablative lasers (e.g. CO_2 and Er:YAG) possess, the use of nonablative lasers (e.g. pulsed dye laser), can also help modulate collagen deposition and alignment and can also address persistent erythema. They offer promising results, especially for patients who are reluctant to undergo any type of surgical intervention.

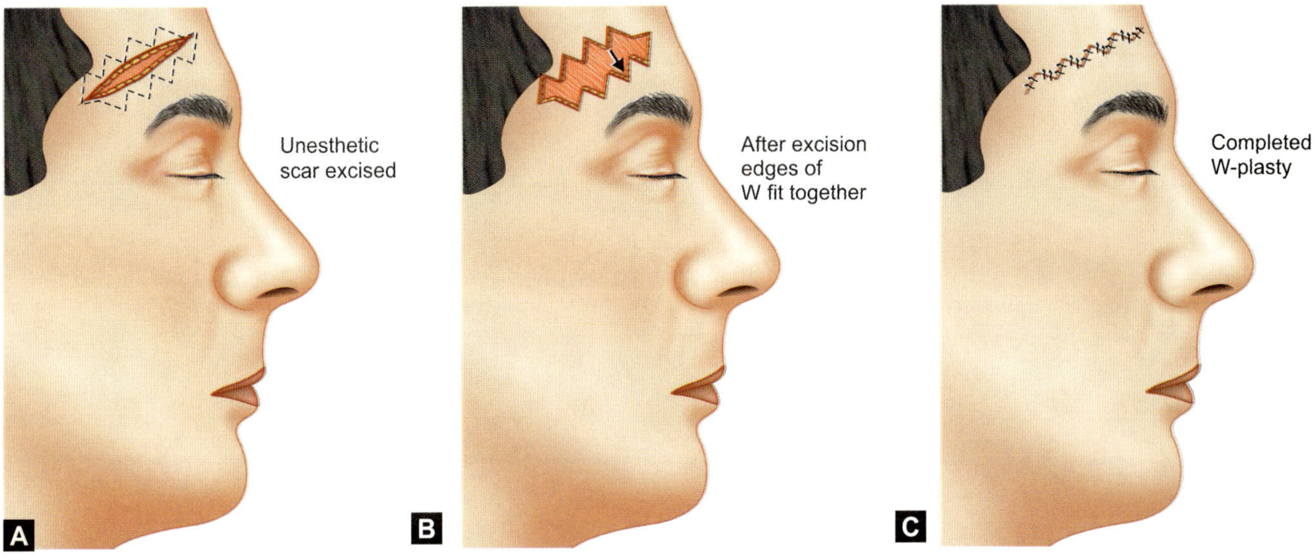

Figs 18.9A to C: W-plasty

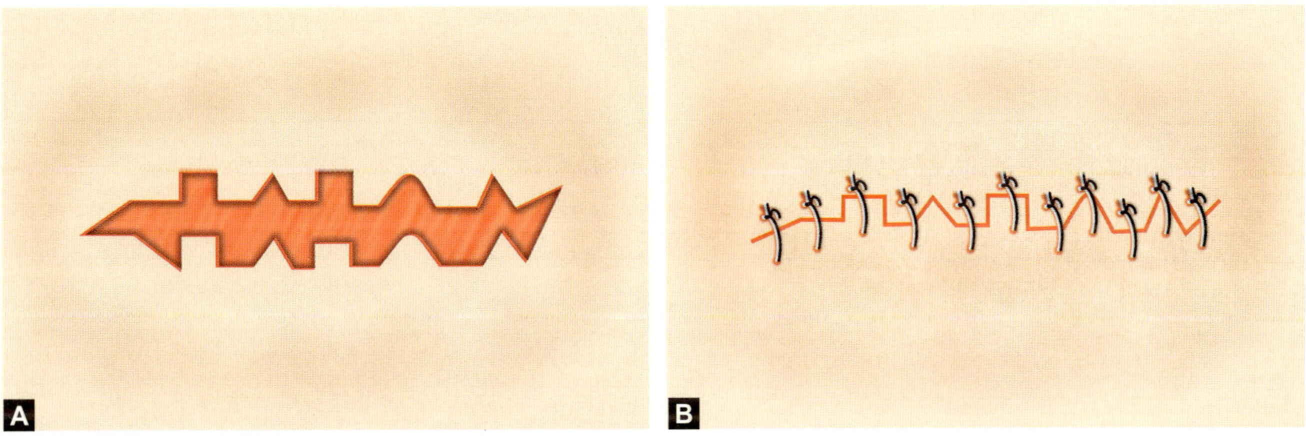

Figs 18.10A and B: Geometric broken line closure

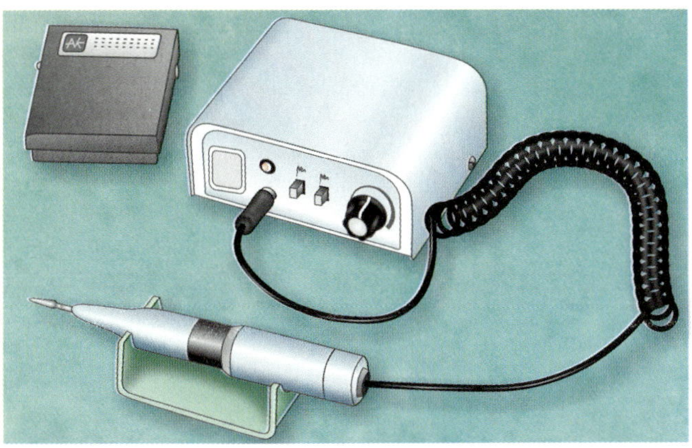
Fig. 18.11: An example of a dermabrader

CONCLUSION

Scar revision is as much art as it is science and there are countless ways in which scars can be improved. Through the techniques discussed in this chapter, the surgeon can gain a foundation in surgical scar revision on which to build. Newer technologies, such as lasers, offer attractive options for difficult scars and for patients in whom further surgery is unwise. Good patient and scar selection and proper patient education can make scar revision an extremely rewarding endeavor.

CHAPTER

19 Reconstruction of Facial Skin Defects

Anthony P Sclafani

OVERVIEW

Repair of skin defects are typically performed after resection of benign or malignant skin lesions, but may be necessary after trauma or in any situation in which local skin is inadequate to cover skin defects. If wide local undermining cannot generate sufficient tissue laxity to close a skin defect, alternatives should be considered and the least complex option, capable of producing an acceptable result, should be used.

SPECIAL CONSIDERATIONS

Relaxed skin tension lines (RSTLs) run perpendicular to facial muscles along which skin folding and wrinkling occurs (Fig. 19.1). To the degree possible, scars should be aligned first along facial unit and subunit junctions (as the change in texture, and often color of skin at these points helps hide scars), within existing creases and lines and along RSTLs.

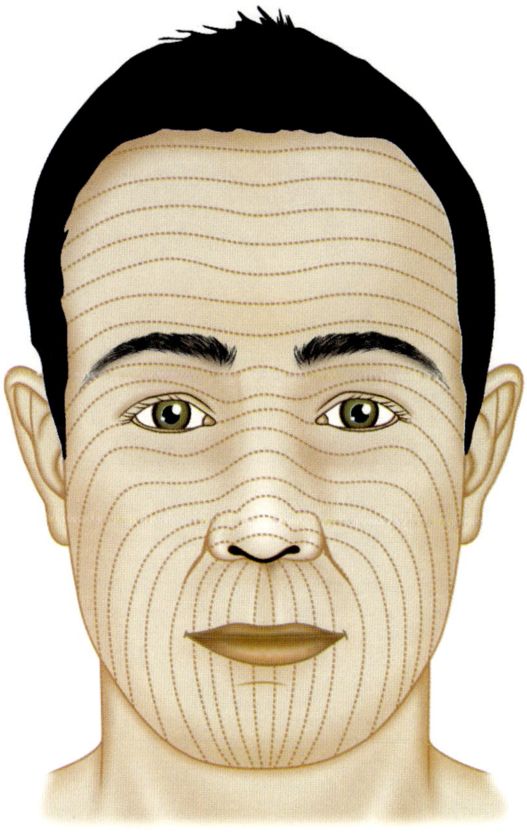

Fig. 19.1: Relaxed skin tension lines

ALTERNATIVES TO PROCEDURE

Malignant skin lesions should be excised with methods that assure a very low rate of recurrence; if this is not possible, consideration should be given to allowing healing by secondary intention or coverage with a split thickness skin graft to allow for monitoring of recurrence for a period of time, after which formal reconstruction can be performed.

TECHNIQUES

Healing by Secondary Intention

Healing by secondary intention involves no incisions, as it is a process whereby the wound is allowed to heal without intervention. The wound is cleaned and kept moist, allowing for development of a wound matrix and migration of epithelial cells inward from the wound edges.

Full Thickness Skin Grafts

Incision Placement

With full thickness skin grafts (FTSGs), no additional incisions are made in the recipient area. However, FTSG harvest requires an incision, which is placed so as to be as

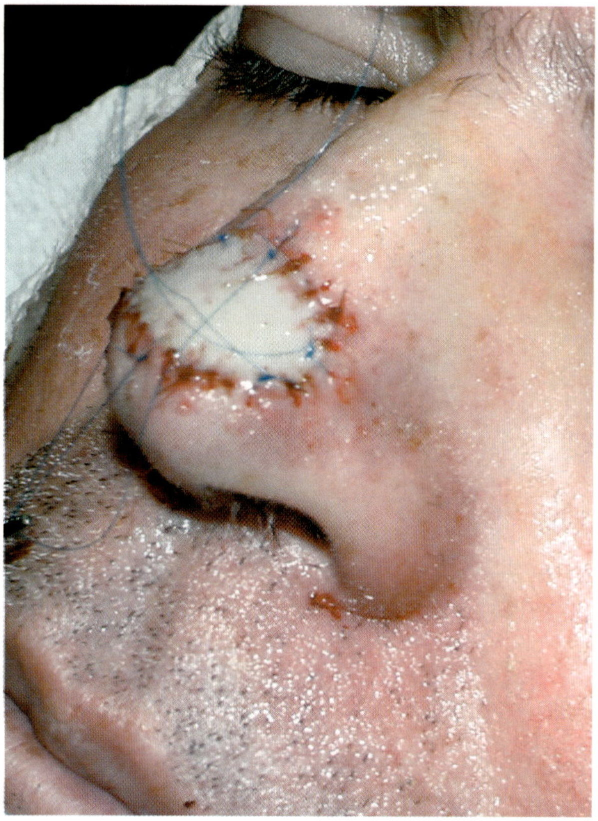

Fig. 19.2: Full thickness skin graft sutured in place, prior to placement of gauze bolster secured with sutures

inconspicuous as possible. Excellent donor sites include the upper eyelid, nasolabial fold, pre or postauricular areas and the supraclavicular fossa. Once the graft is harvested, the donor site is closed primarily. FTSG donor sites are chosen in terms of rough equivalence of thickness and color match. In general, the closer the donor site to the defect, the better the tissue match.

Extent of Undermining/Dissection

Recipient site wound edges are not undermined. Instead, healthy, viable tissue is ensured by debriding any necrotic or devitalized tissue prior to graft placement.

Tissue Modifications

Sutures: Full thickness skin grafts are generally sutured at their periphery with a fine monofilament suture (Fig. 19.2). Additional techniques are necessary to ensure good apposition of the graft to the wound base, as this will be the primary source of vascular buds during healing. Grafts should not move relative to the wound base, or neovascularization will not occur and the graft will fail. A deep "basting" suture can be placed through the graft to secure it to the wound base. More commonly, a bolster dressing of 3% Bismuth Tribromophenate petrolatum gauze (Xeroform, Cardinal Health, Dublin, Ohio, US) is sutured over the graft by tying together over the dressing 3-0 nylon sutures placed at the periphery of the graft. Over the first 48 hours, these grafts survive by a process of serum imbibition, deriving basal nutrient support from serum exuded from the wound base, after which establishment of direct vascular connections to the wound base directly supply the graft (Figs 19.3A to D). It is important to assure a healthy, vascular base for each graft. FTSGs will not survive over cartilage or bone; instead, the outer cortex of bone can be removed with a drill until the vascular diploic space is exposed to serve as a blood supply (Figs 19.4A to D). Likewise, skin grafts will survive on intact and vascularized perichondrium, but exposed cartilage must be fenestrated to allow for vascular access to the grafts.

Composite Grafts

Incision Placement

Composite grafts are composed of two or more distinct tissues, typically skin and cartilage, which are attached and share a mutual blood supply. Common areas for harvesting include the conchal bowl (conchal cartilage with attached anterior or posterior skin) or the helical root (helical cartilage with attached skin and a banner of preauricular skin). A dermis-fat graft can be harvested from an aesthetically unimportant and covered area (e.g. buttocks). The skin is first de-epithelialized manually or by dermabrasion, following which the full thickness of dermis with fat attached on the deep aspect is harvested and the donor site closed primarily. Donor site incisions are placed so as to make the donor site scar as inconspicuous as possible.

Extent of Undermining/Dissection

Dermis-fat grafts are placed in conforming but not constricting pockets in the immediate subdermis for volume augmentation. Skin-cartilage grafts are generally harvested and placed so that the skin edges of the graft match up with the recipient site, while "flanges" of cartilage extend beyond the skin and are used to anchor the graft in place.

Tissue Modifications

Sutures: The "flanges" of composite grafts can be placed into precise pockets at the edges of the recipient sites or sutured directly to the cartilage remnants for additional stability.

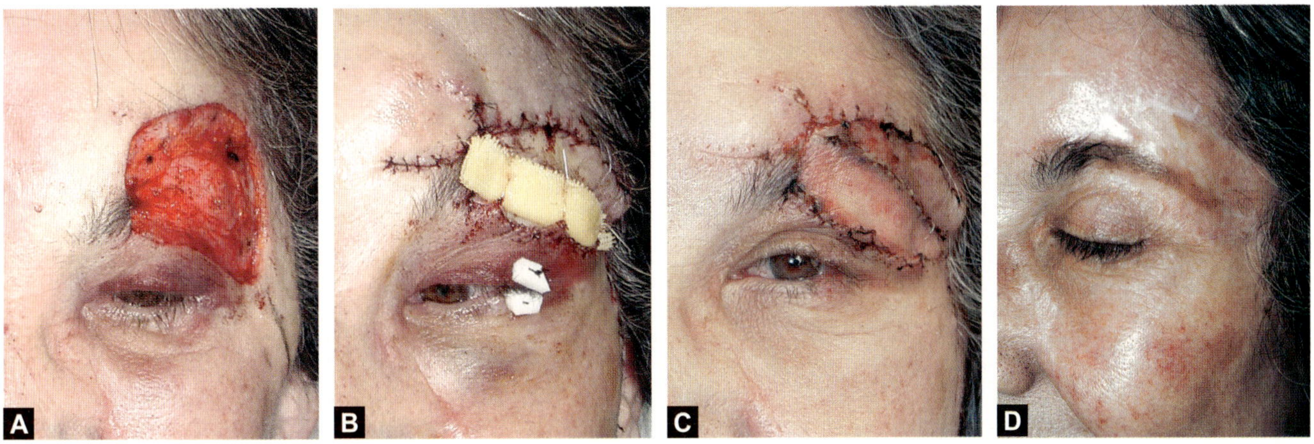

Figs 19.3A to D: Full thickness skin graft and local flaps to reconstruct an extensive defect of the eyelid, eyebrow and temple

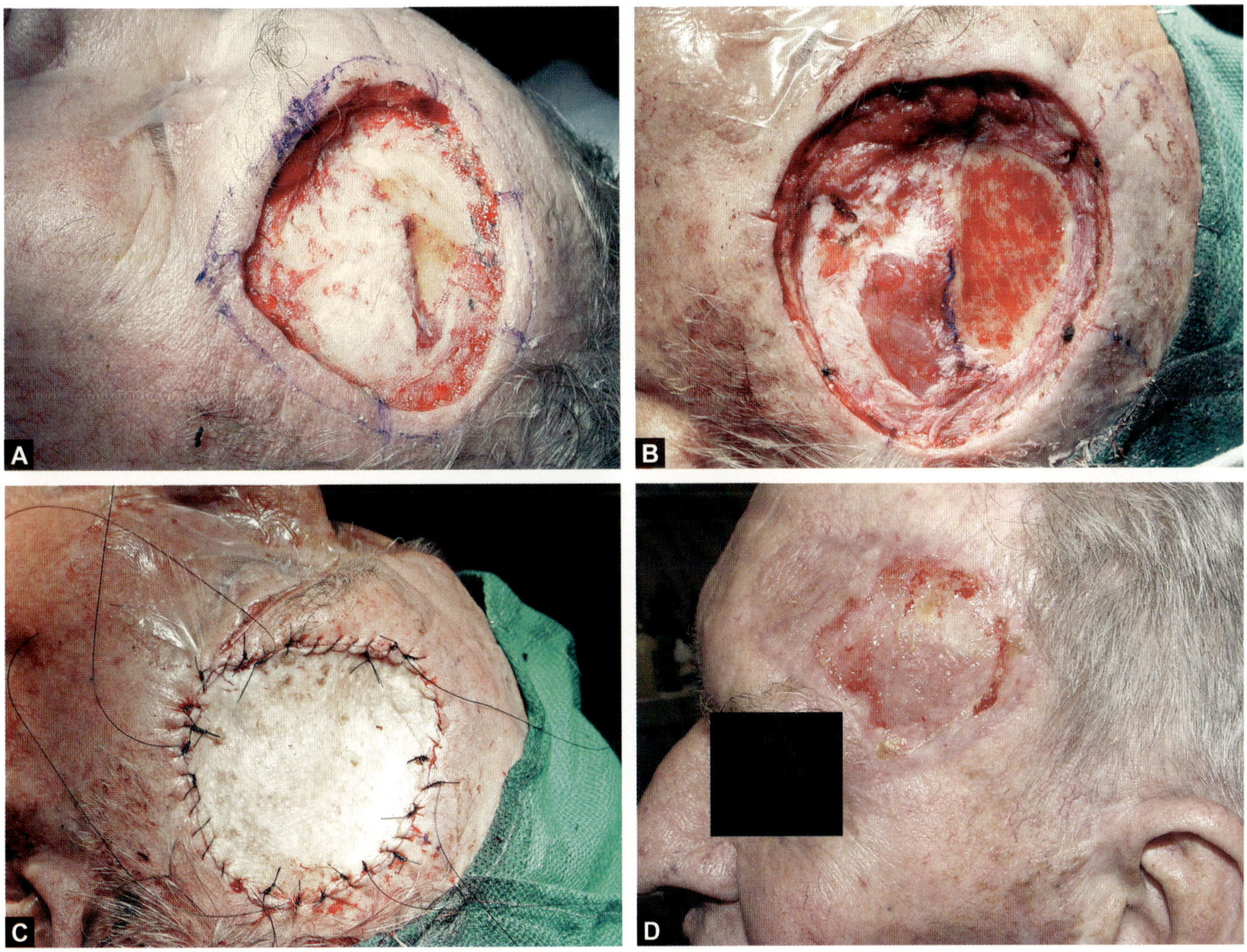

Figs 19.4A to D: Full thickness skin graft placed over left temporalis fascia, temporalis muscle and skull. Since (A) periosteum had been removed in the center of the defect; (B) the outer table was removed with a cutting burr; (C) the graft placed directly on the diploae superiorly; (D) 4 weeks after surgery

Fusiform Excision with or without M-Plasty

Incision Placement

Any defect can be converted into a fusiform shape by excising additional skin. This should be done so that the long axis runs along aesthetic unit borders, existing folds and creases or parallel to RSTLs. The additional skin excised prevents the development of standing cone deformities (dog ears).

Undermining

Surrounding tissues should be undermined sufficiently to allow the wound edges to be advanced together without unacceptable wound tension. In general, wide undermining for up to 4 cm from the wound edge is beneficial, while greater distances do not significantly reduce wound tension and only make the flap blood supply more tenuous. However, in the face it is often difficult to undermine 4 cm without encroaching upon other facial units with mobile structures (e.g. eyelids, nasal ala, lips). Undermining too closely to these structures may distort their position undesirably.

Tissue Modifications

Excision: While a fusiform excision can be planned and marked, it is generally more useful to place some approximation sutures at the center of the defect first and to then judge the amount of skin redundancy present and skin excision needed to avoid a standing cone. The skin is then excised appropriately in the position which best follows aesthetic boundaries and RSTLs. When planned excision of a standing cone deformity will cross an aesthetic boundary, an M-plasty can be incorporated into the design. Rather than continue the edges of the excision smoothly to its apex across the aesthetic boundary, the incision stops at the boundary and is completed by an M shaped incision (Figs 19.5A to C). In general, angles in fusiform excisions and in M-plasties are around 30°.

Tissue advancement: As noted earlier, undermining in a subcutaneous plane decreases the wound closure tension by allowing greater movement of the surrounding tissues. However, tissue advancement may be limited on one side of the defect in order to avoid distortion of mobile structures, such as the eyelid. Differential undermining will assist in directed tissue mobilization.

Closure

Dead space should be eliminated and the dermis should be reapproximated with a resorbable suture. Excess suture material should be avoided, but the dermal sutures should support a relatively tensionless epidermal closure with interrupted or running permanent monofilament sutures.

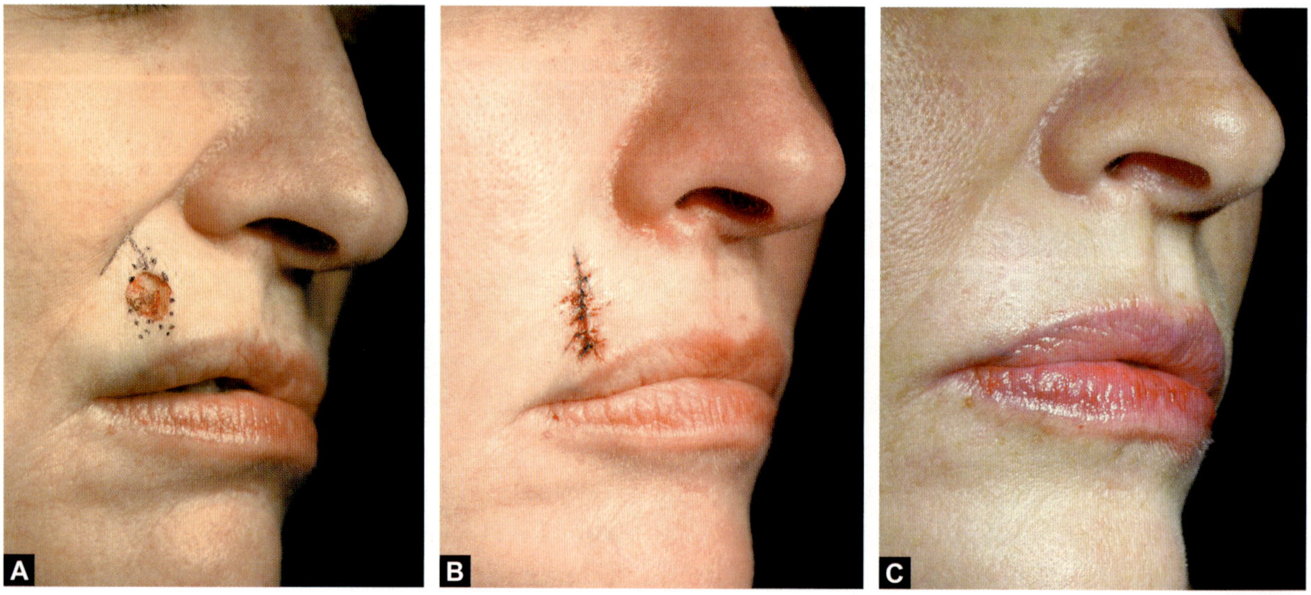

Figs 19.5A to C: (A) Defect of the upper lip near the vermilion border; (B) M-plasty was incorporated into closure inferiorly to avoid crossing the aesthetic boundary of the vermilion border; (C) 1 month after surgery

Advancement Flaps

Incision Placement

Advancement flaps produce a one-dimensional mass movement of tissue. Incisions are placed within or parallel to pre-existing folds and wrinkles extending from an edge of the skin defect.

Extent of Undermining/Dissection

The tissue delineated between these two incisions is elevated in a subdermal plane, and the area is undermined on both sides as well as beyond the base, so that the elevated flap can be advanced into the defect and the skin redundancy of the donor defect site can be distributed along the smaller length of the flap margin.

Tissue Modifications

Tissue advancement: The flap is then advanced into the defect. This necessitates some movement of tissue from the base toward the defect. This movement subsequently generates a standing cone deformity at the junction of the flap base and incisions.

Closure

Closure is generally performed with resorbable sutures placed at the dermal level. It is helpful to place these closer to the base initially, advancing the flap with distributed tension and requiring fewer deep sutures near the distal tip of the flap. Skin is closed with interrupted 4-0 to 6-0 resorbable sutures at the dermal level and smaller monofilament sutures for cutaneous closure. It is prudent to defer any skin resection until the wound tension has been distributed (Figs 19.6A to D).

Burow's Triangles

The movement of the flap into the defect creates standing cone deformities near the base of the flap. These can be treated with Burow's triangle skin excisions that allow the scar to best approximate RSTLs. These are closed in the same way as the flap.

Rotation Flaps

Incision Placement

Rotation flaps produce two-dimensional rotation movement of tissue. Incisions are also placed within or parallel to pre-existing folds and wrinkles extending from an edge of the skin defect, and hence are appropriate in areas with curvilinear RSTLs. As a rule of thumb, the incision length is approximately four times the diameter of the defect (Figs 19.7A to D).

Extent of Undermining/Dissection

The flap as well as some of the intact side of the incision should be undermined to allow the elevated flap to be rotated into the defect and allows most of the skin redundancy of the donor defect site to be distributed.

Tissue Modifications

Tissue advancement: The flap is then rotated into the defect. This creates some redundancy of skin on the non-flap side of the incision and may generate a standing cone deformity.

Closure

Closure is generally performed with resorbable sutures placed at the dermal level, distributing skin redundancy evenly, and external 4-0 to 6-0 monofilament sutures are used for the skin. If skin excess remains, a Burow's triangle can be excised as necessary.

Burow's Triangles

Standing cones generally occur opposite the base of the flap, but Burow's triangles can be placed anywhere along the length of the closure for correction, and are positioned to maximally benefit from aesthetic borders or RSTLs.

Transposition Flaps-Bilobed Flaps

Incision Placement

These flaps which rotate, advance and transpose normal tissue are designed around a central pivot point. A line is then drawn from the pivot point to the distal edge of the defect, and this distance is used to create an arc around the pivot point. The distance from the defect center to the pivot point is measured and used to create a second arc around the pivot point. The primary flap is then created so that its diameter is 75–80% of the defect at the inner arc. A second flap is then created in or near a RSTL so that its width at the inner arc is 75% of the primary flap diameter (Figs 19.8A to E).

Extent of Undermining/Dissection

The entire flap as well as the surrounding tissues are then widely undermined to allow not only transposition of the flap but closure of the secondary flap defect primarily.

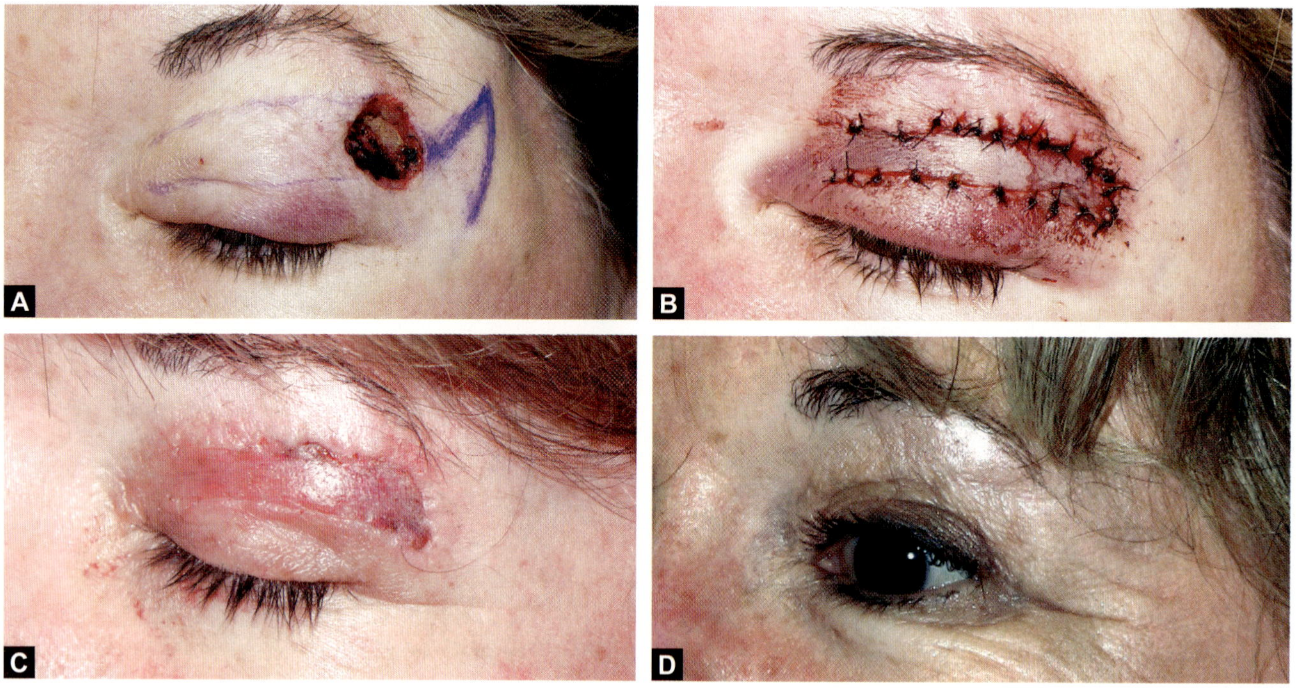

Figs 19.6A to D: (A) Defect of the upper eyelid involving skin and orbicularis oculi muscle and exposing the orbital septum; (B) Musculocutaneous flap elevated and advanced to close the defect; (C) Appearance of flap 1 week after repair; (D) Appearance 9 years after surgery

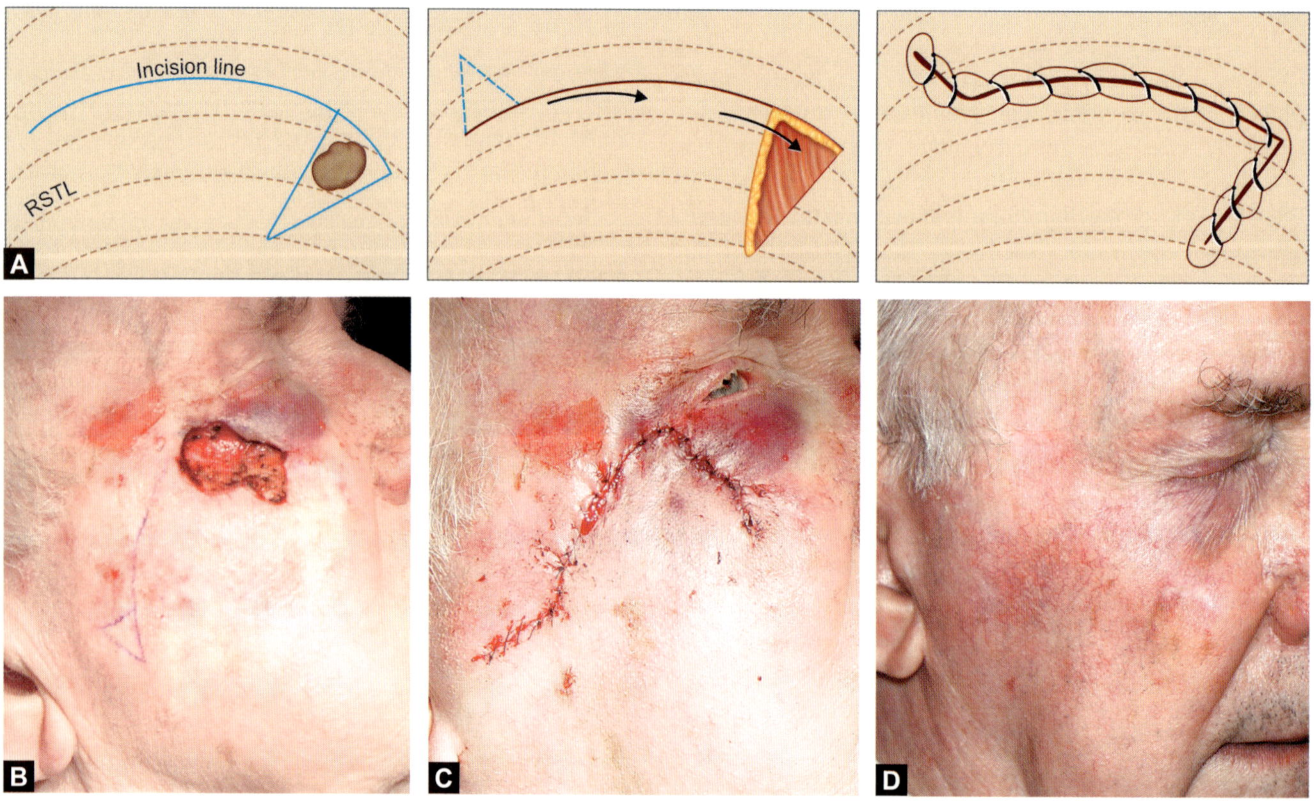

Figs 19.7A to D: Rotation flap. (A) Design extends from one edge of the defect around a pivot point; (B) Defect of the lateral canthal area with rotation flap design shown; (C) The flap is transposed and anchored medially to the periosteum with a resorbable suture; (D) 3 weeks after repair

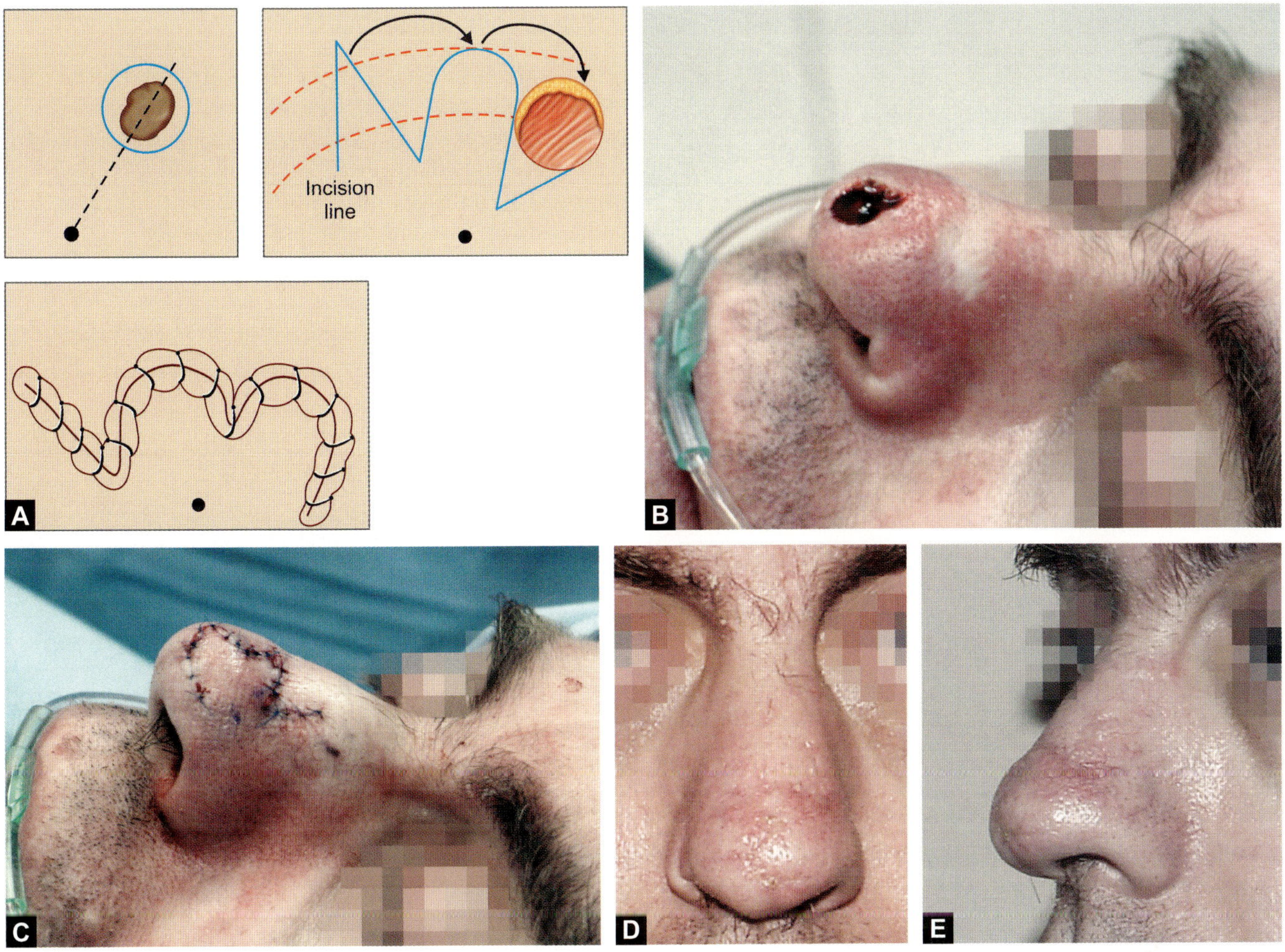

Figs 19.8A to E: Bilobed flap. (A) Flap design includes a primary flap (75–80% of the diameter of the defect) and a secondary flap (75–80% of the diameter of the primary flap), both of which rotate around a common pivot point. Dotted lines intersect the distal aspect and the center of the defect and also rotate about the pivot point and are useful in gauging the size of the flaps; (B) Nasal tip defect; (C) repaired with a bilobed flap; (D and E) Appearance 2 weeks after repair

Tissue Modifications

Tissue advancement: The flap is then transposed into the defect (primary lobe) and the primary flap donor site (secondary lobe). The flaps are trimmed to fit the defects precisely. Flap transposition necessitates some movement of tissue from the base toward the defect. This movement generates a standing cone deformity in between the defect and the pivot point. As some skin redistribution will occur, treatment of these is deferred until after closure.

Closure

Closure is generally performed with resorbable sutures placed at the dermal level. It is helpful to close the secondary flap donor site first, advancing the skin edges together for primary closure. The flaps are then inset as appropriate. Skin is closed with interrupted 4-0 to 6-0 resorbable sutures at the dermal level and smaller monofilament sutures for cutaneous closure.

Burow's Triangles

The movement of the flap into the defect creates standing cone deformities near the base of the flap. These are treated with Burow's triangles as needed.

Rhombic Flap

Incision Placement

A true rhombic flap closes a rhombus with two 60° and two 120° angles. An incision extending from a 120° angle is made parallel to and equal in length to the short axis of the rhombus. A back cut parallel to and equal in length to the rhombus side is made. As can be seen from the diagram, with any given orientation of the rhombus, four flaps can be constructed, and should be planned to allow incisions to lie as close to RSTLs as possible (Figs 19.9A to E). One should keep in mind that the points of maximal tension are located at the junction of the rhombus with the donor site closure and the closure at the distal tip of the flap. For defects that are long and narrow (especially those in which significant lateral skin movement is possible) creation of a traditional rhombus to outline the defect will sacrifice a considerable amount of normal skin. The Dufourmentel modification is useful in such cases (Figs 19.10A to D).

Extent of Undermining/Dissection

The flap is undermined, as is the area around the donor site to reduce wound closure tension.

Tissue Modifications

Tissue advancement: The flap is transposed into the defect, and occasionally needs to be trimmed to fit into the defect precisely. The donor site is closed primarily.

Closure

Closure is generally performed with resorbable sutures placed at the dermal level. The donor site should be closed first. Skin is closed with interrupted 4-0 to 6-0 resorbable sutures at the dermal level and smaller monofilament sutures for cutaneous closure.

Burow's Triangles

When properly planned, standing cones are uncommon after rhombic flap transposition.

Z-Plasty

Incision Placement

Incisions extending from the central limb of the Z-plasty are made. The angle created will affect the final orientation of the scars and will variably lengthen the scar; 30°, 45° and 60° angles will increase the distance between the ends of the original scar by 25%, 50% and 75% respectively. Since Z-plasty alters the relationship between the scar and RSTLs, the Z-plasty limbs should be carefully chosen to produce scars most well hidden (Figs 19.11A to C).

Extent of Undermining/Dissection

The two triangles outlined by the Z-plasty are elevated, but significant undermining peripherally is essential to maximize lateral movement of the surrounding skin.

Tissue Modifications

Tissue advancement: After the flaps are transposed, the overall length of the scar has increased. This is useful in treating contracted scars. This can be demonstrated by pulling the ends of the central limb away from each other prior to flap mobilization; as this distance increases, the flaps will reorient and transpose themselves.

Closure

Resorbable sutures are placed at a dermal level to approximate the tissues, following which the skin is closed with 4-0 to 6-0 monofilament sutures.

Potential Complications

Death of Flap or Graft

Local skin flaps in the face are very hardy due to the robust collateral circulation in the face. In general, flaps should have a length:width ratio of no more than 4-6:1, to ensure adequate arterial supply and venous drainage. Complete flap loss is generally due to compromise of the flap pedicle by internal (hematoma) or external (excessive rotation or narrowing of the flap) factors, and flap elevation should preserve a small amount of subdermal fat to ensure protection of the subdermal plexus. Infection or excessive tension on the wound edges may cause partial flap loss, evidenced by wound dehiscence (see below) or superficial epidermolysis. FTSGs will survive if they are secured in place to prevent micromotion relative to the flap base and any fluid collection between graft and base. This ensures that serum imbibition supports the graft for the first 48 hours, after which endothelial buds develop from the wound base and anastomose with blood vessels within the graft. Generally, flap or graft death should be treated conservatively, allowing the nonviable tissues to demarcate prior to debridement. Once a healthy wound base and edges are assured, primary closure or another flap or graft can be used.

Wound Dehiscence

As noted above, excessive wound tension can lead to early flap dehiscence. Wide undermining and supporting dermal sutures can generally prevent this complication. If this does occur, as with flap death, treatment should be conservation. Generally, with additional undermining the dehiscence can be closed primarily.

Pincushion/Trapdoor

Any flap, but especially those bounded by a concave or curvilinear scar, may develop a pincushion or trapdoor deformity. The natural contractile forces of a scar will be

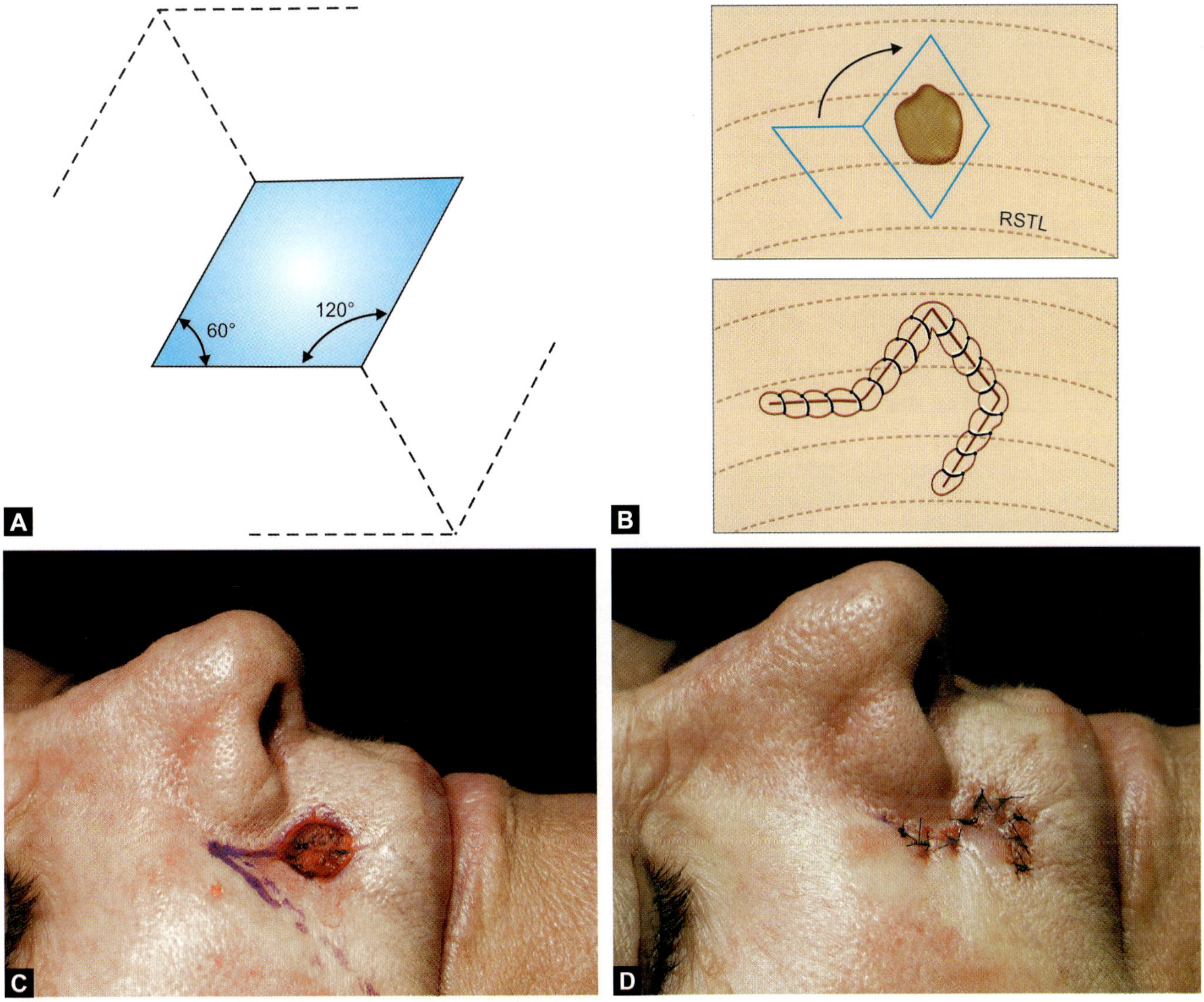

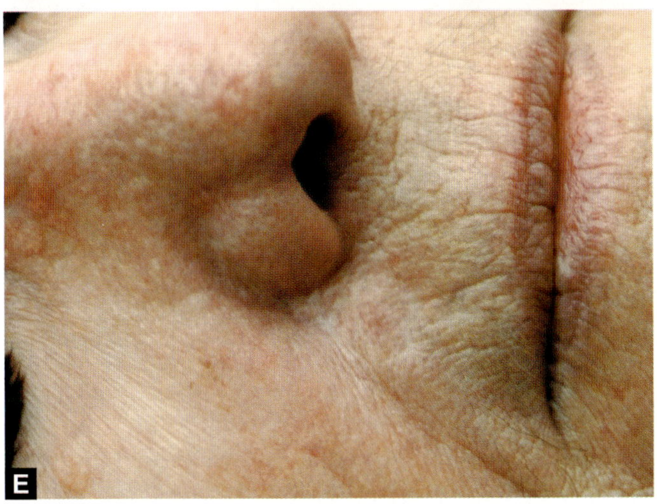

Figs 19.9A to E: Rhombic flap. (A) Once a rhombus is drawn around a defect, four distinct flaps are possible; (B) While predictable, scars of a rhombic flap repair may run against relaxed skin tension lines; (C) Upper lip defect is (D) repaired with a laterally based rhombic flap; (E) 4 weeks after surgery

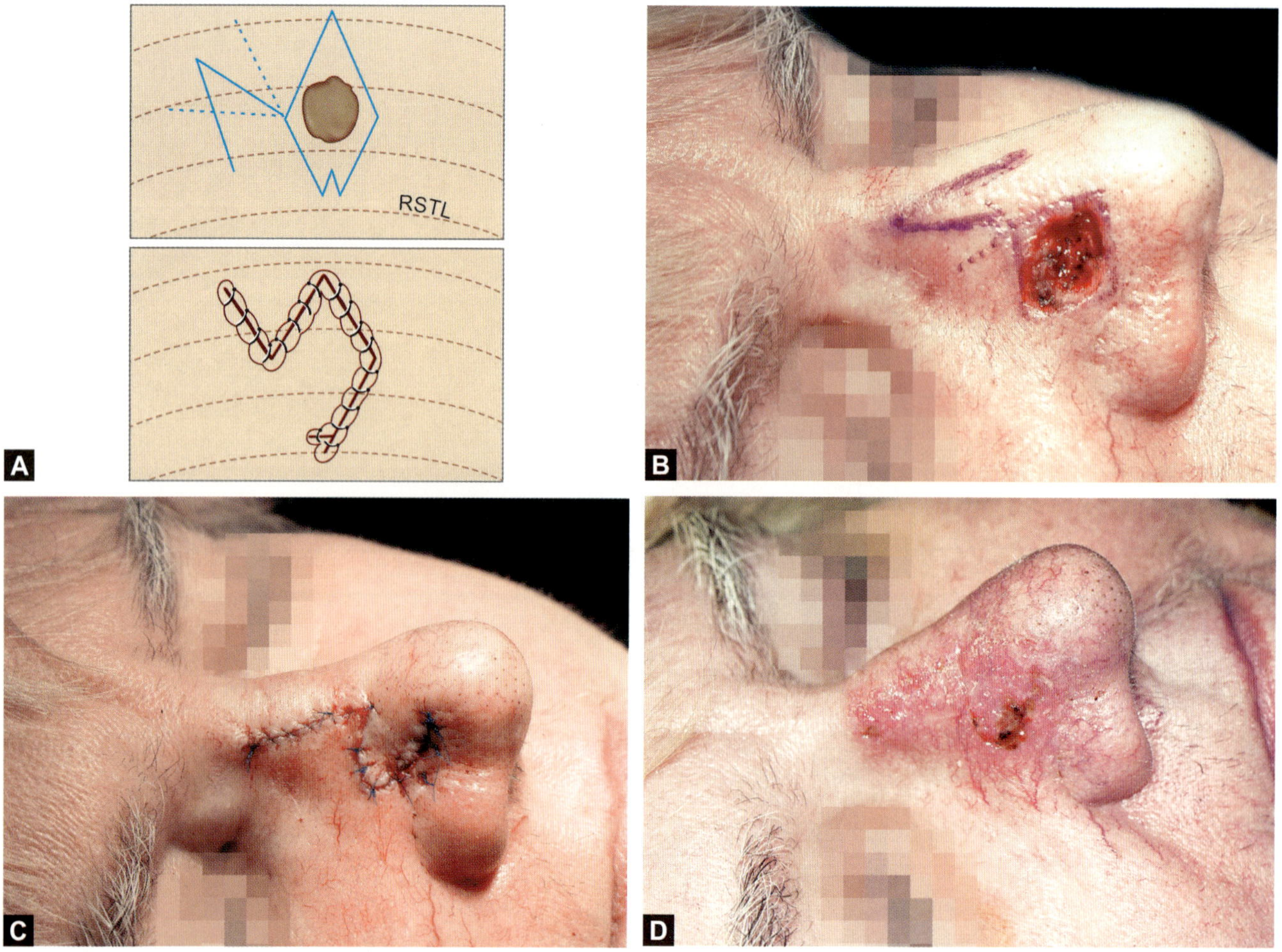

Figs 19.10A to D: (A) Dufourmentel modification of the rhombic flap; (B) Defect of the lateral nasal sidewall. Note the dotted lines extending the side of the rhomboid and the short diagonal; (C) Rotation of the flap to fill the defect is possible because of the lateral movement of skin across the nasal dorsum; (D) 1 week after repair

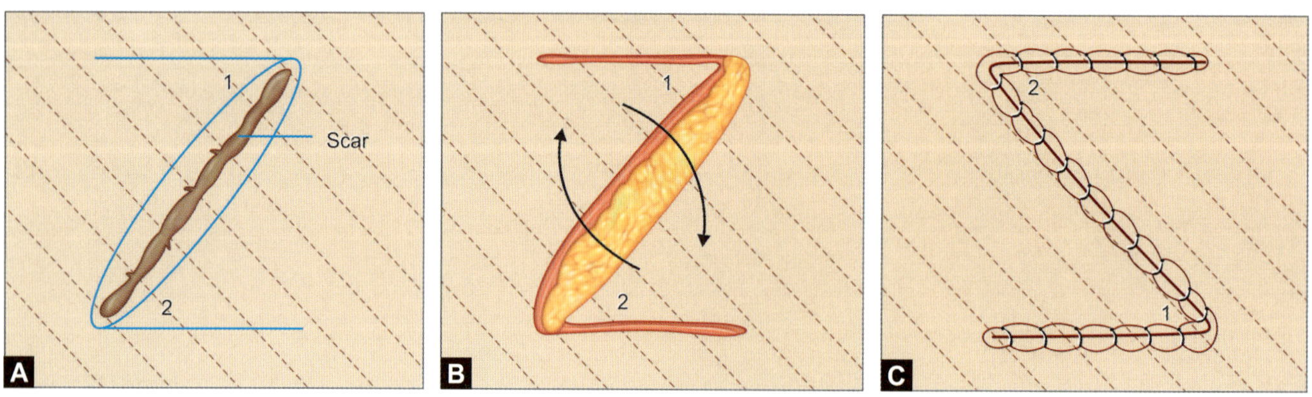

Figs 19.11A to C: Z-plasty

additive toward the center of any flap with a concave scar. Good dermal support with sutures and wide undermining to distribute scar contractile forces generally can prevent the inward contraction and excessive scarring of a pincushion deformity. Injection of small amounts of dilute corticosteroids (triamcinolone acetate, 5–20 mg/cc) into the subdermal scar can usually soften and flatten these deformities, but occasional scar revision with excision of scar tissue, wide undermining and repair with dermal supporting sutures may be necessary.

Unacceptable (Wide/Atrophic, Hypertrophic, Keloid) Scarring

Wide scars are generally associated with excessive wound closure tension and this has also been implicated in the development of some hypertrophic and keloid scars. Scar excision, undermining and layered closure is the preferred treatment, unless contour deformities are mild enough to be treated with dermabrasion alone. Hypertrophic and keloid scars should be treated with serial intralesional corticosteroids.

Distortion of Surrounding Tissues

Surrounding tissues may be distorted in one of two ways: (1) direct distraction of surrounding tissues may occur if flaps are inadequately designed, (2) secondary distortion can occur as a result of postoperative fibrosis. Flaps which are too small or inadequately undermined will exert a pull on the surrounding tissues and may pull mobile structures like the eyelids, lips or alar rim. Additionally, bunching of skin around the flap pivot point may lead to tissue distortion caused by the skin excess.

Telangiectasias or Scar Erythema

Pre-existing telangiectasias may become more prominent after skin defect repair while there is local vasodilatation. Scars will progress through a "red" phase, typically worst at 5–6 weeks postoperatively, after which this erythema will gradually fade. Persistent erythema can be treated with pulsed dye or Nd-YAG laser therapy.

AFTERCARE

Sutures are generally removed at 5–7 days after surgery. Scars can be laser- or mechano-resurfaced after 6 weeks if necessary.

BIBLIOGRAPHY

1. Chu EA, Byrne PJ. Local flaps I: bilobed, rhombic, and cervicofacial. Facial Plast Surg Clin North Am. 2009;17(3): 349-60.
2. Menick FJ. The evolution of lining in nasal reconstruction. Clin Plast Surg. 2009;36:421-41.
3. Siddiqui A, Ditmars DM. Island rotation flap for nasal reconstruction. Plast Reconstr Surg. 2005;116(6):1604-9.
4. Zitelli JA. The bilobed flap for nasal reconstruction. Arch Dermatol. 1989;125(7):957-9.

CHAPTER

20

Myocutaneous and Microvascular Flaps

Grigoriy Mashkevich

OVERVIEW

Myocutaneous and microvascular flaps provide an excellent source of reliable tissue for coverage of various defects involving the head and neck, and upper aerodigestive tract. With meticulous planning, appropriately selected regional and distal flaps can optimally replenish lost tissue volume and diminish the functional impairment of virtually any defect in the head and neck region. Myocutaneous and microvascular flaps are typically reserved for extensive composite wounds that would not be amenable to primary closure, secondary intention healing, or skin grafting. Potentially large surface areas and excellent pliability of flaps allow exact three-dimensional recontouring of complex head and neck defects, which lays the groundwork for optimal rehabilitation of appearance as well as speech and swallowing functions.

Flap reconstruction represents an especially important strategy in patients with previous history or anticipated treatment with radiation therapy for head and neck cancer. It introduces healthy, well-perfused tissue capable of withstanding rigors of wound healing in a compromised and surgically altered environment.

SPECIAL CONSIDERATIONS

Patients undergoing regional and free flap transfer require a complete medical evaluation and optimization in order to withstand potentially long operative times under general anesthesia. Any adverse wound healing risk factors should be assessed during medical clearance, including nutritional status, smoking, previous radiation therapy, connective tissue disorders, peripheral vascular disease, and diabetes.

Determination of the optimal flap donor site depends on the location of the head and neck defect and degree of missing tissue bulk. The majority of soft tissue reconstructions in the head and neck can be achieved with the radial forearm or anterolateral thigh (ALT) free flaps. Pectoralis major myocutaneous flap represents an excellent second choice. It can become a primary option in patients who are poor candidates for free tissue transfer, for anatomical or health reasons. Bony reconstruction of the mandible is best achieved with a fibula free flap. Alternative flap choices include radial osteocutaneous, serratus-rib, scapula, or iliac crest. Each has its pluses and minuses with respect to their bone stock, length of vascular pedicle, and ease of harvest. Facial skeletal and palate defects are best repaired with prosthetics, obturators, or a combination of free bone or cartilage grafts with a soft tissue flap cover.

Physical examination of all potential donor sites focuses on eliciting any evidence of previous trauma or surgery, which may preclude flap harvest due to concerns about potential vascular injury. In addition, assessment of the vasculature can confirm whether safe flap elevation is possible without causing extremity ischemia. Particular to the radial forearm, an Allen's test ensures that the ulnar artery can supply the entire palmar arterial arch. When occluding the radial artery, capillary refill times under 5 seconds indicate sufficient contribution by the ulnar artery to the distal aspect of this arch. Equivocal findings can be clarified with the aid of a pulse oximeter.

Assessment of the ALT as a potential donor site focuses on skin laxity and underlying soft tissue bulk. Excessive subcutaneous fat is a relative contraindication for this site for soft tissue defects involving the upper aerodigestive tract, due to concerns for potential obstruction. However, in defects such as total glossectomy, tissue bulk is typically desirable and can be a positive feature of this site.

For a fibula free flap (FFF), any exam findings with respect to the dorsalis pedis and posterior tibial pulses must be corroborated by vascular imaging. Magnetic resonance angiography (MRA) is the single most important determinant of suitability of FFF harvest.

Certain congenital configurations or peripheral vascular disease involving the peroneal artery are best detected by MRA and would preclude the use of this donor site.

In the initial stages of flap transfer, survival depends solely on perfusion through the vascular pedicle. At about 3 weeks, sufficient circulation is established across flap borders, such that transferred tissue may survive without its pedicle. This time frame does not apply in patients with history of radiation therapy, in whom the recipient tissue bed possesses poor circulation and requires longer time periods to establish a reliable peripheral circulation.

Several anticoagulants can be used for prevention of clot formation in the postoperative setting. These include dextran and aspirin, both of which are equally efficacious. Aspirin 81 mg is continued daily for 4 weeks following microvascular transfer to help maintain vessel patency. Broad-spectrum antibiotics, pain medications, and stool softeners are given in the immediate postoperative setting.

ALTERNATIVES TO PROCEDURE

Healing by secondary intention, skin grafting, and prosthetics represent alternative choices to myocutaneous and free flaps. However, in the majority of settings where significant tissue volume has been removed, these options provide inadequate bulk or vascularity to safely and optimally reconstruct the defect at hand.

Certain external defects, such as total rhinectomy or auriculectomy, represent excellent sites for prosthetic rehabilitation. Prosthetics are also useful in patients with external defects who are not surgical candidates or simply do not prefer to undergo extensive repairs. Prosthetics generally have good compliance and satisfaction rates, and can be attached with adhesives or onto the osseointegrated implants. Adhesives tend to be challenging to older patients who struggle with manual dexterity and poor vision.

TECHNIQUES

Pectoralis Major Myocutaneous Flap

Incision Placement

Flap design takes into account the location of the first two intercostal perforators exiting parasternally (Fig. 20.1). These perforators supply the deltopectoral flap, which spans from the upper sternum to the shoulder. This

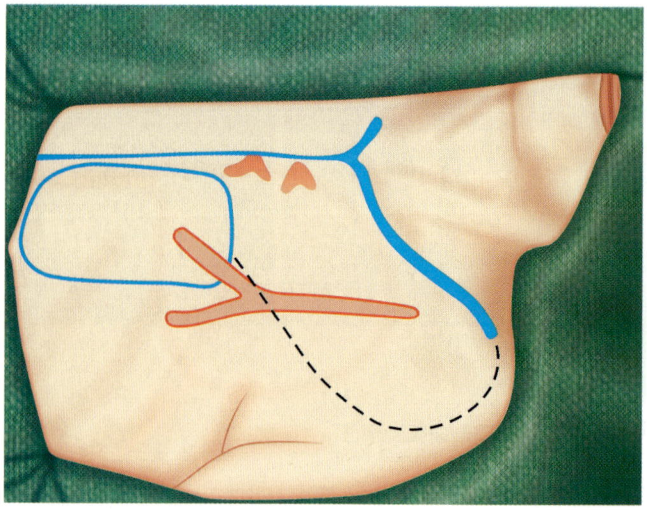

Fig. 20.1: Markings for the pectoralis major flap. The first two intercostal perforators are shown just lateral to the sternum, in the medial aspect of the first two intercostal spaces. The superior border of the skin paddle is marked inferior to the location of the second perforator. The size of the skin paddle reflects the surface area of the defect. A deltopectoral flap is outlined extending to the shoulder. This incorporates three adjacent angiosomes and assists in delay of this flap, should it become needed. Approximate course of the pectoralis major pedicle (pectoral branch of the thoracoacromial artery) is marked along the line between the acromion and xyphoid

cutaneous flap can be used in cases of pectoralis major failure, and its pedicle should be preserved. The skin paddle for the pectoralis major flap is marked below the first two intercostal perforators. The size of the skin paddle is equivalent to the size of anticipated defect. As much as possible, the majority of the skin paddle should be marked over the pectoralis major muscle. While extending the skin paddle beyond the muscle border is acceptable, it increases random blood supply to the skin paddle and raises the probability of partial skin necrosis. An incision from the superior-lateral corner of the skin paddle is marked toward the deltopectoral groove of the shoulder.

Extent of Undermining/Dissection

All incisions are made as marked, down to the level of the pectoralis major muscle. Superiorly, the supramuscular plane is dissected toward the clavicle. A generous communication is made with the neck, to accommodate freely the width and bulk of the flap (Fig. 20.2). Medially, care is taken to stay lateral to the location of deltopectoral flap perforators. At this location, the pectoralis major muscle is incised down to the level of the chest wall.

Laterally, the pectoralis major muscle is exposed on its undersurface and its pedicle (pectoral branch of the thoracoacromial artery) is identified (Fig. 20.3).

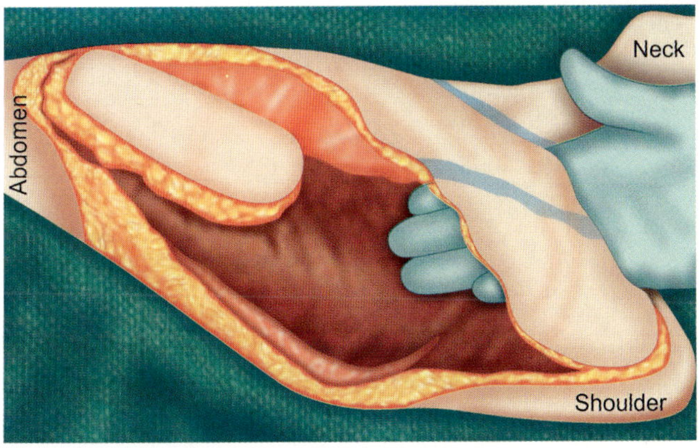

Fig. 20.2: Supramuscular communication with the neck over the clavicle and underneath the central and lateral angiosomes of the deltopectoral flap

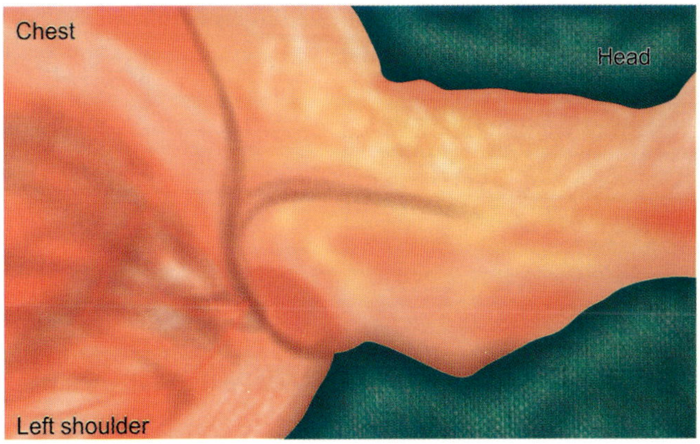

Fig. 20.3: Pectoralis major myocutaneous flap with its pedicle (pectoral branch of the thoracoacromial artery) coursing underneath

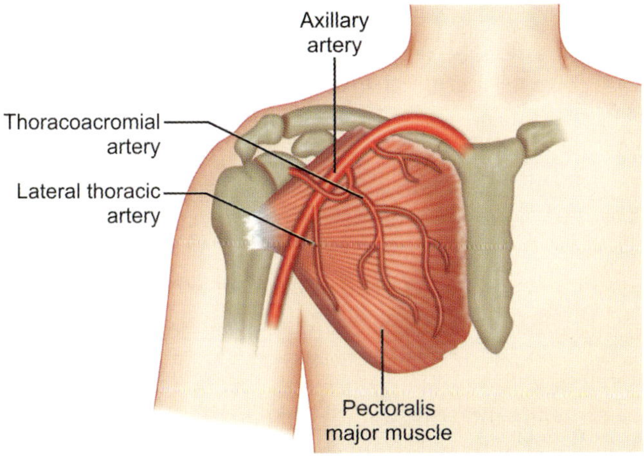

Fig. 20.4: Lateral thoracic artery and muscular attachments to the humerus, requiring transection in order to increase the arc of rotation and reach of the flap

Superolaterally, the attachment of the muscle to the humerus is divided. Similarly, branches of the lateral thoracic artery entering the pectoralis major muscle are divided, increasing the arc of rotation (Fig. 20.4). Once the flap is fully elevated from the underlying rib cage and the pectoralis minor muscle, the skin paddle is introduced into the neck through a previously created tunnel over the clavicle.

Tissue Modifications

- *Tissue advancement*: Great care is taken to handle the skin paddle gently in order to avoid shearing perforating vessels. With good mobilization, the pectoralis major flap can reach as high as ipsilateral zygoma. However, excessive tension on the pectoralis major skin paddle increases the risk of skin ischemia. Partial skin paddle loss can occur in as many as half of all pectoralis major myocutaneous flaps.
- *Suturing*: Securing of the skin paddle is best performed in layers. For external defects, 3-0 Vicryl (Ethicon, Somerville, New Jersey, US) is used for deep layers and 5-0 Nylon is used for skin. For internal resurfacing, transcutaneous horizontal mattress 3-0 Vicryl sutures are utilized for skin paddle fixation to surrounding tissues. Several Vicryl sutures can also be placed to suspend the muscle portion of the flap in order to offset its weight and diminish tension on the perforators. Care must be taken to stay clear of the pedicle situated on the undersurface of the pectoralis major muscle.

Closure

- *Layers/sutures*: The donor defect is closed similarly with a combination of 3-0 Vicryl and 5-0 Nylon sutures.
- *Skin excision*: Skin paddle can be modified depending on the needs of the defect. The resulting chest wall defect can be closed primarily in most situations. Excision of Burrow's triangles is typically necessary to avoid tissue distortion while closing the chest wound.
- *Drains*: A single active drain is placed to evacuate drainage from the chest wound. It may take several days for drainage to sufficiently subside before the drain can be safely removed.
- *Dressings*: Skin staples are covered liberally with bacitracin antibiotic ointment. This continues twice per day for 2 weeks, at which point staples are removed. Patients can shower and clean all incisions with soap and water in 48 hours following surgery.

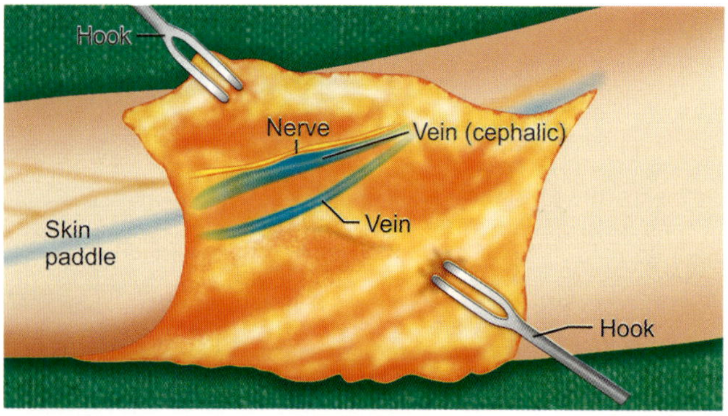

Fig. 20.5: Cephalic vein is identified proximal to the skin paddle in the subcutaneous tissues of the forearm

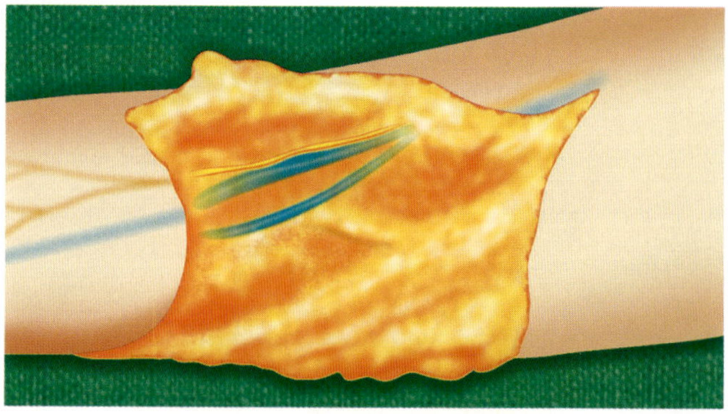

Fig. 20.6: Full course of the cephalic vein is exposed following elevation of the medial and lateral skin flaps in the proximal forearm

Radial Forearm Free Flap

Radial forearm free flap (RFFF) is an ideal soft tissue flap for many head and neck defects. The mid-distal skin of the forearm is highly pliable and can conform to various configurations matching the intricate head and neck anatomy. Common sites for repair with this flap include the tongue and pharynx. The other attractive feature of this flap is its long vascular pedicle and redundant venous drainage. In vessel-depleted necks, the pedicle can reach to the contralateral side for anastomosis with recipient vessels. The venous outflow through the superficial cephalic vein and the deep venous system readily intercommunicates via a number of small vessels. This redundancy allows selection of either vein for the microvenous anastomosis and aids in preventing venous stasis in the flap.

Incision Placement

Skin paddle design is anatomically centered on the radial vasculature of the forearm. The medial border of the skin paddle is restricted to the palmaris tendon in order to avoid potential exposure of ulnar vessels. An incision is marked from the superior border of the skin paddle toward the elbow crease.

Extent of Undermining/Dissection

The anterior surface of the forearm is dissected to expose the brachioradialis muscle laterally and the flexor carpi ulnaris muscle medially. Once the skin paddle is elevated, the dissection proceeds deep along the course of the pedicle.

Tissue Modifications

Incision and flap elevation: Flap elevation is performed under tourniquet compression at 250 mm Hg. Initial incisions are made around the skin paddle periphery and superiorly toward the elbow crease. At the superior border of the flap's skin paddle, cephalic vein is identified by elevating skin edges with double-prong skin hooks and dissecting with tenotomy scissors (Fig. 20.5). This vein is followed along its anterior surface to the level of the elbow crease.

Lateral and medial skin flaps are then developed (Fig. 20.6). The brachioradialis muscle is exposed and fascia lateral to the pedicle is dissected away from this muscle, toward the pedicle (Fig. 20.7). Perforating vessels are divided with either bipolar cautery or harmonic scalpel. In the distal forearm, the superficial branch of the superficial radial nerve is identified as it exits from underneath the brachioradialis tendon (Fig. 20.8). This nerve is sharply dissected away from the undersurface of the skin paddle using a nerve hook and a knife (Fig. 20.9).

Distally, the cephalic vein is identified, ligated, and divided. Radial artery and accompanying venae comitantes are identified next (Fig. 20.10). Medial dissection is completed in a similar fashion by mobilizing fascia toward the pedicle and away from the underlying flexor musculature. The skin paddle is then lifted from the wound and deep perforating vessels are divided in succession, from distal to proximal.

In the proximal forearm, a Weitlaner retractor is placed to improve visualization of proximal forearm vasculature. The flap pedicle is then traced toward its takeoff from the brachial vessels. Care is taken to identify a communicating vein between the deep system and the cephalic vein (Fig. 20.11). All vessels are then circumferentially isolated and the flap is reperfused by releasing the tourniquet.

Suturing: For external defects, 3-0 Vicryl is used for deep layers and 5-0 Nylon is used for the skin. For internal resurfacing, transcutaneous horizontal mattress 3-0 Vicryl sutures are utilized for skin paddle fixation to surrounding tissues.

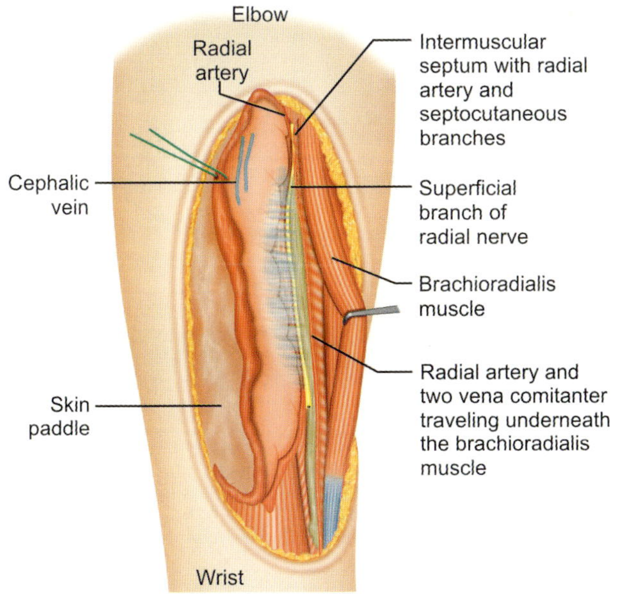

Fig. 20.7: Subfascial dissection along the brachioradialis muscle, exposing the radial artery and venae comitantes. Perforators emanating from the radial artery and entering into the brachioradialis muscle are divided

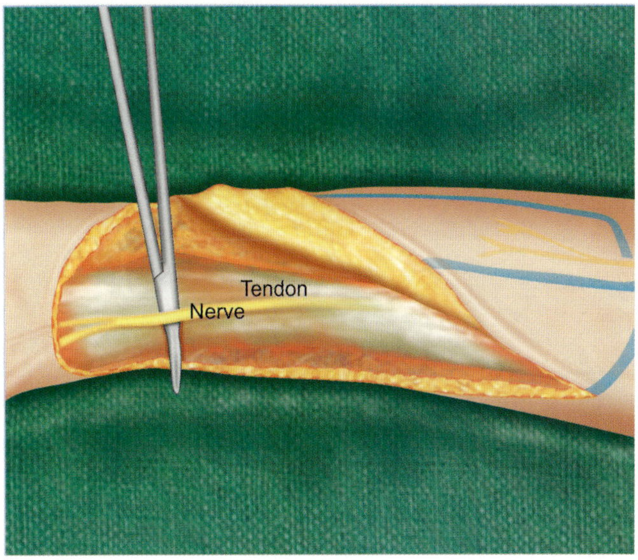

Fig. 20.8: Superficial branch of the superficial radial nerve is identified as it exits laterally from the undersurface of the brachioradialis tendon

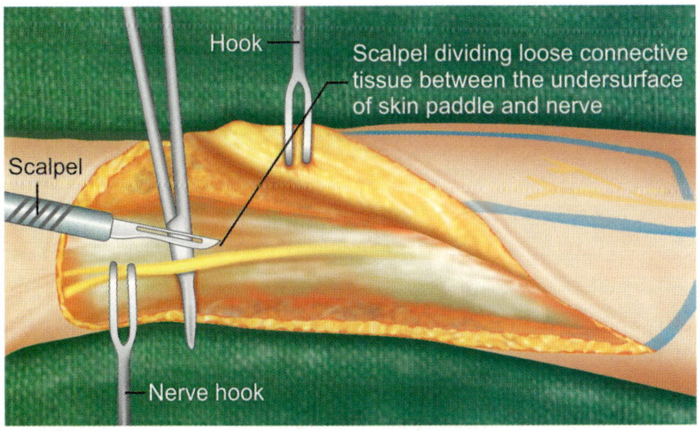

Fig. 20.9: Superficial radial nerve is sharply separated from the undersurface of the skin paddle

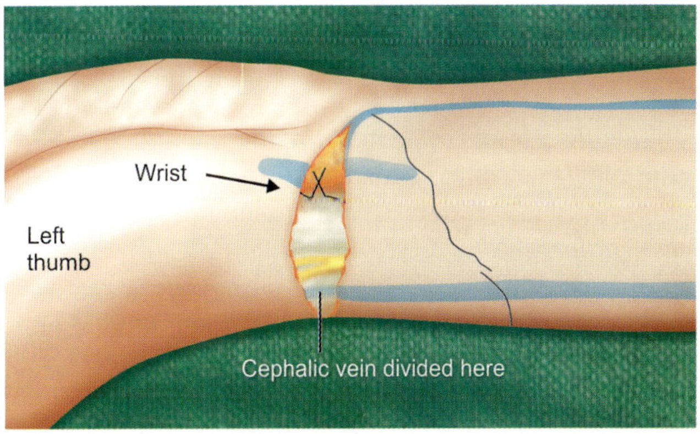

Fig. 20.10: Distal cephalic vein and radial artery with accompanying vena comitantes are identified and divided distal to the skin paddle

Closure

- *Skin excision and grafting*: Excess skin is removed after overlapping medial and lateral skin flaps. The surface area of the wound is diminished by securing wound periphery to the underlying forearm tendons and muscles. A split thickness skin graft is then obtained from the thigh and is perforated with a scalpel in multiple locations. This promotes egress of fluid from underneath the skin graft. A bolster consisting of Xeroform™ (Covidien, Mansfield, Massachusetts, US) wrapped around cotton balls saturated in mineral oil is secured on top of the skin graft.
- *Drains*: No drains are placed in the forearm as perforated skin graft allows passive egress of fluid from the wound.
- *Dressings*: A short arm splint is placed after wrapping the forearm with several layers of Webrill™ cotton padding. The purpose of the splint is to immobilize the forearm and avoid movement around the skin graft. It also provides support against early contracture of the wrist.

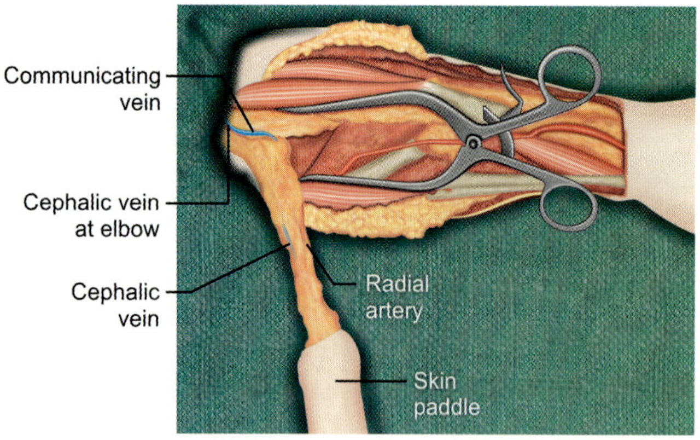

Fig. 20.11: Flap paddle elevation and dissection of the proximal vasculature. Care is taken to identify and preserve a communicating vein between the deep system (vena comitantes) and cephalic vein

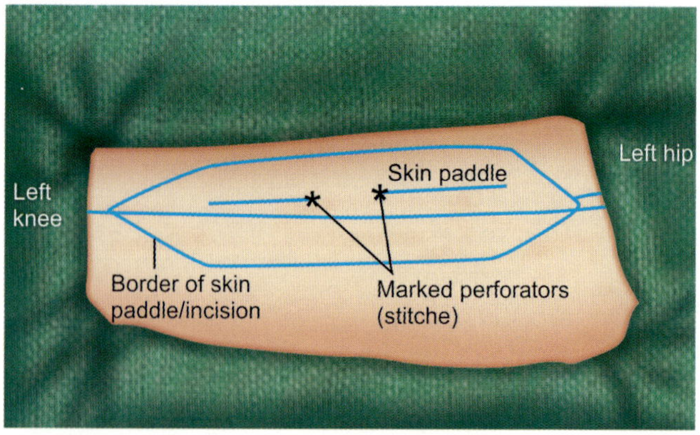

Fig. 20.12: Markings for the anterolateral thigh (ALT) free flap. Perforating branches of the descending branch of the lateral circumflex artery are identified with a Doppler probe along the line connecting anterior superior iliac spine with superolateral patella. The skin paddle is centered on perforators as shown

Anterolateral Thigh Free Flap

The main advantage of the ALT flap over the radial forearm is reduced donor site morbidity. Most thigh defects following flap harvest can be closed primarily, thereby avoiding the need for a skin graft.

Incision Placement

Skin paddle design depends on the identification of perforating vessels from the flap's pedicle—the descending branch of the lateral circumflex femoral vasculature. These perforators lie close to a line drawn between the anterior superior iliac spine and superolateral patella. After pinching redundant skin of the thigh, medial and lateral borders for this flap can be marked (Fig. 20.12).

Extent of Undermining/Dissection

The anterior surface of the thigh is dissected to expose the rectus femoris muscle medially and the vastus lateralis muscle laterally. Following skin paddle elevation, the dissection proceeds deep along the course of the pedicle and between the above muscles.

Tissue Modifications

- *Incision and flap elevation*: Medial incision is performed first, through skin, subcutaneous tissues, and fascia lata. Allis clamps are placed on the fascia lata and identification of perforating vessels is performed in the subfacial plane (Fig. 20.13). Once a sufficient number of perforating vessels is identified, they are dissected toward the pedicle. Musculocutaneous perforators require dissection within the vastus lateralis muscle.

  The vastus lateralis muscle is first divided over the anterior surface of perforators. This can be safely accomplished by dissecting muscle tissue with tenotomy scissors and dividing it with bipolar cautery or harmonic scalpel (Fig. 20.14). Next, a cuff of muscle measuring approximately half a centimeter is dissected on each side of the perforator. This cuff of muscle allows protection and preservation of these fine vessels.

  Once perforators are sufficiently dissected, a posterior incision is made and the skin paddle is elevated from the wound (Fig. 20.15). The distal pedicle is identified, ligated, and divided. A deep retractor is placed in the proximal thigh in order to create space between the rectus femoris and vastus lateralis muscles. The pedicle is then followed proximally and its vessels are circumferentially isolated (Fig. 20.16). Branches of the femoral nerve found within the pedicle are mobilized whenever possible.
- *Suturing*: For external defects, 3-0 Vicryl is used for deep layers and 5-0 Nylon is used for the skin. For internal resurfacing, transcutaneous horizontal mattress 3-0 Vicryl sutures are utilized for skin paddle fixation to surrounding tissues.

Closure

- *Layers/sutures*: The thigh wound is closed in layers after undermining medial and lateral edges in the supramuscular plane and placing a row of towel

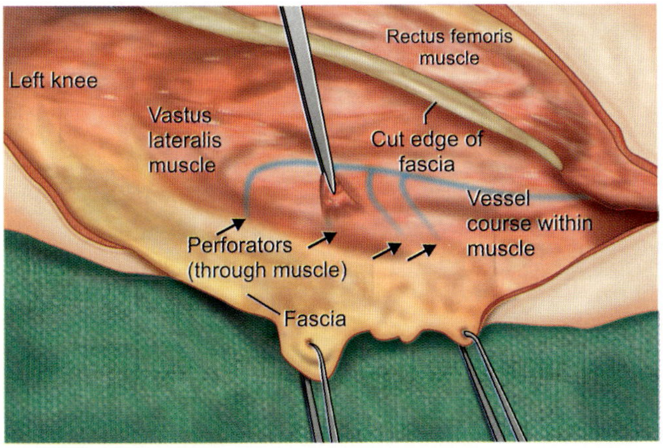

Fig. 20.13: Identification of the perforating vessels in the subfascial plane of the fascia lata. While perforators can follow a septocutaneous course between the rectus femoris and vastus lateralis muscles, most commonly they are found piercing the body of the vastus lateralis

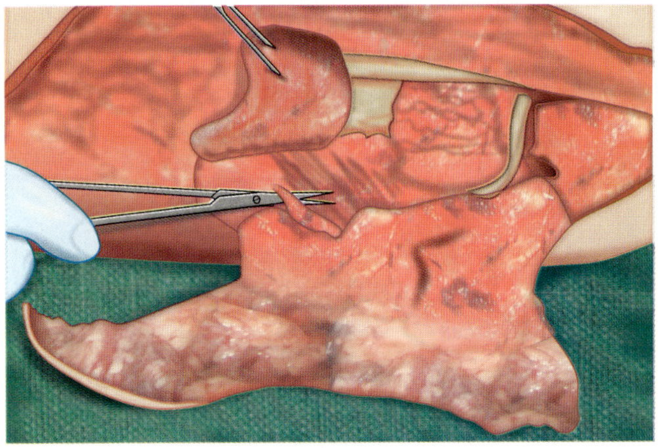

Fig. 20.14: Perforating vessels are dissected by dividing the overlying vastus lateralis muscle. Dissection continues until descending branches of the lateral circumflex femoral artery and vein are encountered

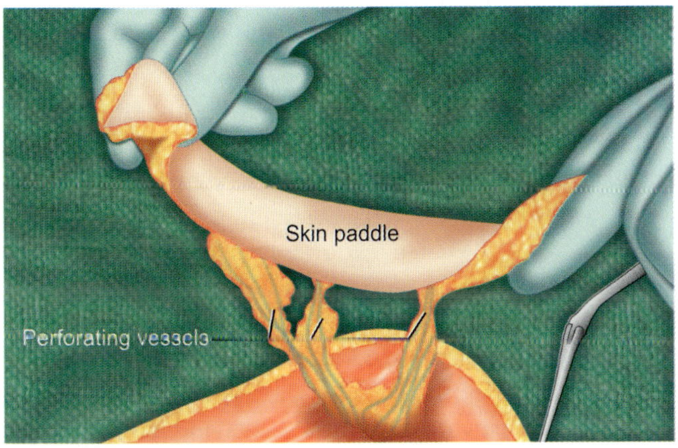

Fig. 20.15: Posterior incision and elevation of the skin paddle, with preservation of perforating vessels. A 1–2 cm cuff of muscle is left around each perforator during dissection

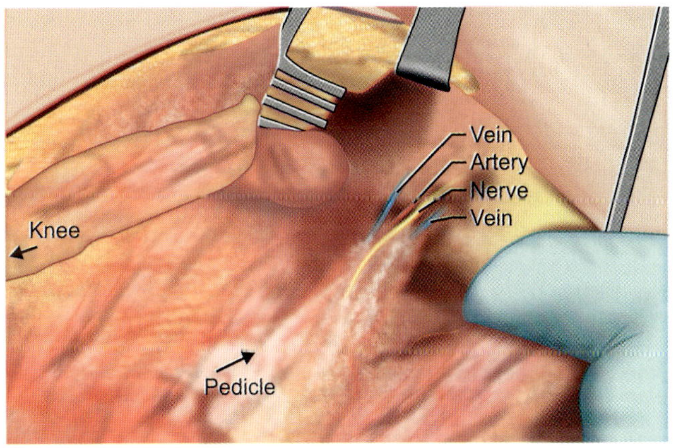

Fig. 20.16: Proximal identification and circumferential dissection of descending branches of the lateral circumflex femoral artery and vein

clamps to assist with intraoperative creep. 3-0 Vicryl sutures are placed into the deep dermal layer and staples are used to close the skin.

- *Drains*: A single active drain is placed to evacuate drainage from the thigh wound. It may take several days for drainage to sufficiently subside before the drain can be safely removed.
- *Dressings*: Skin staples are covered liberally with bacitracin antibiotic ointment. This continues twice per day for 2 weeks, at which point staples are removed. Patients can shower and clean all incisions with soap and water in 48 hours following surgery.

Fibula Free Flap

Fibula free flap represents the most optimal source of tissue for bony reconstruction of the head and neck, especially the mandible. Favorable anatomic characteristics of this flap include available bone length of up to 25 cm, strong cortical bone capable of supporting osseointegrated implants, and a reliable vascular pedicle. In addition, a large area of lateral leg skin can be harvested with this flap, up to 300 cm^2. Harvesting beyond this amount risks partial skin loss. Fibular skin paddle can be used for resurfacing most tongue, cheek, and associated external defects. Fibular bone can precisely reconstitute any segmental mandible defect.

Incision Placement

Proximal and distal ends of the fibula are palpated and marked. 8 cm of bone is marked from each edge for joint preservation. Perforating vessels of the peroneal vasculature, emanating along the posterior surface of the

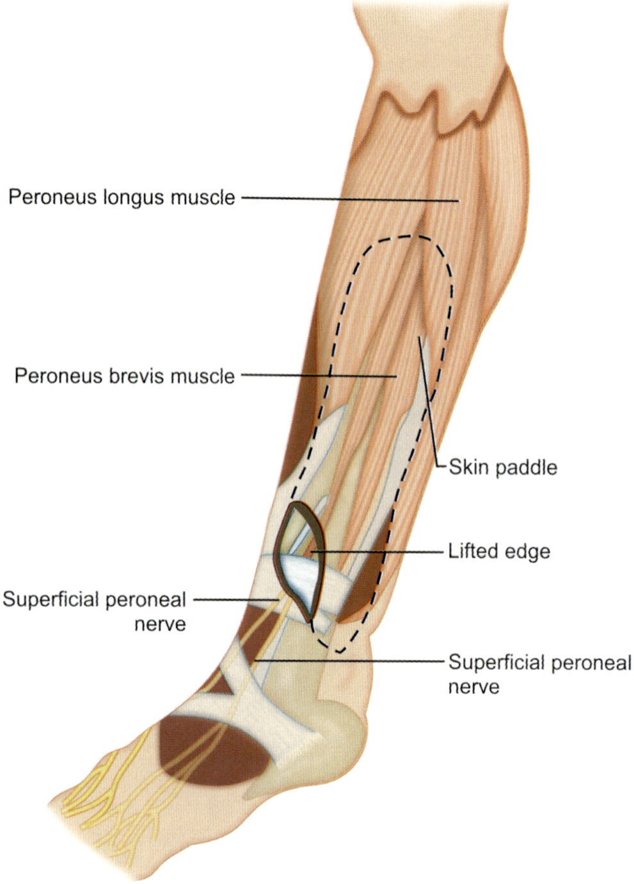

Fig. 20.17: Superficial branches of the peroneal nerve are identified and preserved at the inferior-anterior aspect of the skin incision

fibula, are then identified with a Doppler probe. These are marked with skin sutures. The skin paddle is then drawn centered on perforators.

Extent of Undermining/Dissection

Lateral surface of the lower leg is dissected to expose the anterior and posterior musculature. Following skin paddle and bony elevation the dissection proceeds deep along the course of the pedicle within the lower leg.

Tissue Modifications

- *Incision and flap elevation*: Flap elevation is performed under tourniquet compression at 350 mm Hg. Anterior incision is performed first and the skin paddle is elevated in the suprafascial plane in the posterior direction. Care is taken to identify superficial branches of the peroneal nerve and avoid injuring them (Fig. 20.17). Once the peroneus longus tendon is encountered, a subfascial incision is performed. The

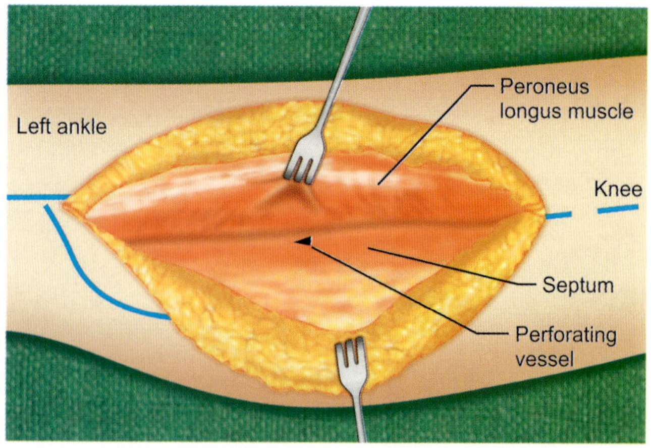

Fig. 20.18: Perforating vessels are identified along the intermuscular septum, lateral to the peroneus musculature, which is reflected anteriorly

intermuscular septum with the perforating vessels is then visualized (Fig. 20.18).

The peroneus musculature is mobilized away from the surface of the fibula in the anterior direction. The anterior compartment musculature is similarly dissected off the medial surface of the fibula while applying good traction and using cautery (Fig. 20.19). Once the interosseous membrane is exposed, it is sharply divided, taking care to avoid injuring the peroneal vasculature in the distal third of the dissection field.

Posterior incision is then made and the skin paddle is elevated from the soleus and gastrocnemius muscles. Inferiorly, sural nerve and saphenous veins are identified and preserved (Fig. 20.20). Care is taken to preserve the perforators as dissection proceeds anterior and deep. Once the skin paddle is isolated on the fibula bone, osteotomies are performed superiorly and inferiorly (Fig. 20.21).

Flexor hallucis muscle and distal peroneal vasculature are identified distally and divided. The pedicle is traced in the superior direction by dividing the overlying tibialis posterior muscle (Fig. 20.22). At their proximal takeoff, all vessels are circumferentially isolated. The tourniquet is released and at this point the flap is reperfused.

- *Suturing and bone contouring*: For external defects, 3-0 Vicryl is used for deep layers and 5-0 Nylon is used for the skin. For internal resurfacing, transcutaneous horizontal mattress 3-0 Vicryl sutures are utilized for skin paddle fixation to surrounding tissues. Contouring of the fibula bone is accomplished with closing osteotomies.

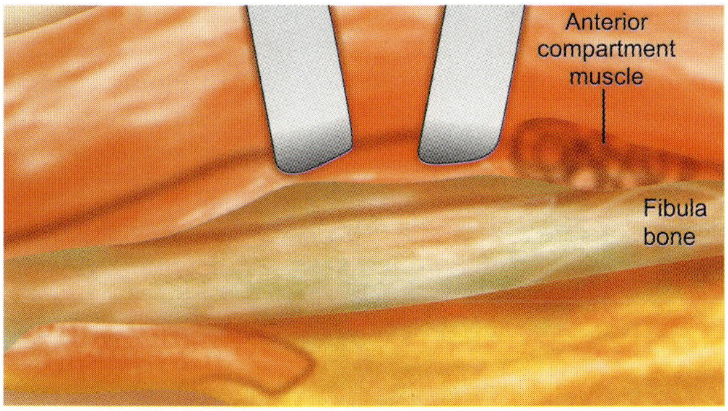

Fig. 20.19: Dissection of the anterior compartment musculature away from the fibula leads to identification of the anterior tibial artery and superficial peroneal nerve. The interosseous membrane is identified deep

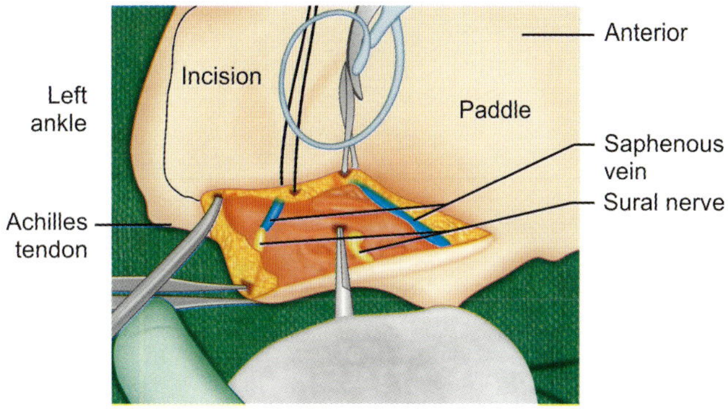

Fig. 20.20: Sural nerve and adjacent saphenous vein are identified in the subcutaneous tissues at the inferior-posterior aspect of the skin paddle. These structures are preserved and dissected away from the Achilles tendon

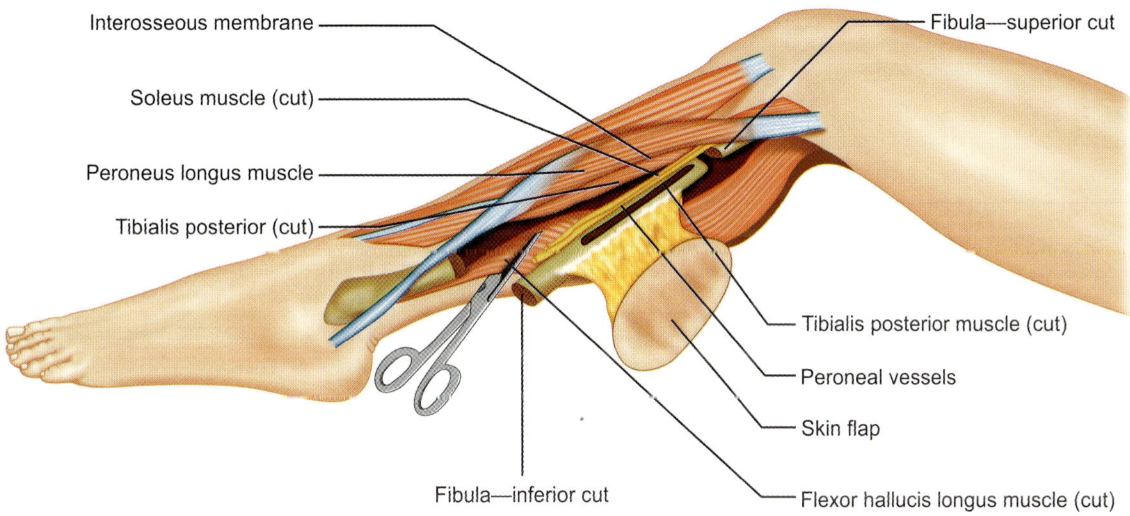

Fig. 20.21: Proximal and distal osteotomies of the fibula bone. A right angle clamp is passed around the fibula shaft, followed by insertion of a malleable retractor, which protects soft tissues against the oscillating saw

Closure

- *Skin grafting*: Most cutaneous defects arising from FFF harvest require skin grafting. The surface area of the wound is diminished by securing wound periphery to the underlying forearm tendons and muscles. A split thickness skin graft is then obtained from the thigh and is perforated with a scalpel in multiple locations. This promotes egress of fluid from underneath the skin graft. A bolster consisting of Xeroform™ wrapped around cotton balls saturated in mineral oil is secured on top of the skin graft. Any remaining incision sites amenable to primary closure are then repaired with 3-0 Vicryl dermal sutures and staples superficially.
- *Dressings*: A short leg splint is placed after wrapping the lower leg with several layers of Webrill™ cotton padding. The purpose of the splint is to immobilize the leg and avoid movement around the skin graft. It also provides support against early contracture of the ankle.

POTENTIAL COMPLICATIONS

Short-term risks related to flap surgery include flap failure and donor site complications such as infection, hematoma, and neurovascular compromise of extremity—all of which are extremely rare. Long-term problems include donor site appearance, scarring and contracture, range of motion impairment and gait disturbance.

Flap Failure

Arterial or venous obstruction of flap vasculature constitutes a flap emergency and requires immediate intervention. The most common cause of vascular

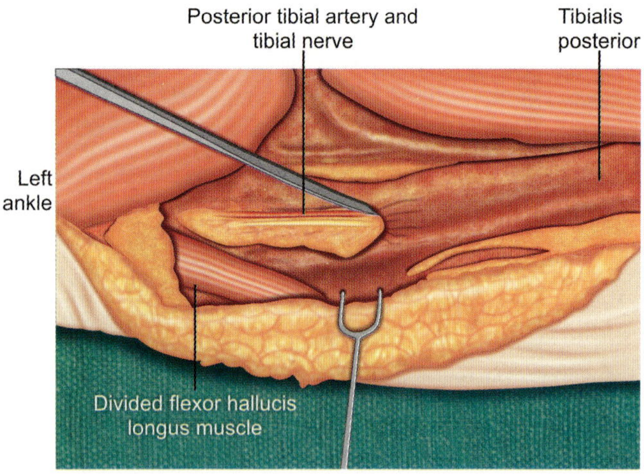

Fig. 20.22: Tibialis posterior muscle is divided exposing the tibial nerve and tibialis posterior vasculature, which joins with the peroneal system superiorly. Peroneal vessels are then circumferentially isolated, concluding the fibula free flap (FFF) harvest

obstruction is thrombus formation. Multiple flap factors can contribute to this event, including poor vessel geometry (kinking or twisting), poorly executed anastomosis (insufficient vessel preparation and cleaning, inadvertently spanning the vessel lumen with sutures), or underlying medical problems predisposing to a hypercoagulable state. Clot formation is most common within 72 hours of performing microvascular anastomosis. Insufficient arterial flow through the flap manifests with paleness of tissue, absent blood flow on needle pricking, and absent arterial Doppler signal. Venous obstruction results in engorged tissues, with continuous dark venous oozing on needle pricking, and a single-phase "water hammer" signal on Doppler ultrasound. These scenarios necessitate urgent return to the operating room for re-exploration of blood vessels, clot evacuation, and revision of anastomosis. If performed within 4–6 hours, revision success rates approach 50%.

Infection

Donor site infections typically manifest at 5–7 days with erythema, pain, and fever. Wound edges may form an eschar. Any suspicion of underlying tissue necrosis and abscess formation require sufficient opening of the wound, culture, irrigation, and daily care. Most open wounds heal with conservative management. However, additional modalities such as hyperbaric oxygen and wound vacuum therapy may be needed to hasten the healing process.

Hematoma

Hematoma formation at the recipient site requires urgent exploration and evacuation. An expanding hematoma may compress flap vasculature and lead to its demise. Hematomas at donor sites are managed in a similar fashion. If not addressed, they may cause compartment syndrome and threaten perfusion of the donor limb.

Neurovascular Compromise

Tight wound closure, tissue swelling, hematomas, and infections can lead to elevated wound pressures and development of compartment syndrome. While extremely rare, serial monitoring of donor limbs with sensory and motor checks guards against missing such a complication. Long-term neurologic deficits related to flap harvest include potential sensory loss in the distribution of the superficial radial nerve (RFFF) and superficial peroneal and sural nerves (FFF).

Scarring

Scar contracture with limitation of hand extension (RFFF), knee flexion (ALT), and ankle dorsiflexion (FFF) are possible. Visible deformity is least in ALT and most in RFFF and FFF owing to skin graft mismatch with surrounding tissue. Grip strength and range of motion can be affected, albeit rarely to any significant extent. Gait disturbances are rare with FFF and ALT.

AFTERCARE

Following flap surgery, donor site care depends on the mode of repair. Primarily closed sites can be washed with soap and water after 48 hours. Twice daily application of bacitracin provides a moist antibiotic environment optimal for wound healing. Skin grafted sites can be washed following bolster removal. Graft perforations tend to seep fluid for 2–3 weeks and require a dressing with Xeroform™ and gauze. All microvascular flap patients continue to take 81 mg of aspirin daily for 1 month after surgery.

BIBLIOGRAPHY

1. Suh JD, Sercarz JA, Abemayor E, et al. Analysis of outcome and complications in 400 cases of microvascular head and neck reconstruction. Arch Otolaryngol Head Neck Surg. 2004;130(8):962-6.
2. Urken ML (Ed). Atlas of Regional and Free Flaps for Head and Neck Reconstruction. Raven Press; 1995.

CHAPTER 21

Nasal, Orbital, and Frontal Sinus Fractures

Thomas C Spalla, Yuan Y Liu

INTRODUCTION

Fractures of the upper third of the face are relatively common with the nose being the most commonly fractured facial bone. This chapter is meant to serve as a guide to the evaluation and management of fractures of the nose, orbital bones and frontal sinus. Each of these fractures may occur in isolation but are not infrequently found concomitantly. The reader is encouraged to seek guidance from numerous sources, as no one source can contain all the variety of management options and pearls which are gained through years of trial and error.

PHYSICAL EXAMINATION

After ensuring that the patient has no life-threatening conditions, the maxillofacial examination can commence. Cervical spine injuries should be considered in the facial trauma patient and ruled out if there is any degree of clinical information pointing towards such an occurrence. The physical examination is not to be overlooked or supplanted by imaging studies. Simply asking the patient where they have pain can be very useful in locating injuries. The key parts to the physical examination of each associated fracture are delineated within each section pertaining to the management of the fracture.

RADIOLOGIC EXAMINATION

Plain films have limited utility in the evaluation of the facial trauma patient. The overlapping structures as well as natural suture lines can make delineation of bony fractures difficult. The only real value of an X-ray in evaluation of a nasal fracture is that it adds to a plaintiff's case should legal counsel be sought.

Computerized tomography (CT) is far superior and can accurately assess all three of the fracture sites mentioned herein. Axial, coronal, and sagittal imaging formats should be obtained in all cases to provide as much information as possible, and when dealing with significant injuries, three dimensional reformats can be beneficial. These models may help plan complex reconstructions and lend themselves to teaching trainees.

When dealing with frontal sinus fractures, if skull base trauma exists (e.g. a cribriform plate defect), magnetic resonance imaging (MRI) can be helpful in determining if neural tissue has herniated into the nasal cavity. Additional studies such as angiography may be necessary if uncontrollable hemorrhage is present.

NASAL FRACTURES

Background and Evaluation

The most common facial fracture is a nasal bone fracture, and Figure 21.1 demonstrates the pertinent nasal anatomy. It is likely that the incidence is underreported because many patients, especially men whom have broken their nose before, may not seek medical treatment. They occur in patients of all ages and have numerous etiologies: sports injuries, interpersonal violence, falls (Figs 21.2A and B), and motor vehicle accidents. When nasal bone fractures present immediately to the emergency department, they are often accompanied by epistaxis that must be addressed prior to the fracture evaluation. Once the bleeding is controlled, a thorough examination of the nose, and any other involved structures, may begin. If it is not likely to interfere with epistaxis control methods, a complete internal nasal examination helps to assess for: septal hematoma, septal fractures, septal deviation, lacerations, foreign material, cerebrospinal fluid (CSF) leak, and exposed bone or cartilage.

Radiologic imaging is seldom necessary in an isolated nasal bone fracture. However, it may add to the evidence if the patient is seeking legal counsel. Physical examination by an experienced facial surgeon is far more useful when it comes to evaluating an isolated nasal bone fracture.

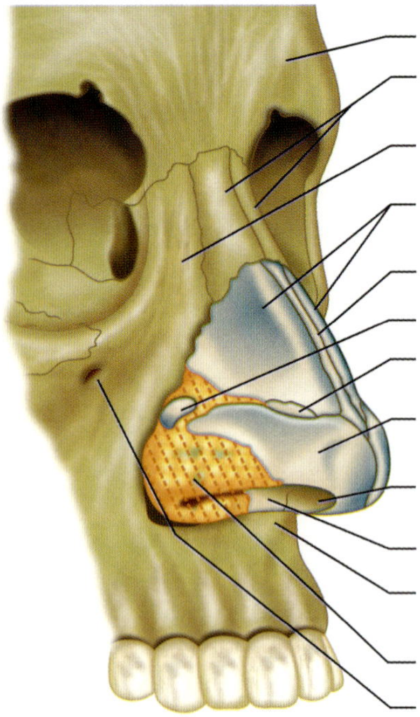

Fig. 21.1: Nasal anatomy

Closed Nasal Bone Fractures

Closed fractures, by definition, do not violate the skin envelope. These are the most common nasal fractures encountered. If they present immediately and the patient is able to be consented, and is amenable, a simple closed reduction may be performed while the patient is still in the emergency department. If the situation does not allow for this, have the patient apply cold compresses to the nose frequently to keep the swelling to a minimum while arrangements are made for the reduction to take place in the operating room where sedation or anesthesia may be administered. The compresses allow for a better evaluation of the injury, or step-off, which may be distorted by edema. This helps the surgeon realign the nasal bones as close to the anatomic position as possible. If severe edema is present, it may be prudent to delay the reduction to allow for an unobstructed view.

Open Nasal Bone Fractures

Open nasal bone fractures present more of an issue due to the skin envelope violation. These injuries are generally more serious and result from more significant force. They also carry the additional risk of foreign material in the wound. The bony repair presents the same challenges as does the closed fracture. However, if the laceration is large, it may be utilized in evaluation of the fracture and subsequent reduction.

Technique

If there is not a significant delay between the time of injury and the time of repair, closed nasal bone reduction is a relatively straightforward procedure. This entire procedure can be done without any sedation, but the choice depends on the patient's comfort and ability to cooperate.

After photodocumentation and consent is obtained, begin by decongesting and topically anesthetizing the intranasal cavity. Suction out any secretions present and then place cotton pledgets soaked with more decongestant and anesthetic (e.g. cocaine or oxymetazoline and 4% lidocaine). It can also be helpful to perform nerve blocks (infraorbital and infratrochlear) to lessen discomfort. Consider a long-acting anesthetic such as bupivacaine to allow for longer term pain control.

Once the patient is comfortable, remove the pledgets and remove any additional secretions and re-examine the intranasal cavity thoroughly to avoid missing any other injuries. Assuming the injury is limited just to the nasal bones, begin by taking an elevator (e.g. Boise or Goldman) and place this externally over the nasal bones to the level of the frontonasal suture line (Fig. 21.2C). Placing the thumb at the nostril allows this insertable length to be constant and acts as a depth gauge to avoid inadvertent trauma to the orbit. Avoid using the instrument in a fulcrum manner. Instead, simply lift the depressed fragment laterally. This can occasionally require significant force. Once the "pop" is felt, atraumatically remove the instrument from the nose and assess the outcome both visually and tactilely. Repeat this maneuver until the desired reduction is obtained. If overcorrection is performed, simply manually replace the displaced fragment to the desired position.

Some form of external splint is helpful in reducing postoperative edema. It may also act as a very light protection against a gentle brush or bump. The nasal splint is not to be used as a "reminder" that surgery occurred. He or she is very aware that the nose was reset as it can be quite tender for some time. To place the splint, first degrease the nasal skin with isopropyl alcohol. Allow it to dry and then place, with mild tension to decrease edema, adhesive strips (or a liquid adhesive followed by surgical tape). Follow this with the desired splint (generally some form of plastic or metal). Reinforce this with additional tapes to avoid slippage.

For most fractures additional stabilization is unnecessary. However, some fractures may be quite unstable and comminuted. In these situations, splinting the fractures, through the use of packing, from inside the nasal to prevent inward collapse may be warranted.

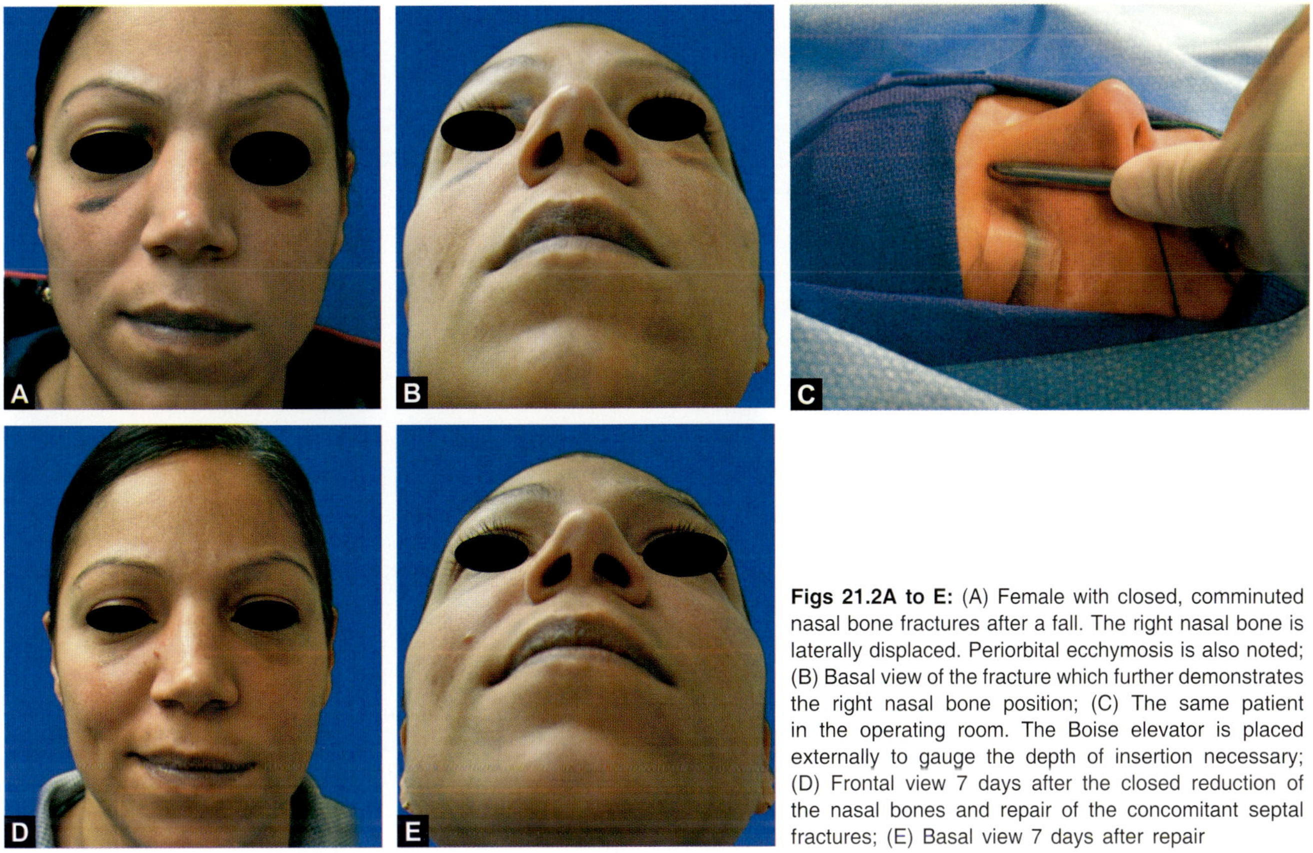

Figs 21.2A to E: (A) Female with closed, comminuted nasal bone fractures after a fall. The right nasal bone is laterally displaced. Periorbital ecchymosis is also noted; (B) Basal view of the fracture which further demonstrates the right nasal bone position; (C) The same patient in the operating room. The Boise elevator is placed externally to gauge the depth of insertion necessary; (D) Frontal view 7 days after the closed reduction of the nasal bones and repair of the concomitant septal fractures; (E) Basal view 7 days after repair

Any packing or external splints should be removed around postoperative day 7 (Figs 21.2D and E). Thoroughly clean out the inside of the nose with suction after decongesting and topically anesthetizing the nose. Look for any internal complications of the procedure. Atraumatically remove the external splint with the aid of adhesive remover. Palpate the bones. If any shift has occurred, gentle replacement can be performed, and if severe instability is present, consider re-taping the nose for support.

Open fracture repair is managed in a similar fashion except techniques for soft tissue repair should of course be abided by as well. Occasionally the lacerations may allow direct access to, and assessment of, the fracture lines. It is not recommended to increase the size of these traumatic lacerations for the sake of a nasal fracture repair unless the situation justifies access for advanced plating techniques and stabilization.

ORBITAL FRACTURES

Background

Fractures of the orbit are commonly seen as a result of trauma and motor vehicle accidents. The orbit is made up seven bones: the frontal bone, maxilla, zygoma, ethmoid, lacrimal bone, greater and lesser wings of the sphenoid, and the palatine bone. These bones vary in thickness and in strength. In approaching a patient with an orbital fracture one must remember that visual preservation is the first concern, prevention of diplopia is second, and restoration of form is third.

This chapter addresses the more commonly seen types of orbital fracture and seeks to elucidate some of the more common approaches and repairs of the orbit. The chapter is not meant to stand as a fully comprehensive guide. The reader is encouraged to seek out as many sources as possible and continue to track the ever-evolving management of these fractures.

Evaluation

The reader is directed to the proceeding bony trauma evaluation section for a general overview and assessment. However, it bears worth repeating that ruling out a globe injury and a comprehensive ophthalmologic examination is critical. If there is an injury to the globe or ophthalmic nerve, these injuries take precedence and will need to addressed and stabilized before any attempt to correct the orbital fracture is undertaken. Orbital fractures are by definition in a delicate and critical area, and therefore a team approach (e.g. ophthalmology, plastic surgery and neurosurgery) is encouraged.

History and Physical

After the patient is stabilized, a history and physical examination may take place. A full comprehensive history with particular attention to vision (prior injury, use of corrective lenses, dry eyes, medications, etc.) should be undertaken. Once this is complete, the physical examination can proceed. It can be helpful to examine the remainder of the head and neck last. This is done to ensure no other concomitant injuries are overlooked by the other caregivers. It also allows the patient to gain trust in the facial surgeon as the whole of the patient is being treated and not just one site. A gross visual fields test must be done with particular attention to diplopia and changes in visual acuity.

Thorough documentation of the vision and sensation around the orbit is mandatory. Neglect to document the preoperative status of vision and sensation could lead to an indefensible case against the surgeon.

Some of these patients may be under the influence of illicit substance or may be intoxicated, incoherent or even combative. It is imperative that there is good communication with the ophthalmology service so that there is as much reliable information as possible regarding the patient's visual status; also the ophthalmology team will need to give clearance that no contraindications to surgical intervention are present.

Radiologic Imaging

Computerized tomography (CT) of the maxillofacial skeleton with cuts less than 1 mm can adequately assess all of facial fractures. Three dimensional reconstructions are not mandatory but may play role in education of the patient as well as trainees. Postoperative CT is useful to determine bony alignment and should be obtained when possible. The key to preventing late enophthalmos and other sequelae is to maintain and restore the pre-traumatic orbital volume.

Early Intervention

The repair of orbital fractures can be an emergency in instances of muscle entrapment or nerve impingement. However, the majority of these fractures can be treated after stabilization and evaluation by other services. Some

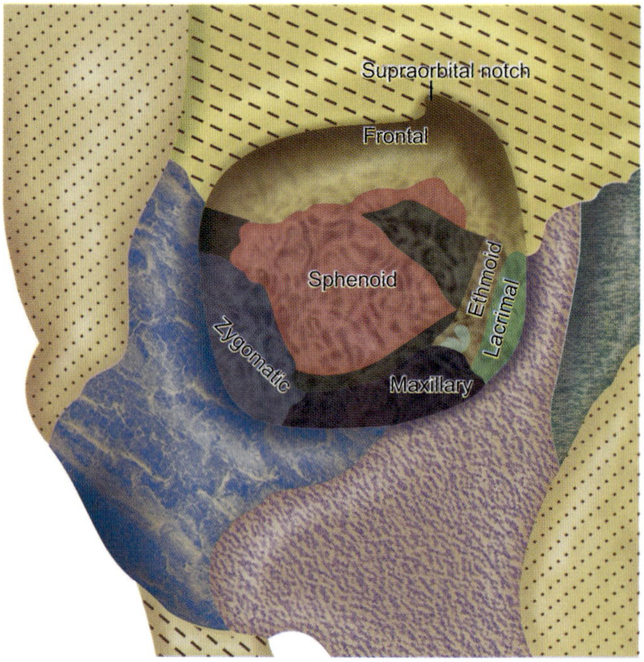

Fig. 21.3: Anatomy of the orbit

surgeons even insist on waiting until the edema and swelling has gone down which may take days to weeks. Repair at the earliest opportunity before adhesions have formed is generally advisable. The explanation of risks, both immediate and long-term, especially pertaining to vision is a necessary part of patient management. Risks include: loss of vision (partial or complete), diplopia, hematoma, infection, problems with the hardware placed (e.g. palpability or cold sensitivity), scar and need for further surgery. The patient also needs to understand that there are risks with not operating as well with enophthalmos and diplopia being of primary concern.

If the surgery is to be delayed, pain medication should be prescribed and antibiotics should be considered in the face of an open fracture. Also, remind patients not to sniff or blow their nose as this can lead to subcutaneous and intraorbital emphysema further distorting the physical examination. Patients will need to follow up concurrently with ophthalmology.

Anatomy

Figure 21.3 illustrates the anatomy of the orbit.

Classification

The classification of orbital fracture is as follows and the orbital fracture may be a part of other fracture complexes[1] such as zygomaticomaxillary complex (ZMC), nasoorbitalethmoid (NOE) and LeFort fractures, or it can be a pure orbital fracture. This chapter focuses on purely orbital fractures. Pure orbital fractures are classified and described by their location. Their management and treatment are also generally differentiated by their location.

Principles of Management

The following goals should be kept in mind when managing orbital fractures:

- Preservation of visual acuity
- Accurate bony reduction
- Fracture immobilization
- Avoid long-term diplopia and enophthalmos, preservation of orbital volume
- Ophthalmology follow-up.

The following steps are followed prior to the majority of orbital surgeries:

- Check tetanus status and administer booster, if necessary
- Ophthalmology
  - Complete evaluation and documentation of visual acuity, visual fields, and ocular muscle mobility
  - Clearance for surgery
- Radiology studies should be readily available in the operating room for review
- Postoperative reduction CT is obtained.

Management by Site

Orbital Floor (Blowout Fracture)

Isolated orbital blowout fractures are relatively common and usually result from a mixture of force directed into the globe (hydraulic forces)[2,3] and a blow to the orbital rim (bone conduction mechanism). Clinical findings include diplopia and enophthalmos. Surgery may be an emergency if one suspects entrapment of ocular muscles. The general size cutoff for surgical intervention is greater than or equal to 1×1 cm[2].[4]

Orbital floor fractures may easily be accessed through a subconjunctival incision thus sparing an external scar. While elevating the orbicularis oculi off the septum, care must be taken not to enter the septum which obscures the field with blood and makes the dissection more difficult. It can be useful to release the lower lid 5 mm from the lateral canthus and extend the incision through the crow's feet wrinkles, if needed, and to use a titanium plate for the fixation.

Steps through the use of plate (Figs 21.4A to D):

1. Release of the tarsal plate 5 mm from the lateral canthus.
2. Elevate the conjunctiva 1–2 mm below the tarsal plate.
3. Dissect to the orbital rim, staying on the orbital septum.
4. Elevate the periosteum of the orbital floor.
5. Dissect and reduce the herniated orbital contents.
6. Expose the posterior step-off of the orbital floor.
7. Place and fixate the plate.
8. Close the wound in layers:
   - Close the conjunctival layer with 6-0 plain gut interrupted sutures.
   - Close the tarsal plate with 3-0 polydioxanone sutures.
   - Close the lids with 5-0 silk sutures.
9. Perform a forward traction test.

Orbital Roof Fractures

Orbital roof fractures are rare and are usually associated with severe fractures of other facial bones. Unless the fracture is large and inferiorly displaced, conservative treatment is usually adequate. If reduction is needed, it will need to be done in conjunction with neurosurgery as it will require a craniotomy and reduction and repair from above the orbital roof.

Medial Orbital Wall Fractures

These fractures may involve nasal and ethmoid bone and may be a part of NOE fractures. Isolated medial wall fractures usually do not require surgical intervention unless there is entrapment of the medial rectus or significant loss of intraconal volume.

Follow-up

Close follow-up with the surgical team and ophthalmology is necessary after surgery. During these visits the surgeon needs to evaluate gross visual acuity, extraocular movements, healing of incisions, and other concerns and questions the patient and caregivers may have. Also, ensure that the patient is following instructions regarding: limitations, medications, and wound care.

Late outpatient visits several weeks to months later is necessary to evaluate the patient once surgical swelling has subsided and late enophthalmos and diplopia may occur. Radiologic imaging may be obtained to document hardware placement or an untoward outcome.

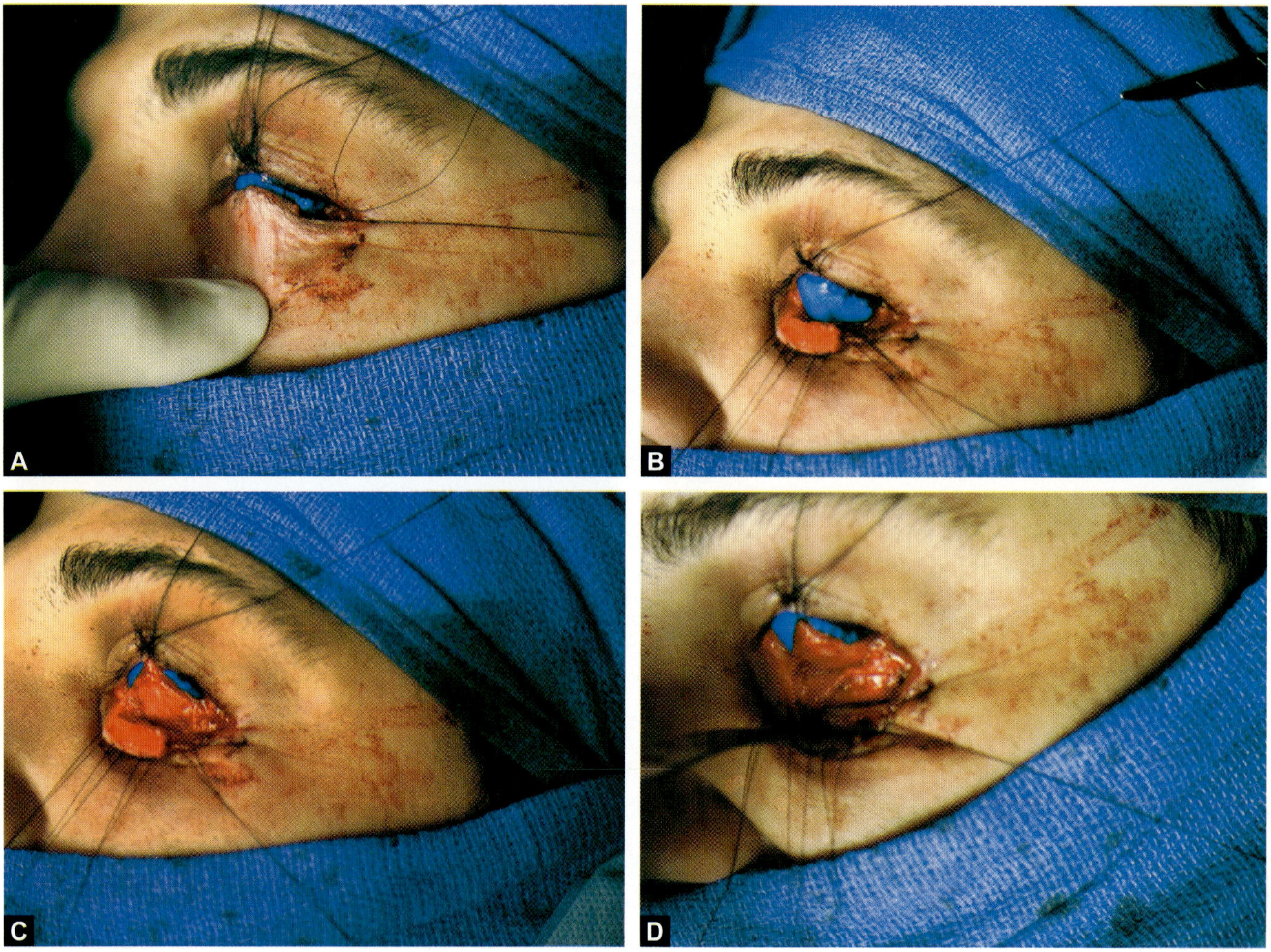

Figs 21.4A to D: (A) Release of the tarsal plate 5 mm from the lateral canthus; (B) Elevation of the conjunctiva 1–2 mm below the tarsal plate; (C) Dissection to the orbital rim on top of the orbital septum; (D) Elevation of the periosteum off the orbital floor

FRONTAL SINUS FRACTURES

Introduction

Fractures of the frontal sinus require a tremendous amount of force to occur and are often associated with motor vehicle accidents or interpersonal violence. Therefore, simultaneous intracranial injury should be assumed until proven otherwise and cervical spine injury ruled out as well. Fractures of the frontal sinus can involve the anterior wall, posterior wall or both. Enlisting the help of neurosurgical colleagues is warranted if any involvement of the posterior table occurs. The management of each injury pattern varies and is detailed herein. Figures 21.5A and B demonstrate the frontal sinuses and their relation to adjacent structures. Keep in mind that the nasofrontal ducts are situated posteromedially in the sinus.

Physical Examination

After the patient is stabilized and the rest of the head and neck is examined, the key points of the physical examination in regards to a frontal sinus fracture are to look for an open fracture, endoscopically evaluate for a CSF leak, perform a detailed neurologic examination (supraorbital nerve, supratrochlear nerve, mentation), and perform a gross ophthalmologic examination since up to 59% of these patients have concomitant orbital injuries.[5] Once these are completed, the radiologic imaging will help to guide the reconstructive options. Do not hesitate

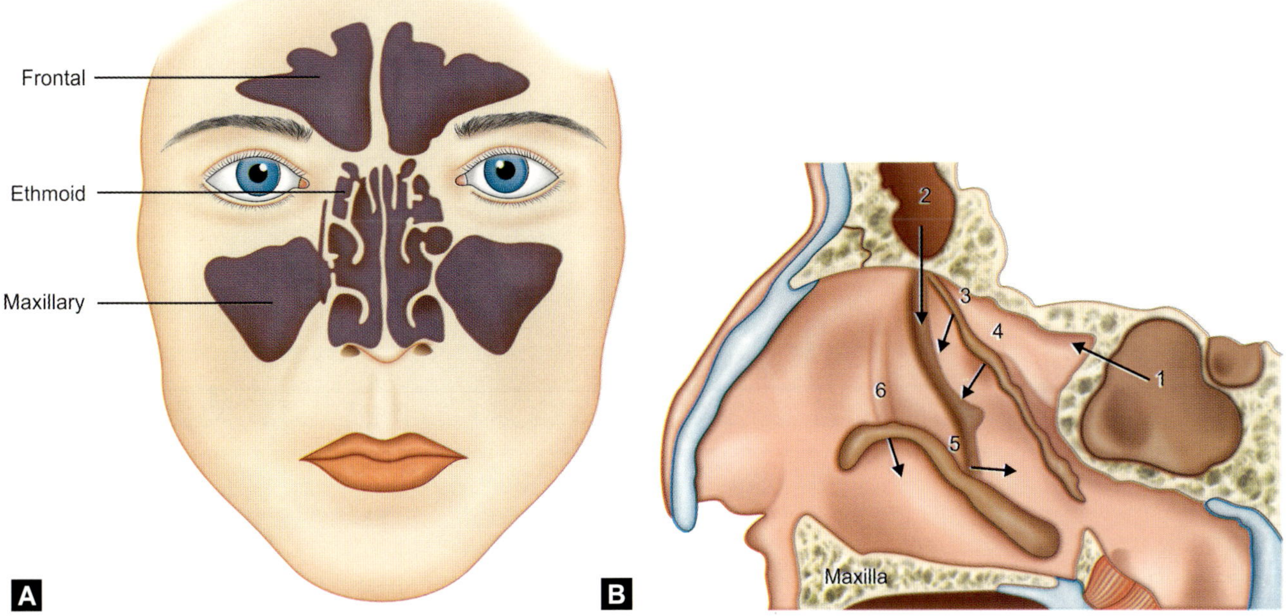

Figs 21.5A and B: (A) Frontal sinus anatomy, coronal view; (B) Frontal sinus anatomy, sagittal view

to re-examine the patient should the radiologic findings reveal something that was not apparent on the physical examination such as a suspected skull base defect.

Radiologic Examination

Computerized tomography is the imaging study of choice for the evaluation of frontal sinus fractures. Axial, coronal and sagittal formats should be obtained in all cases to provide as much information as possible, such as nasofrontal duct evaluation. Postoperative CTs are beneficial in assessing reduction of fractures. In the situation in which the nasofrontal duct is questionably involved and repair is done on or around it, yearly CT scans are warranted for the early detection of mucoceles which may occur decades after the incident.[6]

When dealing with frontal sinus fractures, if skull base trauma exists (e.g. a cribriform plate defect), MRI can be helpful in determining if neural tissue has herniated into the nasal cavity.

Anterior Table Fractures

Fractures limited to the outer table represent 43–61% of frontal sinus fractures.[7-9] Figure 21.6 represents a young male who was struck in the forehead during an altercation by a male with brass knuckle with injury limited to the anterior table. Anterior table fractures which are limited in size and do not cause a loss of form and those which do not result in significant loss of anterior skull protection (unlike Fig. 21.6), do not require intervention. They can simply be observed. However, when significant displacement or comminution occurs, intervention is required.

Technique for Repairing Isolated Anterior Table Fractures

Barring the cases in which open lacerations allow access to the sinus, the optimal approach is generally a bicoronal approach. The bicoronal approach allows for good cosmesis since the incision is hidden behind the hairline while affording ample exposure.

Steps:

1. Part the hair and secure back with rubber bands if it is long.
2. Demarcate the incision (a gentle gull wing design can be used) approximately 4 cm posterior to the hairline (Fig. 21.7).
3. Infiltrate with 0.5–1% lidocaine and 1/200,000 to 1/100,000 epinephrine.
4. Incise to the pericranium and bluntly elevate in this plane.
5. Incise the pericranium a few centimeters anterior to the bicoronal incision in the coronal plane and then create sagittal incisions in the pericranium and

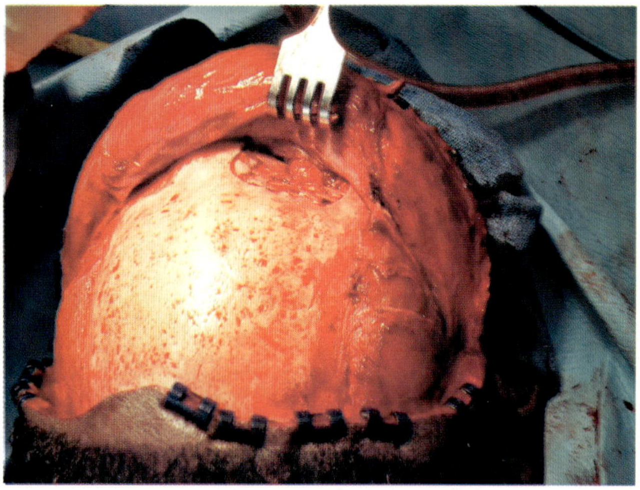

Fig. 21.6: Comminuted anterior table fracture after an altercation

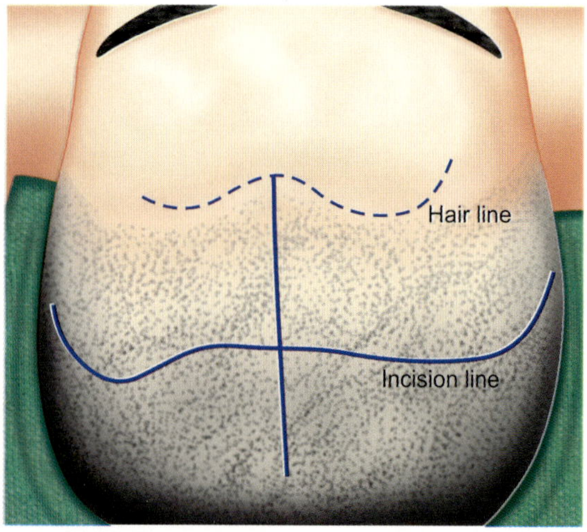

Fig. 21.7: Delineation of the bicoronal incision

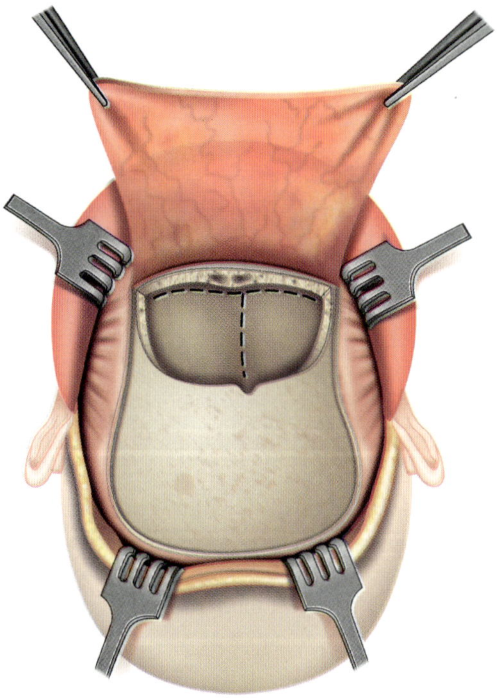

Fig. 21.8: Creation of a pericranial flap

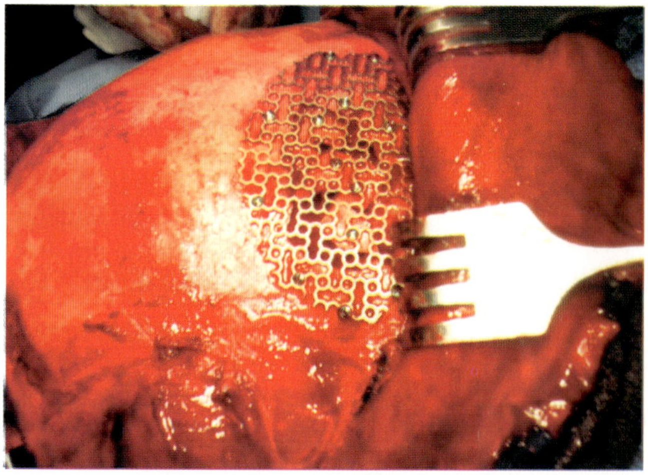

Fig. 21.9: Plating a comminuted anterior table fracture

carry them anteriorly. This creates the pericranial flap (Fig. 21.8). The pericranial flap can be used to line anterior skull base defects. Even if it is not used during this reconstruction, preserving it for future needs is prudent.

6. Continue to elevate along the skull until the supraorbital nerve is reached. It may come out of a foramen or a notch in the supraorbital rim. It can be skeletonized to allow additional inferior retraction and exposure, especially in cases of orbital or nasal fracture repair.
7. Gently explore the fracture. Irrigating any clots away to examine the sinus is helpful. Take care not to unnecessarily explore the sinus and put the nasofrontal duct at risk of scarring.
8. Elevate the depressed bony pieces.
   - If they are of limited size and cannot be stabilized, they may be discarded.
   - If they are a reasonable size, support the piece and using a high speed drill, create a 1.0 or 1.5 mm hole in the bony piece for screw placement.
9. Using either miniplates or mesh, stabilize the fracture to the remaining frontal bone (Fig. 21.9).

10. Closure can now occur.
    - Lay the pericranial flap back in place.
    - Close the pericranial layer with dissolvable suture (3-0 polyglactin 910).
    - Close the scalp with staples.
    - Drains are not necessary.
11. Perioperative antibiotics are reasonable for a short time (< 24 hours), but longer courses should be considered if gross contamination is present.

Follow-up after Isolated Anterior Table Fracture Repair

A follow-up CT scan should be performed to assess the adequacy of the reduction. Have the patient return in 7 days after surgery for staple removal and a wound check. Edema will have improved quite a bit by this point and the ability to assess contour should be possible. However, stress to the patient that continued improvement is likely to occur over the following weeks. Follow-up yearly CT scans should be performed to ensure that mucocele formation has not occurred.

Anterior Table Fractures with Involvement of the Nasofrontal Duct

The nasofrontal duct is located at the posterior-medial aspect of the sinus and significant frontal sinus trauma may involve this region. Controversy exists as to the most appropriate way of managing these injuries. Some authors routinely address these injuries as a terminal event to the sinus and feel that it is best to perform sinus obliteration. Others feel that this may be unnecessary and frontal sinus stenting can be used or endoscopic frontal sinus surgery to create and help to ensure long-term patency can be performed. The steps for obliteration are detailed below. The reader should seek appropriate endoscopic sinus techniques for advanced frontal sinus rescue surgery.

Technique for Frontal Sinus Obliteration

Steps:

Follow steps 1 through 6 for repairing isolated anterior table fractures.

7. An osteoplastic flap should be created to fully expose the entire frontal sinus cavity.
8. Take down the intersinus septum.
9. Carefully remove all sinus mucosa using elevators and high-speed diamond burrs.
10. Irrigate copiously and inspect to ensure total mucosal removal.
11. Plug the nasofrontal duct to ensure that it is not patent. Several options may be used and are mentioned herein as described by Haug and Cunningham:[10]
    - Invert the mucosa around the nasofrontal duct downward into the duct to plug it.
    - Place a tissue sealant.
    - Use muscle (frontalis) or fascia (temporalis) to layer over this.
    - Harvest a small piece of inner calvarium and fashion it to plug the duct.
    - Use a tissue sealant around these autologous materials.
    - Once things are felt to be secure, test the seal by gently irrigating the sinus and looking for a leak into the nasal cavity.
12. Harvest fat from the abdomen. A periumbilical incision can be used and is more aesthetic than one near the lower waistline.
13. Rinse the fat of the free fatty acids with saline.
14. Pack the fat into the frontal sinus cavity.
15. Replace the osteoplastic flap and close as detailed above.
16. Placement of an abdominal binder may help with preventing a seroma and with discomfort.

Follow-up after Frontal Sinus Obliteration

A follow-up CT scan should be performed. Have the patient return in 7 days after surgery for staple removal and check of the scalp, forehead, and abdomen. As above, the appearance is not finalized but is improving. Yearly CT scans should be performed.

Posterior Table Fractures

When a posterior table fracture is identified, the neurosurgical team should be consulted for input on management. Dural tears, CSF leaks, and frontal lobe injury are not uncommon and the neurosurgical team's assistance is valuable. A posterior fracture without associated dural tear, CSF leak, and a patent frontal duct, does not necessarily need repair. However, when a complication exists, the posterior table should be addressed. When persistent CSF leaks or posterior table displacement resulting in neurologic injury are present, cranialization should be considered. Cranialization is the process by which the posterior wall of the frontal sinus is removed which increases the cranial cavity and allows the brain to expand into the volume of the frontal sinus.

Technique for Frontal Sinus Cranialization

Steps:

Follow steps 1 through 11 for frontal sinus obliteration.

12. With the assistance of neurosurgery, carefully remove the fractured sites of the posterior table.
13. Examine for dural tears.
14. Inspect the brain for necrotic tissue which will be removed by the neurosurgical team, if present.
15. Perform dural closure.
16. Replace the osteoplastic flap and close as detailed above.

Follow-up after Frontal Sinus Cranialization

The patient should be kept in a neurosurgical intensive care unit, at least overnight, and serial neurologic examinations performed along with a CT scan. After the initial healing period, follow-up is as above.

CONCLUSION

When a patient presents with a fracture of the upper third of the maxillofacial skeleton, concomitant intracranial and orbital injuries must be considered. Nasal fractures are extremely common and generally very straight forward to manage. Early management, while the bones are still mobile, is recommended to avoid osteotomies which introduce more variables into the healing process.

Orbital fractures are more involved and have the potential for devastating sequelae. Therefore, a team approach with ophthalmology is recommended. Unless, the fracture is very small without entrapment or significant loss of orbital volume, intervention is warranted. The facial plastic surgeon should be facile with a variety of approaches to handle these fractures. Follow-up in these patients is important to detect issues such as diplopia or enophthalmos.

Frontal sinus fractures require significant force to occur and early neurosurgical consultation is warranted. Thorough assessment of the nasofrontal duct is important and the potential need for obliteration should be considered. Regardless of the fracture site of the frontal sinus, yearly CT scans are indicated to detect the potential for mucocele formation.

Each of these fractures can occur in isolation or as a complex of injuries, and therefore the facial plastic surgeon should be adept at the repair of each injury site.

REFERENCES

1. Crumley RL, Leibsohn J, Krause CJ, et al. Fractures of the orbital floor. Laryngoscope. 1977;87:934-47.
2. Erling BF, Iliff N, Robertson B, et al. Footprints of the globe: a practical look at the mechanism of orbital blowout fractures, with a revisit to the work of Raymond Pfeiffer. Plast Reconstr Surg. 1999;103:1313-6.
3. Smith B, Regan WF. Blowout fractures of the orbit: mechanism and correction of internal orbital fractures. Am J Ophthalmol. 1957;44:733-9.
4. Raskin EM, Millman AL, Lubkin V, et al. Prediction of late enophthalmos by volumetric analysis of orbital fractures. Ophthalmic Plast Reconstr Surg. 1998;14:19-26.
5. Levin SB, Rowe LD, Keane WM, et al. Evaluation and treatment of frontal sinus fractures. Otolaryngol Head Neck Surg. 1986;95:19-22.
6. Godin DA, Miller RH. Frontal sinus fractures. J La State med Soc. 1998;150:50-5.
7. Gerbino G, Roccia F, Benech A, et al. Analysis of 158 frontal sinus fractures: current surgical management and complications. J Craniomaxillofac Surg. 2000;28:133-9.
8. Xie C, Mehendale N, Barrett D, et al. 30-year retrospective review of frontal sinus fractures: the Charity Hospital experience. J Craniomaxillofac Trauma. 2000;6:7-15.
9. Onishi K, Nakajima T, Yoshimura Y. Treatment and therapeutic devices in the management of frontal sinus fractures: our experience with 42 cases. J Craniomaxillofac Surg. 1989;17:58-63.
10. Haug RH, Cunningham LL. Management of fractures of the frontal bone and frontal sinus. Selected Readings in Oral and Maxillofacial Surgery. 2002;10(6).

CHAPTER

22

Mandibular Fractures

Thomas C Spalla

BACKGROUND

Fractures of the mandible are frequently encountered, particularly in urban trauma hospitals where the number and complexity of facial injuries is the greatest. Mandibular fractures may result from a variety of causes: interpersonal violence, motor vehicle accidents, falls, sports-related injuries or iatrogenic (e.g. during a difficult tooth extraction). Also, pathologic fractures arising from malignancy or even certain medications (e.g. bisphosphonates and bevacizumab)[1-4] and radiation may occur. Each etiology should be assessed carefully prior to management as certain causes may need to be managed uniquely.

Therefore, a cookie-cutter approach to fractures is not wise. The variability in regions, training and backgrounds of the surgeons performing repairs can make a literature review daunting for the novice surgeon. This chapter seeks to elucidate some of the more common approaches and repairs of the mandible and is not meant to stand as a fully comprehensive guide to the management of such fractures. The reader is encouraged to seek out as many sources as possible and speak with other facial trauma surgeons to gain insight into the ever-evolving management of these problems.

HISTORY AND EVALUATION

The reader is directed to the preceding bony trauma evaluation section for a general overview and assessment. However, it bears worth repeating that ruling out a cervical spine injury and concomitant intracranial injury is of the utmost importance. Additionally, when bilateral mandibular body fractures occur, the loss of genioglossus support anteriorly may lead to airway loss due to tongue base collapse posteriorly. In this unique situation, the surgeon or assistant may need to perform a gentle distraction of this segment anteriorly to prevent loss of the airway. If other injuries permit, head elevation and even a tripod position may help the patient breathe more comfortably. If airway compromise begins to occur, transoral intubation could be considered, but an awake, fiberoptic intubation may be safer given the circumstances. The surgical team should be prepared to perform a tracheotomy if imminent loss of the airway is possible.

After the patient is stabilized, a history and physical examination may take place. The obtainment of a history as detailed previously should be undertaken. Once this is complete, the physical examination should proceed. Thorough documentation of the injury and any associated sequelae such as mental nerve hypoesthesia or mandibular branch weakness is mandatory. Neglect to document the preoperative status of a nerve injury may lead the patient to erroneously believe that it was an iatrogenic injury, and this could lead to an indefensible case against the surgeon. Carefully examine the teeth for acute injuries, but also note chips, cracks, missing teeth, etc. to avoid a similar situation.

RADIOLOGIC IMAGING

If concomitant facial fractures are present, or suspected, a CT of the maxillofacial skeleton should serve to adequately assess all of the facial fractures. In cases of significant comminution, the ability to render three-dimensional images can be useful in understanding the necessary reconstruction, and it serves as a tool for medical education. If an isolated mandibular fracture is found based on history and physical examination, plain film radiographs or panoramic imaging may be sufficient. Regardless of the image type initially taken, follow-up radiography is useful to determine bony alignment.

EARLY INTERVENTION

The repair of mandibular fractures is rarely an emergency and therefore stabilization and correction of any underlying abnormalities can, and should, take place prior to repair. This will likely afford a better surgical

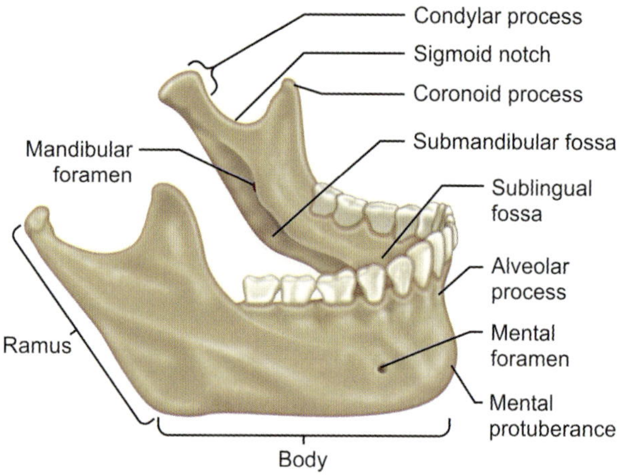

Fig. 22.1: Anatomy of the mandible

outcome. In open fractures, ensure that the patient's tetanus status is current. To decrease the risk of additional contamination prior to surgery, the patient's mouth should be kept clean. Consider a chlorhexidine rinse at the time of initial evaluation and, if the patient is not going to be nil per os (NPO) due to a delay in going to the operating room, this solution can be used after meals (a liquid diet at this time). If this is not feasible, dilute mouthwash or saline may be used.

If the surgery is to be delayed, consider some form of elastic splint around the jaw to allow for some immobilization to decrease the pain. Pain medication should be prescribed and antibiotics should be considered in the face of an open fracture. The author routinely puts any open fracture on antibiotics in the perioperative period.

Anatomy

Figure 22.1 illustrates the anatomy of the mandible.

Classification

A strong suspicion for more than one fracture site must always be kept in mind, because mandibular fractures typically occur in at least two places due to the inherent ring-like shape of the mandible. However, a sharp direct blow may produce a single fracture site.

As with any bony fracture, standard nomenclature such as greenstick, compound/open, comminuted, etc. exists. However, it is useful to attach this nomenclature to the specific mandibular fracture site. This serves to produce a mental picture to those who have yet to see the radiography and also creates the platform for understanding the necessary approach and reconstructive method.

PRINCIPLES OF MANAGEMENT

The following goals should be kept in mind when managing mandibular fractures:

- Re-establish dental occlusion
- Accurate bony reduction
- Fracture immobilization
- Avoid long-term maxillomandibular fixation (MMF) to prevent temporomandibular joint (TMJ) ankylosis
- Dental follow-up

The author utilizes the following steps prior to any mandibular surgery:

1. Check tetanus status and administer booster, if necessary
2. Administer antibiotics
   - Given in the emergency department if an open fracture is detected, or suspected.
   - Continued on a standard schedule until the time of repair. May require redosing just prior to incision depending on the timing of the repair.
   - Continue antibiotics in the postoperative period. This may not be standard of care and is debatable.
3. Perform dental blocks
   - The author will perform these at bedside if there is going to be a delay before the operating room (e.g. NPO status), if there is no contraindication, to give the patient much needed pain relief. This may allow for a more thorough examination. Of course, sensory status must be documented prior to the administration of local anesthesia.
   - These are repeated in the operating room with a long-acting anesthetic (e.g. 0.5% bupivacaine).
4. Nose preparation
   - With some exception, the patients are electively intubated for the procedure. This is done transnasally (Fig. 22.2A) to allow for MMF and to allow for exposure during surgery, when necessary. Therefore, the nose should be examined by the head and neck surgeon to rule out any potential problems (e.g. septal deviation, intranasal trauma, skull base fracture) with transnasal intubation.
   - Once the optimal side is chosen, topically decongest the nose (although this should have ideally been performed for a thorough nasal examination). Oxymetazoline works well and has a low systemic profile. Even if the anesthesia team does this, the time that is allowed for effect is generally insufficient in the author's experience when administered only by the anesthesia team. Repeat this a few minutes prior to the intubation. The time spent preventing epistaxis will save time, trouble and patient morbidity.

- Topically anesthetize the nose. The author tends to use 4% lidocaine for this purpose. This step is often supplanted by the anesthesia team through the use of viscous lidocaine. However, the author has found the following steps incredibly helpful to both the patient and the anesthesia team.
    - Spray the nose with oxymetazoline and 4% lidocaine, and allow time for effect.
    - Slowly introduce a soft nasal trumpet copiously lubricated with viscous lidocaine in the more patent nasal cavity.
        - Allow this to sit in the anterior cavity to allow the patient to adjust to this.
        - Then, slowly advance the trumpet until it is fully inserted.
    - The trumpet stays in place until the intubation is ready to be performed.

5. Be available for the anesthesia team. Not every anesthesiologist is adept with transnasal intubations, so be prepared to assist, because the surgeon will be the one managing a lacerated nose or oral cavity, or a tracheotomy if the airway cannot otherwise be established. Also, the unified team and care approach is always superior to a bunch of providers acting in isolation.
6. Mouth preparation
    - Some surgeons administer a fluoride treatment to help prevent demineralization.
    - In the operating room, the author likes to prepare and clean the mouth with a chlorhexidine solution and a toothbrush. This helps to remove dried blood and potential foreign bodies while decreasing the bacterial load, and potentially decreasing postoperative infections.
7. Radiology studies should be readily available in the operating room for review.
8. Postoperative reduction films are obtained. Plain radiographs may be sufficient, but CT imaging ±3D reconstructions may be preferred in complex cases.

MANAGEMENT BY SITE

Symphysis

Isolated symphyseal fractures are relatively uncommon and usually result from a blow directed upward toward the submental region such as from a fall onto the chin. These upward blows may also commonly cause a subcondylar fracture, so this should be assumed until proven otherwise.

Symphyseal fractures may easily be accessed through a gingivolabial sulcus incision thus sparing an external scar. While elevating the periosteum, care must be taken to avoid injury to the mental nerves as they are spared in a pure symphyseal fracture.

Steps through the use of plate(s):

1. Achieve MMF
    - Arch bars with interdental fixation (Fig. 22.2B)
    - Intermaxillary fixation (IMF) screws
    - Ivy loops
2. Make a gingivolabial incision (see Fig. 22.4B)
    - Leave at least 1 cm along the gingival to allow for closure
    - Once the incision is made, take care not to continue dissecting in this direction, as the direction is 90° toward the mandible.
    - Perform enough subperiosteal dissection to make room for the plates, but excessive elevation is unnecessary and deprives the outer cortex of this blood supply.
    - Take care not to injure the mental nerves. They may be traced and dissected to gain additional mobility while minimizing the risk of tearing or stretching the nerves.
3. Reduce the fracture manually and have the assistant maintain this alignment
4. Check occlusion (if present) to ensure proper alignment
5. *Achieving compression*: Utilize a 4–6 hole 2.0 compression plate along the inferior border of the mandible
    - Fashion it with plate-benders to the appropriate mandibular contour
    - Ensure that a minimum of two screws are used on each side of the fracture
    - Drill bicortical holes for the screws
    - Use a depth gauge to ensure proper screw length
    - Tighten one screw on each side of the plate at a time, but do not overtighten
        - This allows for slight adjustments without the need to redrill a hole
        - It also prevents stripping of the hole (i.e. a screw will simply spin and not gain any further purchase). A rescue screw (i.e. a screw with a larger diameter secondary to deeper threads) should be used if this occurs or else osseointegration (i.e. the bind of screw to bone on a molecular level) will not occur.
    - Continually recheck fracture reduction during this portion of the procedure.
6. Achieving tension
    - If arch bars were utilized, they may serve as the source of tension across the fracture and be left in place. The time that patients are left in arch bars varies considerably from surgeon to surgeon.

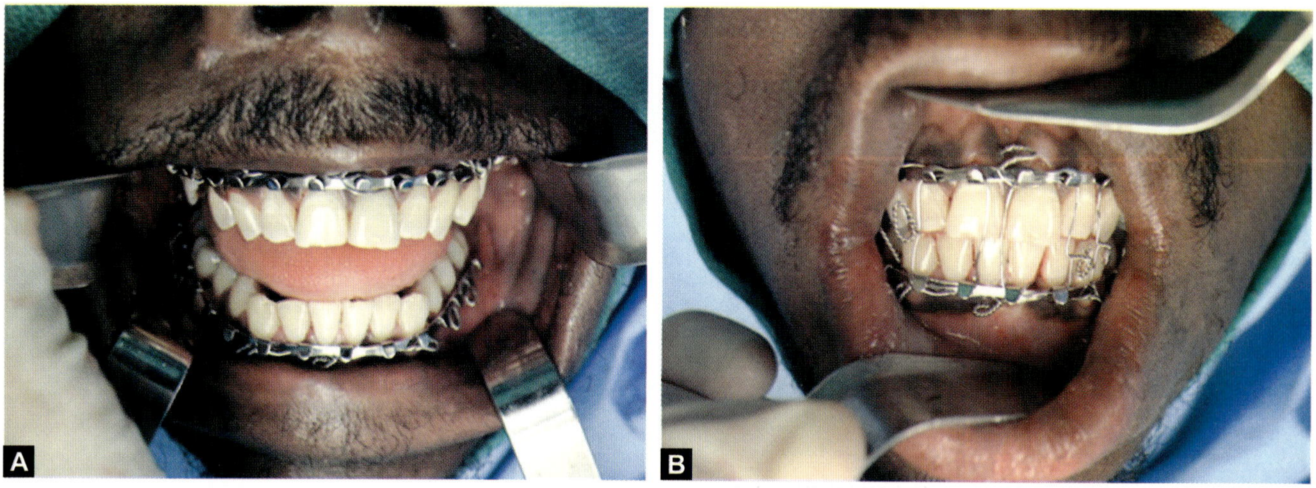

Figs 22.2A and B: (A) Arch bar placement for maxillomandibular fixation; (B) Box wire placement to secure the maxillomandibular fixation

However, it is outdated, and likely of no benefit, to leave a patient completely immobilized through the use of arch bars until complete fracture healing has occurred (approximately 6 weeks). The wires across the arch bars may be switched to guiding elastics to allow mobilization of the TMJs while still preventing fracture line motion.

- Intermaxillary fixation screws and Ivy loops are a rapid way to gain IMF thereby re-establishing occlusion. However, they are not intended as long-term management. Therefore, a tension plate should be fashioned toward the upper aspect of the mandible. The same steps should be followed as above for plate placement except that the screws are monocortically placed to lessen the chance for tooth root injury. If a tension plate is used, and the surgeon is confident of the alignment and occlusion, the IMF screws and Ivy loops may be removed. This prevents the patient from going home with a jaw "wired shut".

7. Wound closure should occur in layers.
   - Close the transected mentalis muscle with resorbable sutures
   - The author's preference is to close the mucosal layer with large bites with a 3-0 gut in a running locked fashion followed by a simple running 4-0 gut suture through the remaining everted mucosa. It may be overkill, but dealing with plate exposure can be problematic.

The symphyseal region also lends itself well to a lag screw repair technique. The following diagram (Figs 22.3A and B) illustrates the methods with which lag screws reduce fractures. Due to the necessity of placing the lag screws perpendicular to the fracture segments for ideal compression, this technique ideally suits fractures which are oriented vertically.

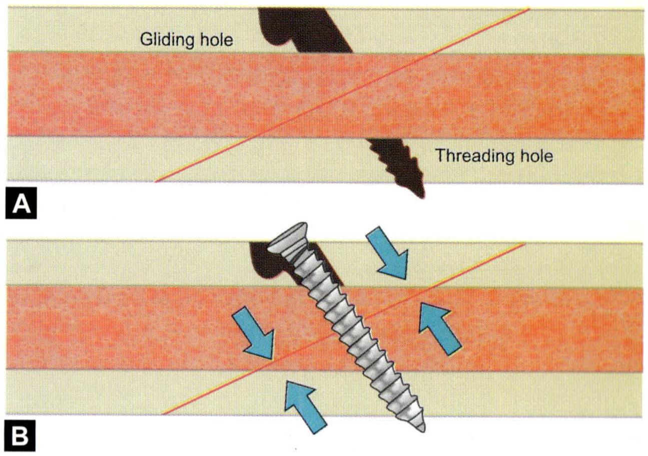

Figs 22.3A and B: Lag screw technique

Steps in the lag screw technique:

1. Exposure and closure is the same as above.
2. Ensure that the sites chosen for the screws do not violate tooth roots or the mental nerve.
3. The proximal segment is drilled using a drill with a diameter equal to the external diameter of the screw.
4. Make sure the fragments are reduced.
5. Drill through the distal segment using a drill guide with an extension on its tip equal in diameter to the external diameter of the screw.
6. Countersink the hole to allow a better seating of the screw head.
7. Using a depth gauge, determine the necessary screw length.

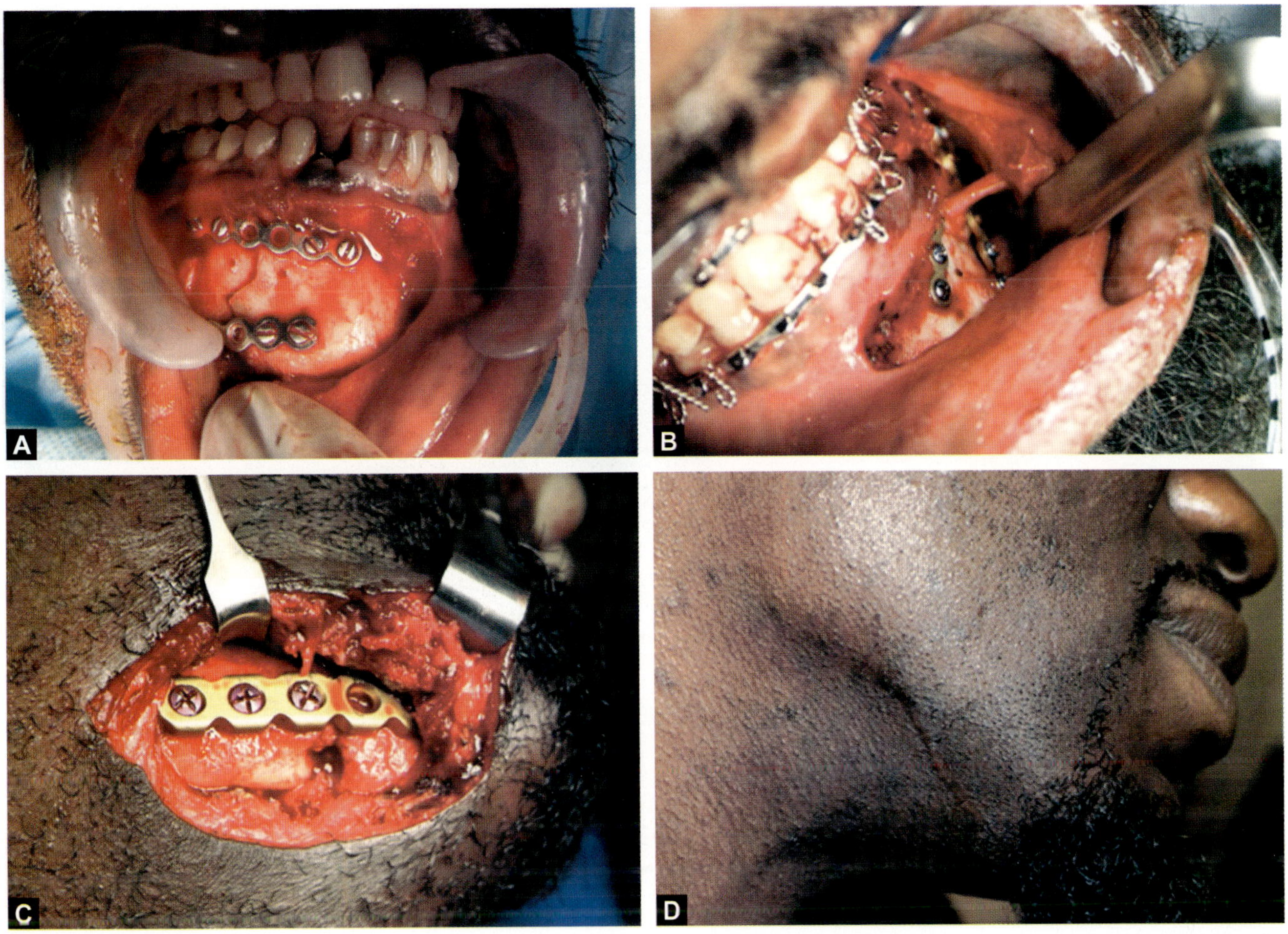

Figs 22.4A to D: (A) Compression and tension plates; (B) Demonstration of the gingivolabial approach to a parasymphyseal fracture with an inferior compression plate, a superior tension plate and interdental fixation through the use of arch bars. The mental nerve is dissected free, preserved and shown between the plates; (C) This patient also has a parasymphyseal fracture, but he presented with an open wound and therefore an external approach was taken; (D) Postoperative scar after external approach in the above patient

Photo Courtesy: Yuan Liu, MD

8. While maintaining reduction, insert the screw and feel the purchase into the distal segment. The segments will become compressed.
9. A second lag screw several millimeters from this one should be created. Some authors prefer to orient this opposite of the first screw (i.e. each segment will serve as the distal segment for one screw).

Parasymphysis and Body

These regions of the mandible can be addressed similarly to the plating techniques described in the symphyseal repair section. However, a lag screw technique is not utilized in these sites. Figures 22.4A to D demonstrates both an internal as well as external approach to the parasymphyseal site and demonstrates the relation of these fractures to the mental nerve.

Angle

There are many techniques to address the angle. Similar plating techniques as described above may be utilized. Additionally, some surgeons have used the lag screw technique in angle repair. One further method of repair bears mentioning, the use of a single miniplate for maxillofacial repair as described by Champy.[5] Figures 22.5A and B demonstrates the Champy technique through the use of monocortical plating. Plating techniques are detailed above.

Ramus

Monocortical miniplates may be used in repair of fractures of the ramus. Intraoral exposure is usually adequate. However, the surgeon may choose a parotidectomy

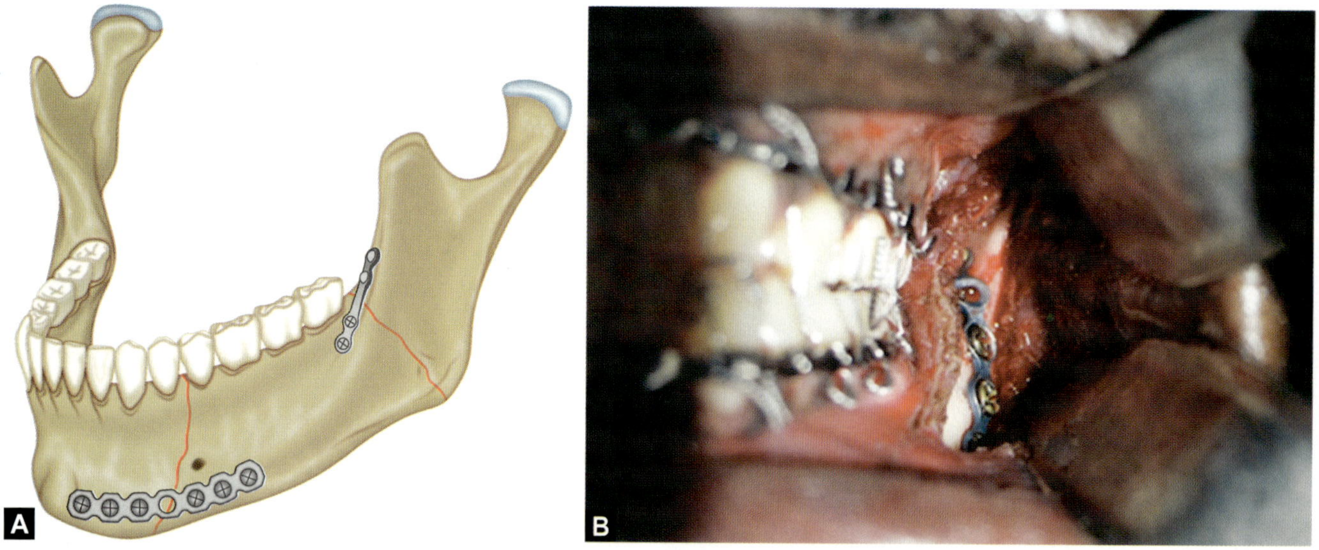

Figs 22.5A and B: (A) Champy technique; (B) Intraoperative picture showing the Champy plate technique using 1.5 mm screws

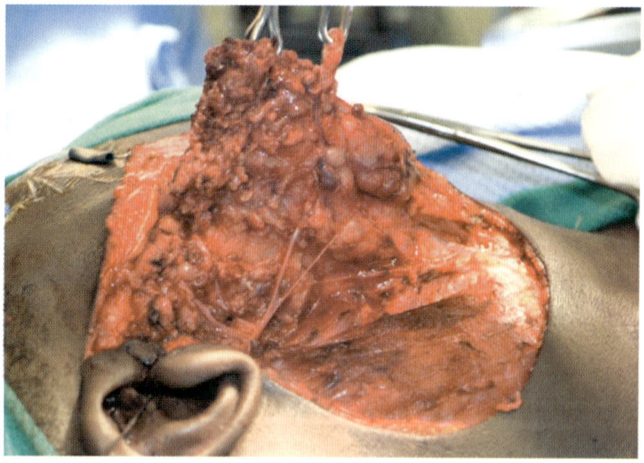

Fig. 22.6: Demonstrating exposure of the facial nerve and its ramifications in a patient undergoing a parotidectomy

approach to this as well as complex fractures of the subcondylar region and mandibular condyle. Surgeons inexperienced with parotid surgery should take caution as the facial nerve traverses the gland and may vary considerably in its anatomic course. If transaction of the facial nerve occurs, immediate, tension-free neurorrhaphy should occur. Figure 22.6 illustrates the facial nerve during a parotidectomy. This degree of exposure of the nerve and its divisions is rarely seen outside of parotid surgery.

Subcondylar Region

Many surgeons take a closed approach to management of subcondylar fractures. A liquid/soft diet, oral rehabilitation and close follow-up may be all that is necessary. However, in the author's experience, interdental fixation is warranted. Complete immobilization may be unnecessary, but guiding elastics help to minimize motion while maintaining occlusion. In cases of significant displacement (especially laterally or into the middle cranial fossa), loss of facial symmetry or failure of conservative treatment, an open approach may be undertaken. A facelift/parotidectomy approach can be used.

Condyle

The condyle is also generally approached in a closed fashion. When undertaking repair, an open approach via a facelift incision is typically utilized.

Coronoid Process

Isolated fractures of the coronoid are uncommon. Unless they are causing significant problems with occlusion, a closed approach is usually advisable. A liquid/soft diet, oral rehabilitation and close follow-up may be all that is necessary. In more significant cases, closed treatment with interdental fixation may be necessary.

FOLLOW-UP

No matter what method of management is chosen, follow-up is necessary. During these visits the surgeon and his/her team should be assessing for: occlusal problems, infections, fluid collections, hardware exposure, loose interdental fixation (if present), pain, and other concerns and questions the patient and caregivers may have. Additionally, enquire about nutrition as this may be difficult. High calorie and protein shakes can be helpful. Do not hesitate to consult with a dietician if concern for malnutrition exists. Also, ensure that the patient is following instructions regarding limitations, medications and wound care. In some situations, it may be beneficial to ask about the patient's social situation. This is to open this topic of conversation in cases of assault or abuse which led to this injury. Even in purely accidental cases this may be necessary such as a patient in an unsafe home environment (e.g. elderly patient with ambulatory difficulties in an ill-equipped house for such a person).

Repeated outpatient visits which are slowly spread out are warranted until the patient has fully demonstrated complete recovery, or if he or she demonstrates the need for further intervention. Radiologic imaging should be obtained to document proper reduction, hardware placement, or to seek for a cause for any suspected untoward outcome. Referral to other care providers such as dentistry, oral surgery, or occupational therapy should be considered early if any issues are suspected.

CONCLUSION

Patients with fractures of the mandible must first be managed as a trauma patient, and other injuries and medical conditions must not be overlooked. Once stabilized, repair of the mandible may begin. These fractures may be managed in a variety of ways depending on the surgeon's training, past experience and current trends. Although these patients often do not have a good alternative in management, informed consent must not be overlooked. The explanation of risks, both immediate and long-term, as well as expectations is a necessary part of patient management. These frank discussions will serve to allow the surgeon to take better care of the patient as a whole. Close follow-up is mandatory to manage any potential untoward outcomes. Restoring both form and function to these patients can be rewarding and the facial surgeon would be remiss to allow these cases to routinely pass by him or her.

REFERENCES

1. Kamoh AK and Ogle O. Bisphosphinate-related osteonecrosis of the jaws - a case report. Compend Contin Educ Dent. 2012;33(5):e74-7.
2. Akintoye SO and Hersh EV. Risks for jaw osteonecrosis drastically increases after 2 years of bisphosphonate therapy. J Evid Based Dent Pract. 2012;12(3 Suppl):251-3.
3. Ebker T, Rech J, von Wilmowsky C, et al. Fulminant course of osteonecrosis of the jaw in a rheumatoid arthritis patient following oral bisphosphonate intake and biologic therapy. Rheumatology (Oxford). 2013;52(1):218-20.
4. Pakosch D, Papadimas D, Munding J, et al. Osteonecrosis of the mandible due to anti-angiogenic agent, bevacizumab. Oral Maxillofac Surg. 2012.
5. Worthington P, Champy M. Monocortical miniplate osteosynthesis. Otolaryngol Clin North Am. 1987;20(3):607-20.
6. Kellman RM, Cienfuegos R. Endoscopic approaches to subcondylar fractures of the mandible. Facial Plast Surg. 2009;25(1):23-8.
7. Kellman RM. Endoscopic approach to subcondylar mandible fractures. Facial Plast Surg. 2004;20(3):239-47.

CHAPTER

23

Maxillary and Zygomatic Fractures

Thomas C Spalla

BACKGROUND

After nasal bone fractures, zygomatic fractures are the second most common facial fractures encountered. Therefore, the facial surgeon should have a thorough understanding of the relevant anatomy and methods with which these injuries can be managed. Intimately linked with fractures of the zygoma are fractures of the maxilla, and therefore will be covered in this chapter.

HISTORY AND PHYSICAL EXAMINATION

The reader is directed to the proceeding bony trauma evaluation section for a general overview and assessment. However, it bears worth repeating that ruling out a cervical spine injury and concomitant intracranial injury is of the utmost importance.

After the patient is stabilized, a history and physical examination may take place. The obtainment of a history as detailed previously should be undertaken. Once this is complete, the physical examination should proceed. Thorough documentation of the injury and any associated sequelae such as infraorbital nerve hypesthesia is mandatory. Neglect to document the preoperative status of a nerve injury may lead the patient to erroneously believe that it was an iatrogenic injury, and this could lead to an indefensible case against the surgeon. Carefully examine the teeth for acute injuries, but also note chips, cracks, missing teeth, etc. to avoid a similar situation.

Due to the fact that fractures of the maxillary sinus are connected to the nasal cavity, this may lead to subcutaneous emphysema. This can present as massive, soft facial swelling with inability to open the ipsilateral eye, or it may be subtle. Subcutaneous emphysema is palpable as a crispy sensation beneath the skin. It is also seen radiographically with almost a delicate honeycomb appearance. The patient should be instructed not to vigorous sniff or blow his/her nose.

Midface fractures are often described using the LeFort classification (Fig. 23.1) as this has been well known to facial surgeons for decades. While this can be useful to help rapidly describe the injury, fractures often do not follow these exact patterns. Therefore, describing each of the involved segments is preferable. As is evident by Figure 23.1, each of the increasing patterns of injury leads to increasing instability of the lower face. In fact, a LeFort III is complete craniofacial dissociation. Therefore, the surgeon must respect the amount of force required for such injuries and thus be thorough in his/her evaluation of these patients. Angiography may be necessary in evaluating bleeding from these injuries with a low threshold for embolization. If the surgeon has a co-operative patient, the second and third digits may be placed intraorally along the hard palate while the thumb braces on the upper lip. By gently pulling away from the face or rocking the palate, the surgeon can evaluate for midface mobility. If this is present, a fracture extending all the way through the pterygoid plates, a LeFort fracture, is likely present. Do not be fooled by a simple alveolar ridge fracture. The surgical trainees should get a feel for this while in the operative room repairing such injuries.

The zygomatic arch creates the lateral width of the face. With a depressed arch fracture, this may be lost, thereby leaving the patient with asymmetry. This asymmetry can be difficult to evaluate in the early stages due to edema. However, it should be sought out as early as feasible and reevaluated after healing or repair has taken place.

Some of these patients may be under the influence of illicit substance or may be intoxicated, incoherent or even combative. If this situation presents itself and the injuries are not life threatening, a repeat evaluation after the patient has gained better control of his/her faculties and had his/her pain controlled is warranted. While this simple consideration may be overlooked by some, gaining the patient's trust may make him/her more likely to follow-up, follow recommendations and have the best outcome.

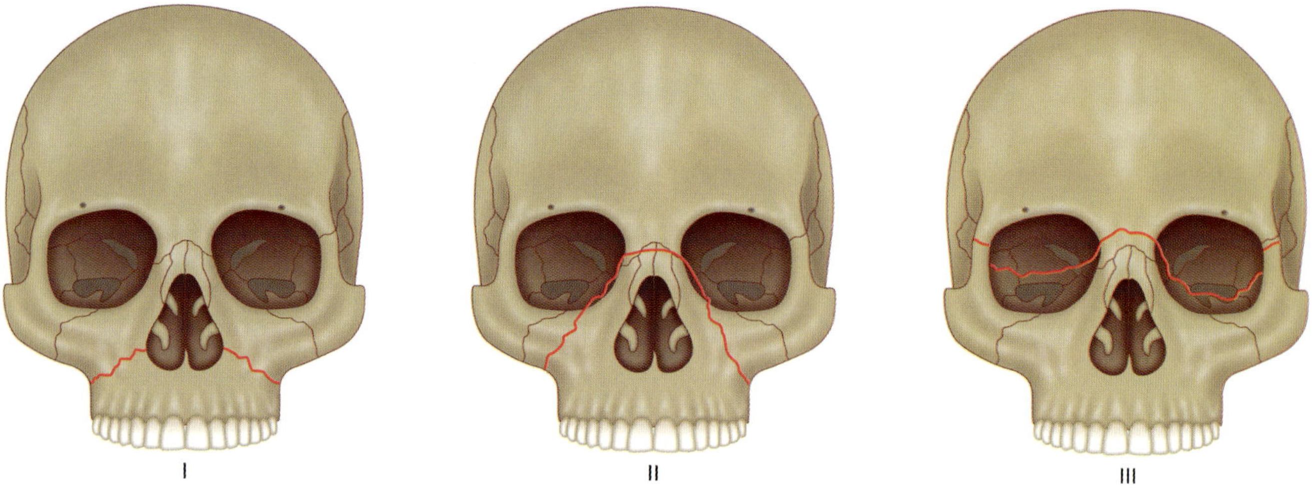

Fig. 23.1: Demonstration of the LeFort fracture classification

RADIOLOGIC IMAGING

If concomitant facial fractures are present or suspected, a computerized tomography (CT) of the maxillofacial skeleton should serve to adequately assess all of the facial fractures. In cases of significant comminution, the ability to render three-dimensional (3D) images can be useful in understanding the necessary reconstruction, and it serves as a tool for medical education. Regardless of the image type initially taken, follow-up radiography is useful to determine bony alignment after intervention.

ANATOMY

Figures 23.2 and 23.3 illustrate the maxilla and zygomatic arch with the bony relationships to the remainder of the facial skeleton.

PRINCIPLES OF MANAGEMENT

The following goals should be kept in mind when managing zygomatic and maxillary fractures:

- Re-establish/maintain dental occlusion.
- Accurate bony reduction.
- Fracture immobilization.
- Avoid long-term maxillary-mandibular fixation to prevent temporomandibular joint ankylosis.

The author utilizes the following steps prior to most midface surgery:

1. Check tetanus status and administer booster, if necessary.
2. Antibiotics:
   - *If open fracture*: Given in the emergency department and continued on a standard schedule until the time of repair.
   - *If closed fracture*: Perioperative antibiotics as dictated by hospital operating room protocol.
   - Short postoperative course. This is debatable.
3. Perform dental blocks:
   - The author performs these at bedside if there is going to be a delay before the operating room [e.g. nil per os (NPO) status], if there is no contraindication to give the patient pain relief. This may allow for a more thorough examination. Of course, sensory status must be documented prior to the administration of local anesthesia.
   - These are repeated in the operating room with a long-acting anesthetic (e.g. 0.5% bupivacaine).
4. Nose preparation (if transnasal intubation is deemed necessary):
   - With some exception, the patients are electively intubated for the procedure. This may be done transnasally to allow for maxillomandibular fixation (MMF), when necessary. Therefore, the nose should be examined by the head and neck surgeon to rule out any potential problems (e.g. septal deviation, intranasal trauma, skull base fracture) with transnasal intubation.
   - Once the optimal side is chosen, topically decongest the nose (although this should have ideally been performed for a thorough nasal examination). Oxymetazoline works well and has a low systemic profile. Even if the anesthesia team does this, the time that is allowed for effect is generally insufficient in the author's experience when administered only by the anesthesia team. Repeat this a few minutes prior to the intubation. The time spent preventing epistaxis will save time, trouble and patient's morbidity.

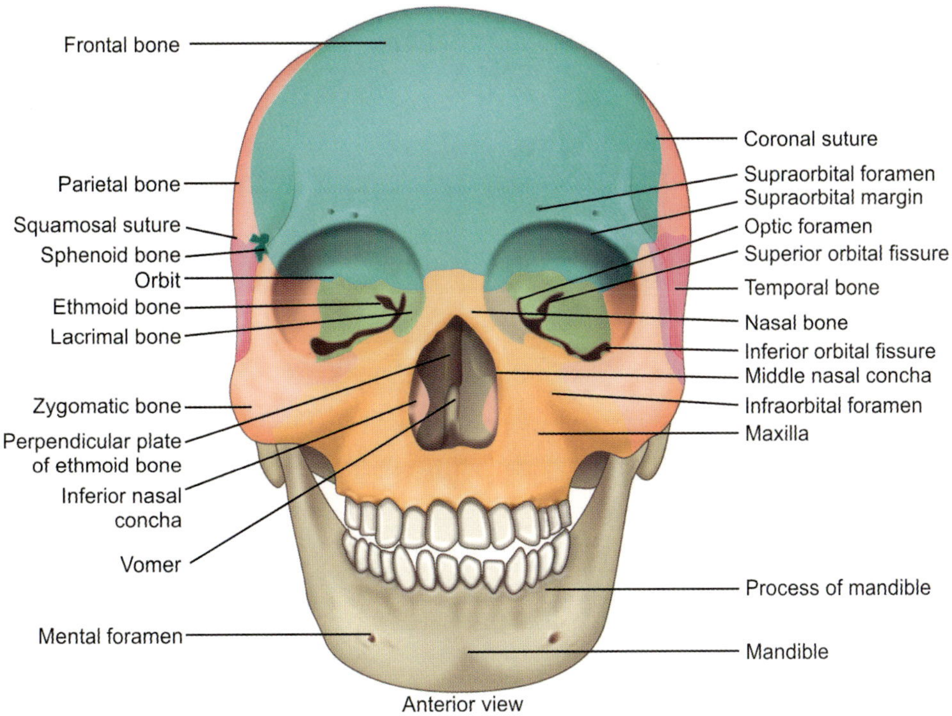

Fig. 23.2: The facial skeleton

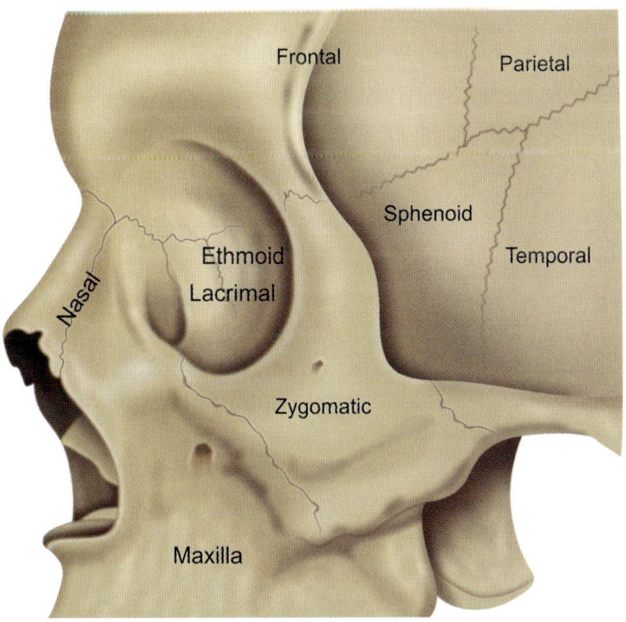

Fig. 23.3: The zygomatic arch

- Topically anesthetize the nose. The author tends to use 4% lidocaine for this purpose. This step is often supplanted by the anesthesia team through the use of viscous lidocaine. However, the author has found the following steps incredibly helpful to both the patient and the anesthesia team.
  - Spray the nose with oxymetazoline and 4% lidocaine, and allow time for effect.
  - Slowly introduce a soft nasal trumpet copiously lubricated with viscous lidocaine in the chosen nasal cavity.
  - Allow this to sit in the anterior cavity to allow the patient to adjust to this.
  - Then, slowly advance the trumpet until it is fully inserted.
- The trumpet stays in place until the intubation is ready to be performed.

5. Be available for the anesthesia team. Not every anesthesiologist is adept with transnasal intubations, so be prepared to assist, because the surgeon will be the one managing a lacerated nasal or oral cavity! Plus, a unified team is always superior to a group of lone providers.
6. Mouth preparation:
   - Some surgeons administer a fluoride treatment to help prevent demineralization.
   - In the operating room, the author likes to prepare and clean the mouth with a chlorhexidine solution and a toothbrush. This helps to remove dried blood and potential foreign bodies while decreasing the bacterial load and potentially decreasing postoperative infections.

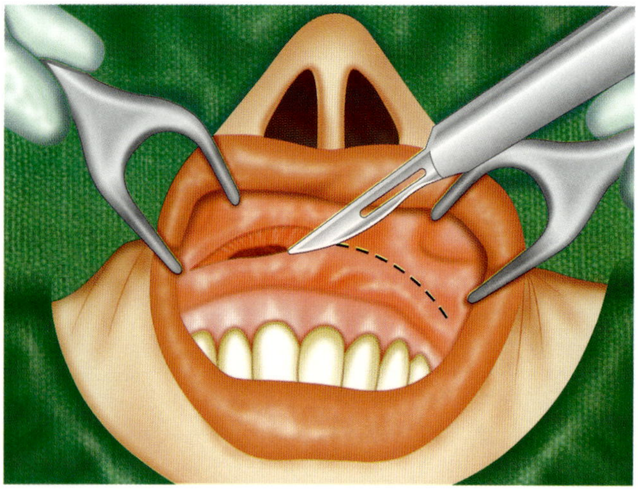

Fig. 23.4: Gingivolabial incision for access to the midface

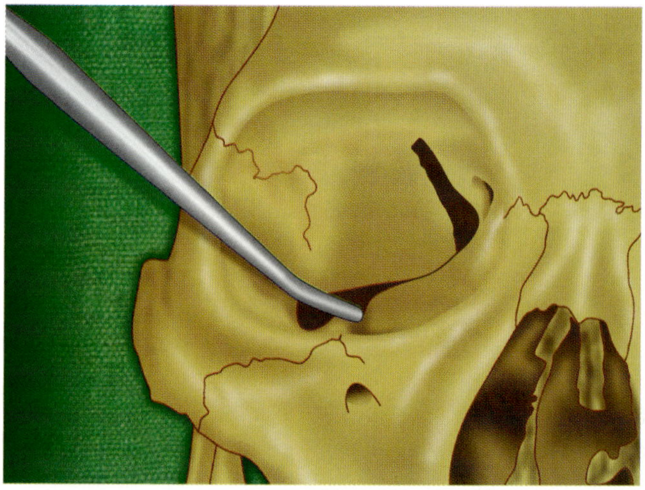

Fig. 23.5: The infraorbital nerve pathway along the orbital floor with its associated foramen seen on the anterior maxilla

7. Radiology studies should be readily available in the operating room for review.
8. Postoperative reduction films are obtained. Plain radiographs may be sufficient, but CT imaging ± 3D reconstructions may be preferred in complex cases.

MANAGEMENT OF MAXILLARY SINUS FRACTURES

Isolated maxillary sinus fractures generally do not require operative intervention. They rarely produce significant deformity or morbidity. However, if the maxillary sinus mucosa is violated, there exists a potential for subcutaneous emphysema. To minimize this, instruct the patient to avoid blowing his/her nose as well as vigorous sniffing. If this occurs, reassure the patient that it will slowly reabsorb. There will likely be blood in the sinus and subsequently in the nose. Gentle saline sprays may help in clearing this. If significant nasal congestion occurs, which disrupts sleep or activities of daily living, a short course of oxymetazoline nasal spray may be beneficial.

If significant deformity exists, or if bony fragments are loose in the maxillary sinus, it may be preferable to remove the fragments and plate the anterior face of the sinus.

Steps in Operative Management

1. Plan the placement of the gingivolabial incision (Fig. 23.4) and infiltrate local anesthesia containing epinephrine (barring any contraindication). Allow 10 minutes for this to take effect. This is a good time to prepare the mouth with chlorhexidine.
2. The incision may be made with a #15 blade or with cautery. Ensure that enough mucosa (~ 1 cm) is left toward the gingival to allow for adequate closure (i.e. good suture purchase). Once the incision is made, the direction of further dissection should be perpendicular to the face of the maxilla.
3. Blunt periosteal elevators are then used to elevate in a subperiosteal plane. Care must be taken to avoid the infraorbital nerve (Fig. 23.5).
4. The fracture(s) should be readily apparent.
5. Retrieve any pieces out of the maxillary sinus. If they appear to be of a suitable size for replacement, preserve them. Otherwise, discard the small shards of bone.
6. A small titanium mesh may be used to rebuild the anterior sinus wall. Fashion it to adequately cover the defect and allow room for screw placement outside the defect. If the recovered pieces are large enough, small screws can be placed through the plate and into the pieces on the back table prior to fixating the plate in vivo.
7. Once the plate has been secured, layered closure of the incision may commence.
8. Close the transected muscle with resorbable sutures.
9. The author's preference is to close the mucosal layer with large bites with a 3-0 gut in a running locked fashion followed by a simple running 4-0 gut suture through the remaining everted mucosa.

MANAGEMENT OF FRACTURES OF THE MAXILLA

The LeFort fracture patterns as shown in Figure 23.1 have been discussed below. As stated previously, fractures often do not follow these patterns, but they do serve a useful guide for fracture management. When posed with a complex situation, it is generally best to begin with establishing and securing occlusion such as through the use of MMF. This stabilization acts as a stable framework from which to begin. Many surgeons take an outside-to-inside approach when dealing with complex facial fractures. This means that the facial buttresses are addressed and stabilized first which helps to ensure craniofacial support and form.

The LeFort I fracture pattern bears special attention as it can be utilized as an approach for maxillary-mandibular advancement procedures (e.g. for facial dysmorphism or obstructive sleep apnea). Additionally, it can be used for access to a juvenile nasal angiofibroma (JNA).

Steps in Operative Management of LeFort I Fractures

1. Prepare the mouth with chlorhexidine.
2. If the midface needs to be accessed as in a LeFort I or II fracture pattern, then plan the placement of the gingivolabial incision and infiltrate local anesthesia containing epinephrine (barring any contraindication).
3. Place the patient in MMF.
4. The incision may be made with a #15 blade or with cautery. Ensure that enough mucosa (~ 1 cm) is left toward the gingival to allow for adequate closure (i.e. good suture purchase). Once the incision is made, the direction of further dissection should be perpendicular to the face of the maxilla.
5. Blunt periosteal elevators are then used to elevate in a subperiosteal plane. Care must be taken to avoid the infraorbital nerve. Fully expose the fracture(s).
6. See Figures 23.6 and 23.7A and B as examples of plate placement. Note that at least two miniplates with two screws on each side of the fracture are used for maximum security.
7. Once the plate has been secured, layered closure of the incision may commence.
8. Close the transected muscle with resorbable sutures.
9. The author's preference is to close the mucosal layer with large bites with a 3-0 gut in a running locked fashion followed by a simple running 4-0 gut suture through the remaining everted mucosa.

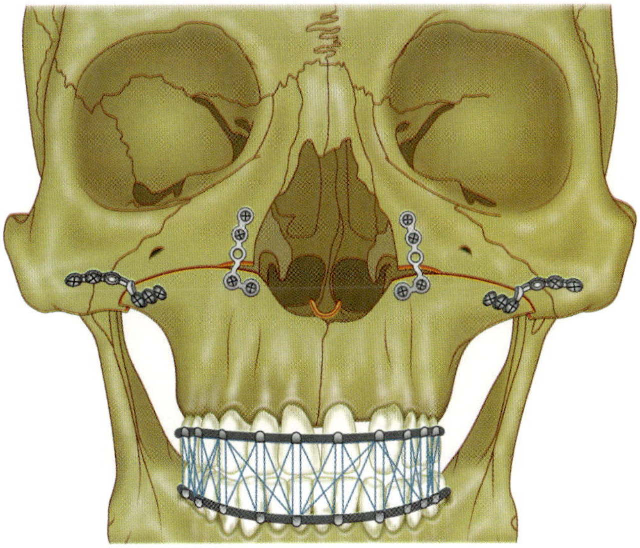

Fig. 23.6: Diagram demonstrating plate fixation for repair of a fractured maxilla

Steps in Operative Management of LeFort II Fractures

LeFort II fractures require the sublabial approach to the lower aspect of the fracture. Exposure of the superior aspect of the fracture along the region of the nasomaxillary and nasofrontal regions becomes more difficult. Midface degloving techniques through intranasal releasing incisions may yield enough exposure to accurately reduce and fixate these fracture lines. If this technique cannot be utilized or if other injury patterns or surgeon comfort dictate otherwise, a bicoronal approach (Figs 23.8A and B) combined with the sublabial approach will allow for the necessary subperiosteal dissection and exposure of the fractures.

1. Follow Steps 1 to 6 as above.
2. See Figures 23.9 and 23.10 as examples of plate placement.
3. Closure is as above.

Steps in Operative Management of LeFort III Fractures

1. Prepare the mouth with chlorhexidine.
2. If the midface needs to be accessed as in a LeFort I or II fracture pattern, then plan the placement of the gingivolabial incision and infiltrate local anesthesia containing epinephrine (barring any contraindication). Address the midface as described above, if necessary after placing the patient in MMF.
3. Place the patient in MMF.

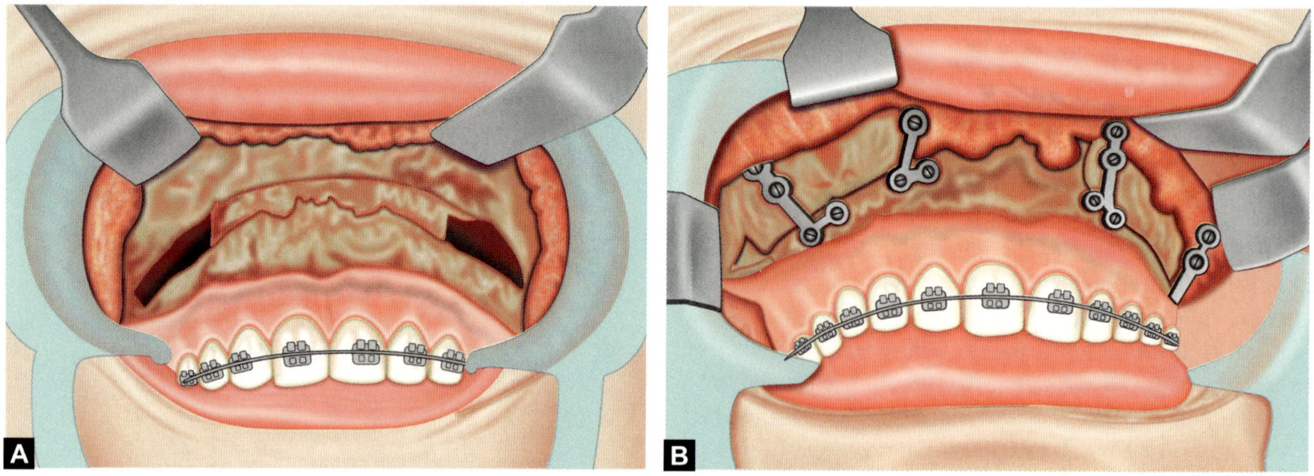

Figs 23.7A and B: Demonstration of (A) midface exposure of the maxillary fracture and (B) subsequent fixation

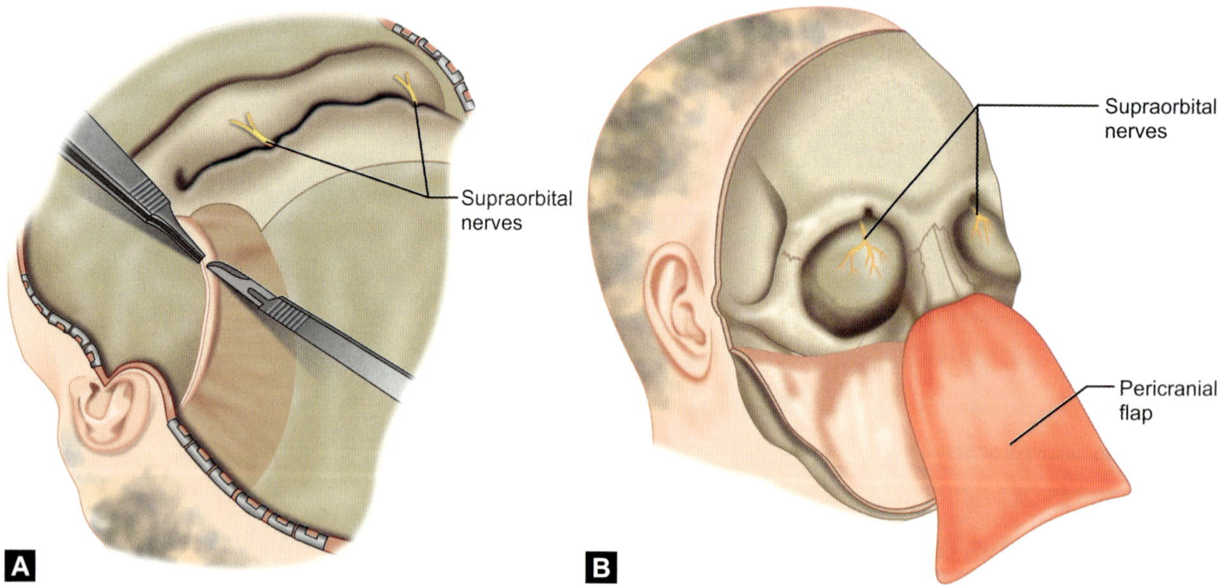

Figs 23.8A and B: (A) The bicoronal approach to access the midface; (B) Continued dissection of the bicoronal approach to expose the nasal bones

4. A lateral brow incision (Fig. 23.11) can be made to access the lateral orbital rim and plate fixation can then occur. However, stabilization of the nasofrontal region is necessary and the lateral orbital fractures can be addressed with the exposure of the bicoronal flap (see Figs 23.8A and B).
   - A bicoronal flap can be designed to go from the pretragal to the pretragal region to gain adequate inferior retraction of the flap.
   - Preservation of the supraorbital neurovascular bundle as well as the temporal branch of the facial nerve is critical. Dissection in the subperiosteal plane (thereby preserving the pericranial flap) should be performed.
   - Dissection just beneath the deep temporal fascia helps to protect the facial nerve.
5. Secure the plates as shown in Figure 23.9.
6. Layered closure of the incisions may commence.
   - The facial portion of the incision can be closed in layers using a 4-0 polyglactin 910 suture in the deep layer and a 5-0 polydioxanone suture superficially.

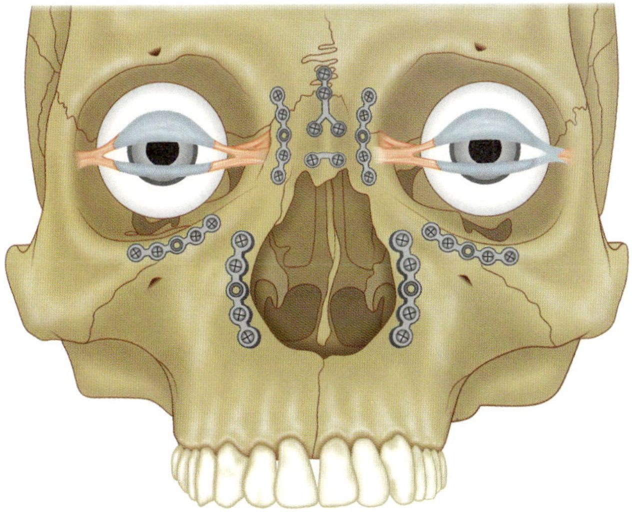

Fig. 23.9: An illustration demonstrating plate placement in a complex midface fracture

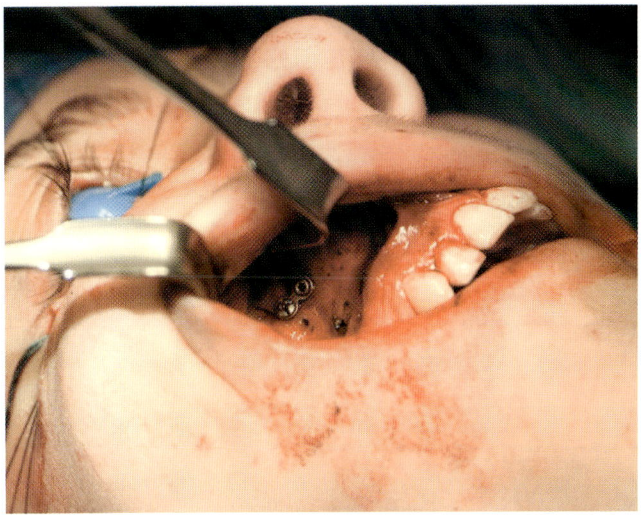

Fig. 23.10: Intraoperative photo demonstrating plate placement
Courtesy: Yuan Liu, MD

- In the hair, a deep suture such as 3-0 polyglactin 910 suture is helpful followed by staples.

MANAGEMENT OF ZYGOMATIC ARCH FRACTURES

Percutaneous Treatment

One method of addressing the zygomatic arch involves percutaneously reducing the arch through the use of a bone hook (Fig. 23.12).

Steps

1. Use a #11 blade and made a stab incision through the cheek skin.
2. Place the bone hook, as shown in Figure 23.12, beneath the arch.
3. Using the nondominant hand and an assistant, stabilize the head while significant lateral traction is made. Take care to ensure that the hook stays engaged to the bone, or else it could slip and tear the skin and a branch of the facial nerve.
4. A palpable (sometimes audible) "pop" will be felt when reduction occurs.
5. Close the stab wound.

Open Treatment (Gillie's Approach)

This technique is rather easy to teach and avoids a scar, albeit small, on the face unlike the percutaneous approach described above.

Steps

1. Part the hair (if applicable) and design a 3–4 cm incision just behind the hairline at the temporal hair tuft.
2. Infiltrate with 1% lidocaine + 1/100,000 epinephrine and allow time to take effect.
3. Use a #15 blade and cut straight down through the skin and to the deep temporal fascia.
4. Incise the deep temporal fascia sharply which exposes the temporalis muscle.
5. A blunt elevator is slid between the deep temporal fascia and the temporalis muscle to lie just beneath the zygomatic arch (Fig. 23.13).
6. Roll a gauze pad and place this between the skin and the elevator to act as a fulcrum and protect the skin.
7. Use the nondominant hand over the arch to palpate while the dominant hand uses the elevator in a lever-like fashion to elevate the depressed segment.
8. A "pop" should be felt indicating reduction.
9. Close the incision in layers and do not use cautery near the hair to prevent alopecia.

Hemicoronal Approach

The hemicoronal approach can be used to expose the arch in situations of severe comminution which requires plating, or if the more conservative techniques fail to achieve adequate reduction. The hemicoronal approach (Figs 23.14A to C) is approached in a similar fashion to the bicoronal approach as shown above. Care to preserve the supraorbital neurovascular bundle as well as the temporal branch of the facial nerve is critical.

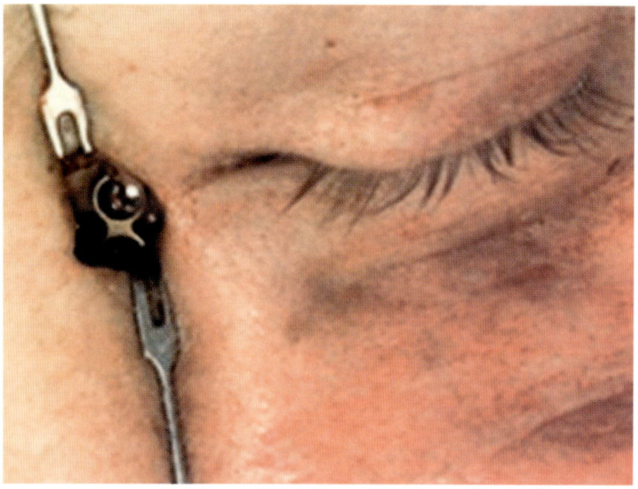

Fig. 23.11: A lateral orbital incision to access the lateral orbital rim

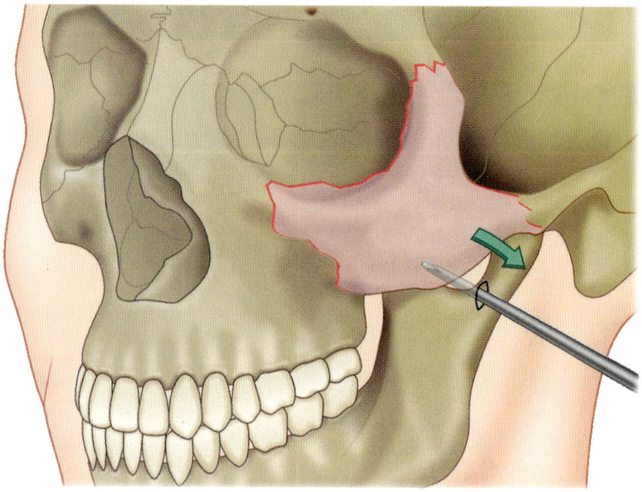

Fig. 23.12: Bone hook reduction of the zygoma

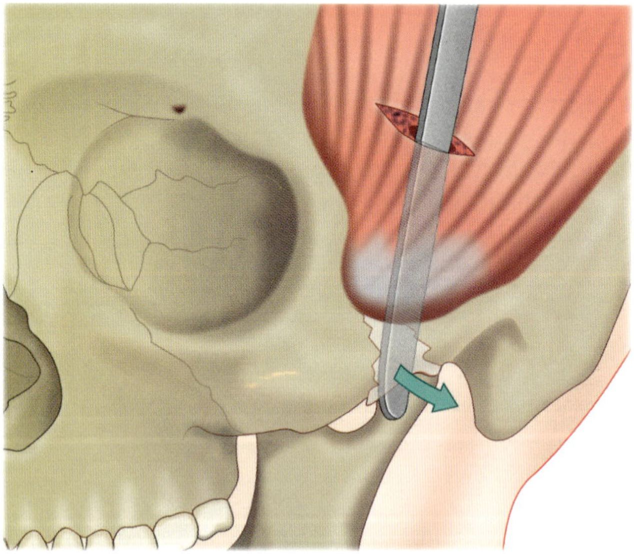

Fig. 23.13: The Gillie's approach to zygomatic arch reduction

Steps

1. See the coronal approach for exposure.
2. Once the fragments are reduced, 1.5 or 2.0 mm plates can be used to fixate the segments.
3. Wound closure is detailed above.

Follow-up

No matter what method of management is chosen, follow-up is necessary. During these visits the surgeon and his/her team should be assessing for occlusal problems, infections, fluid collections, hardware exposure, loose interdental fixation (if present), pain and other concerns, and questions the patient and caregivers may have. Have the patient start on a liquid diet so as not to cause excessive masseter muscle pull on the zygomatic arch. Enquire about the ability to do this, as this may be difficult for some patients. High calorie and protein shakes may be helpful. Do not hesitate to consult with a dietician if concern for malnutrition exists. Also, ensure that the patient is following instructions regarding limitations, medications and wound care. In some situations it may be beneficial to ask about the patient's social situation. This is to open this topic of conversation in cases of assault or abuse which led to this injury. Even in purely accidental cases, this may be necessary such as a patient in an unsafe home environment (e.g. elderly patient with ambulatory difficulties in an ill-equipped house for such a person).

Repeated outpatient visits which are slowly spread out are warranted until the patient has demonstrated complete recovery, or if he or she demonstrates the need for further intervention. Radiologic imaging may be obtained to document proper reduction, hardware placement, or to seek for a cause for any suspected untoward outcome. Referral to other care providers such as dentistry, oral surgery or occupational therapy should be considered early if any issues are suspected.

CONCLUSION

Patients with fractures of the maxilla and zygoma must first be managed as a trauma patient, and other injuries

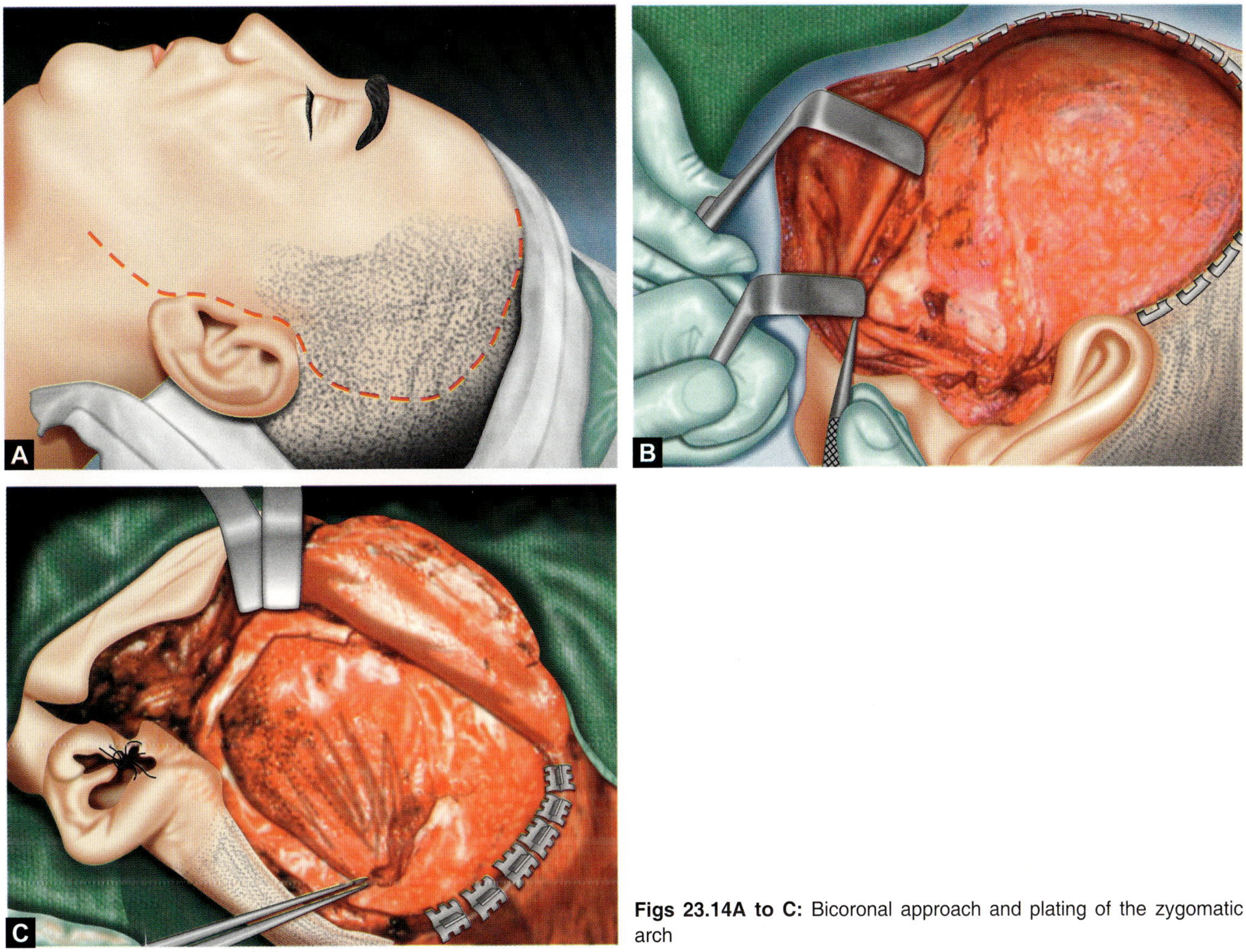

Figs 23.14A to C: Bicoronal approach and plating of the zygomatic arch

and medical conditions must not be overlooked. Once stabilized, repair of the fractures may begin. These fractures may be managed in a variety of ways depending on the surgeon's training, past experience and current trends. Carefully study the preoperative CT scans to help plan for the proposed incisions, but have alternatives in mind in case of unforeseen intraoperative issues. Close follow-up is mandatory to manage any potential untoward outcomes. Restoring both form and function to these patients can be rewarding and the facial surgeon would be remiss to allow these cases to routinely pass by him or her.

BIBLIOGRAPHY

1. Ellis E, Zide MF. Surgical Approaches to the Facial Skeleton, 2nd edition. Baltimore: Lippincott Williams &Wilkins; 2005.
2. Loré JM, Medina JE. An Atlas of Head & Neck Surgery, 4th edition. Philadelphia: Elsevier Saunders; 2005.

CHAPTER

24

Surgical Management of Facial Paralysis

Thomas C Spalla

INTRODUCTION

Facial paralysis may result from a number of factors: Bell's palsy, trauma (laceration, temporal bone fracture, forceps compression during a difficult birth), iatrogenic (surgery: parotid, skull base, mastoid, middle ear), Lyme disease, sarcoidosis, Mobius syndrome, cerebrovascular accident, malignancy (parotid, skull base) and tumors (schwannoma, meningioma). The resultant deficit can be disfiguring and lead to significant functional deficits. Additionally, the psychological trauma associated with facial paralysis can be severe enough to lead to social withdrawal.

Through an understanding of the functional loss secondary to facial paralysis, one may gain insight into the means with which reconstructive efforts can be successful. Going from superior to inferior, the deficits encountered are as follows:

- *The brow*: Ptosis leading to forehead asymmetry, a heavy-appearing eye and potential visual field deficit.
- *The eye*:
  - Incomplete closure leading to corneal exposure, irritation, blurry vision, pain and blindness.
  - Inadequate tear pumping mechanism leading to epiphora.
- *The nose*: Nasal valve collapse leading to restricted nasal airflow.
- *The mouth*:
  - Oral incompetence with resultant difficulties in articulation and eating.
  - Buccinator weakness resulting in food trapping in the cheek.
- *The face as a whole*:
  - Visible asymmetry resulting in a disturbed aesthetic.
  - Lack of animation limiting expression.

EXAMINATION

After a complete history, the physical examination should include a thorough head and neck evaluation with particular attention paid to the cranial nerves and the resultant deficits secondary to the facial nerve injury. If the cause of paralysis is not clear from the history, the head and neck surgeon should attempt to narrow down potential causes. Outside of the deficits mentioned above, some important portions of the physical examination are detailed below.

Neurologic

Mental status is ascertained while speaking with the patient. Examining the limbs for any gross motor or sensory deficit helps to rule out cerebrovascular accident in the differential. A detailed cranial nerve examination is of paramount importance. Do not forget to include corneal sensation and the blink reflex.

Dermatologic

The skin of the head and neck should be examined looking for any cutaneous malignancies. If the history is suspicious, checking the remainder of the body for abnormal rashes or bites may be warranted.

Ophthalmologic

Look for signs of irritation or frank ulceration. Look for Bell's phenomenon, the upward protective rotation of the globe with eye closure, as shown in Figure 24.1. A referral to an ophthalmologist is beneficial.

Head and Neck

Examine the parotid glands to rule out a mass lesion.

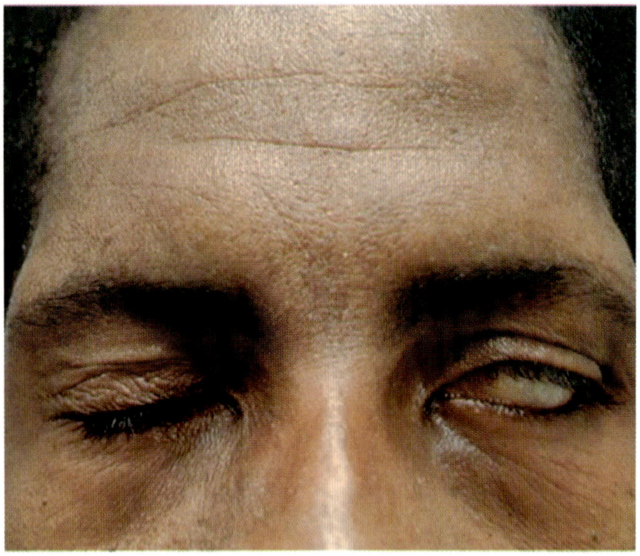

Fig. 24.1: Complete left-sided facial paralysis from a canal wall down mastoidectomy many years ago. Bell's phenomenon is present in this patient

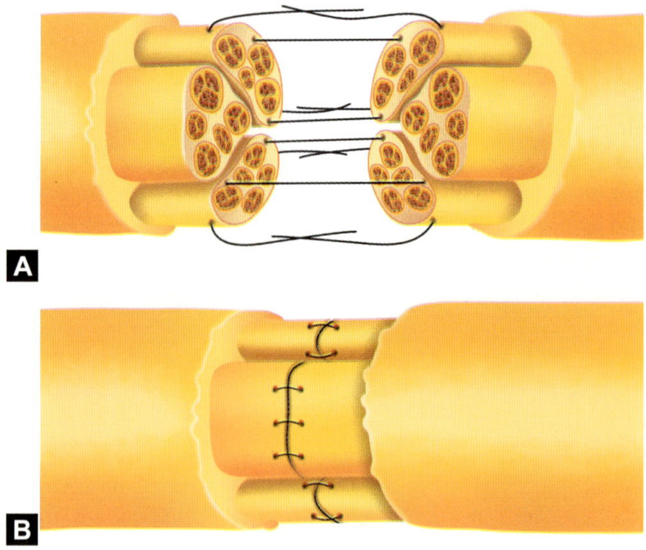

Figs 24.2A and B: Nerve preparation for end-to-end anastamosis. The diagram illustrates stripping away of epineurium to allow direct perineural anastamosis

Otologic

Obtain an audiogram, tympanometry and acoustic reflex testing. Thorough inspection of the ears for effusion, mass and vesicles is required.

PATIENT EDUCATION

Patient education is extremely important when dealing with facial paralysis. First and foremost, the patient must understand how crucial meticulous eye protection is in this situation. Referral to an ophthalmologist to rule out corneal irritation and abrasion is warranted early in the course of paralysis and ensuring corneal exposure is minimized to prevent this problem. Also, providing the patient with realistic expectations of recovery is necessary so that he or she understands the rationale for the reconstruction, and it also helps him or her to come to some degree of acceptance in cases in which complete recovery is unlikely.

RECONSTRUCTIVE CONSIDERATIONS

The role of this chapter is in managing patients who present with a facial nerve paralysis. If the nerve is iatrogenically injured, immediate tension-free neurrorhaphy (Figs 24.2A and B) is recommended. If the ends cannot be brought together in a tension-free manner, then an interposition nerve graft (e.g. auricular, sural) should be used to achieve this.

The status of the facial nerve must be considered prior to undertaking any reconstruction which may put it at risk if there is any chance for spontaneous recovery.

A thorough history is essential to determine:

- When the nerve dysfunction occurred.
- Why the paresis/paralysis occurred.
- Progession—sudden, gradual, any improvement.
- Past history—prior episodes, medical comorbidities, surgical history.
- Interventions—any medical or surgical attempts at improvement.

Attempt to acquire any operative reports if these prior operations could have put the nerve at risk. It may be helpful, particularly in a traumatic setting, to obtain records in which evaluating medical personnel may have documented the facial nerve status upon presentation. In these situations, the facial plastic surgeon is usually involved later in the course, and the patient may be sedated making an accurate nerve examination impossible, so having this information can be invaluable.

Laboratory work-up should be directed toward patient's comorbidities (e.g. diabetes) as well as suspected diagnoses such as Lyme disease. A shotgun ordering approach is rarely helpful and is not cost effective. Radiologic imaging should be treated in the same manner. Electrophysiologic work-up of the facial nerve's status is beyond the scope of this chapter, but the reader is strongly encouraged to seek out this information prior to undertaking facial nerve reconstruction in a situation where the nerve status is questionable or unknown.

STATIC RECONSTRUCTION

Lid Loading

Since protection of the eye is the most important goal in treating a patient with facial nerve paralysis, correction of corneal exposure should be considered early. Even in situations in which the nerve is expected to recover, a reversible procedure, such as gold or platinum weight implantation should be considered if the time to recovery is estimated to be prolonged.

The two most common implant materials used for lid loading are gold and platinum. Gold is generally used due to its lower cost. However, in patients with known gold sensitivity, platinum should be used. Also, due to the higher density of platinum, the implants are smaller which makes them less conspicuous.

By placing a weight in the upper eyelid, the eyelid is able to passively close with the aid of gravity. The patient must be made aware that when lying supine, due to the inherent convexity of the globe, the eyelid may be pulled more open as the weight will shift superiorly. Elevating the head of bed should correct this. The proper weight must be selected. One which is too light will insufficiently close the aperture while one which is too heavy will cause ptosis when the eye is open and may also be felt on the globe. It is recommended that a sizing kit be used preoperatively. These alternative sizes allow the patient to tape sequential weights to the eyelid to find the optimal amount to achieve closure while minimizing the aforementioned problems. Figure 24.3 demonstrates a small amount of visibility in bright light in a thin-skinned individual with the eyes closed.

Risks are minimal but include hematoma, infection, extrusion, allergic reaction, visibility, palpability, corneal abrasion and ptosis.

Benefits include good cosmesis, low risk, reliability and reversibility.

Steps in gold or platinum weight implantation (Figs 24.4A to D) are as follows:

1. Select the proper weight, typically around 1.0 gm. Maintain sterility throughout the case. Do not open or touch the weight until it is ready to be placed.
2. Using a fine-tipped marking pen, plan the incision in the upper eyelid in the tarsal-supratarsal crease (Fig. 24.4A). The weight should be centered over the medial one-third of the eye for maximal benefit.
3. Prepare the eye by placing a couple drops of tetracaine for topical anesthesia.
4. Place a cornea shield.
5. Infiltrate with a small amount of local anesthesia containing epinephrine and allow time for the effect.

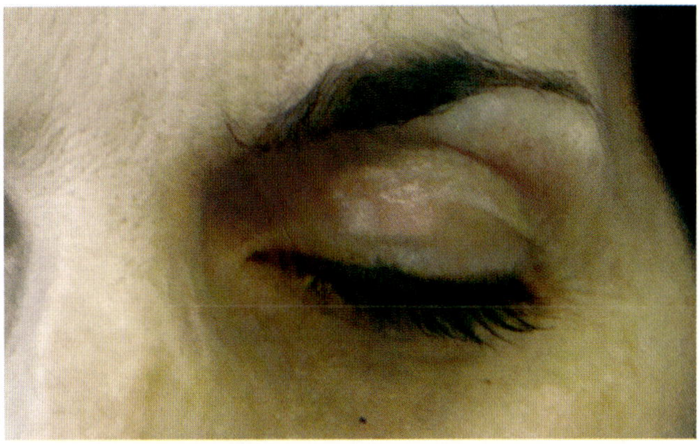

Fig. 24.3: Demonstration of visibility of gold weight implant in a thin-skinned individual

6. Prepare the skin with an antibacterial solution safe for ophthalmologic use and drape in a sterile fashion.
7. Sharply incise the skin and dissect down to the tarsal plate. The pocket created for implant should be large enough to accommodate the implant without fear of extrusion, but it should be small enough to prevent migration. Also, ensure that the superior aspect of the implant will not lie directly under the suture line. This will help to prevent extrusion.
8. Dissect to within 3 mm of the lid margin.
9. Obtain meticulous hemostasis.
10. Place the implant directly in the pocket with the two holes facing upwards (Fig. 24.4B).
11. Secure the implant to the fascia over lying the tarsal plate with a nonabsorbable suture such as 7-0 or 8-0 clear Nylon through the inferior hole to the tarsal plate. Secure the superior holes to the orbital septum.
12. Irrigate the wound and ensure hemostasis.
13. Layered closure is recommended followed by an ophthalmic ointment over the incision.
14. Remove the corneal shield and examine the eye for any injury. If the patient is verbal, a quick visual check can be performed.

Postoperatively, a short course of antibiotics directed toward skin flora is typically prescribed. Cool compresses, pain medication as needed and head of bed elevation is recommended. Avoidance of straining and exertion for at least 1 week is advisable and make sure the patient calls with any untoward swelling, bleeding, increasing pain, or visual disturbance.

Tarsorrhaphy

The indications for performing a tarsorrhaphy are the same as those for a lid loading procedure. A tarsorrhaphy is a reversible procedure which aids in eye closure

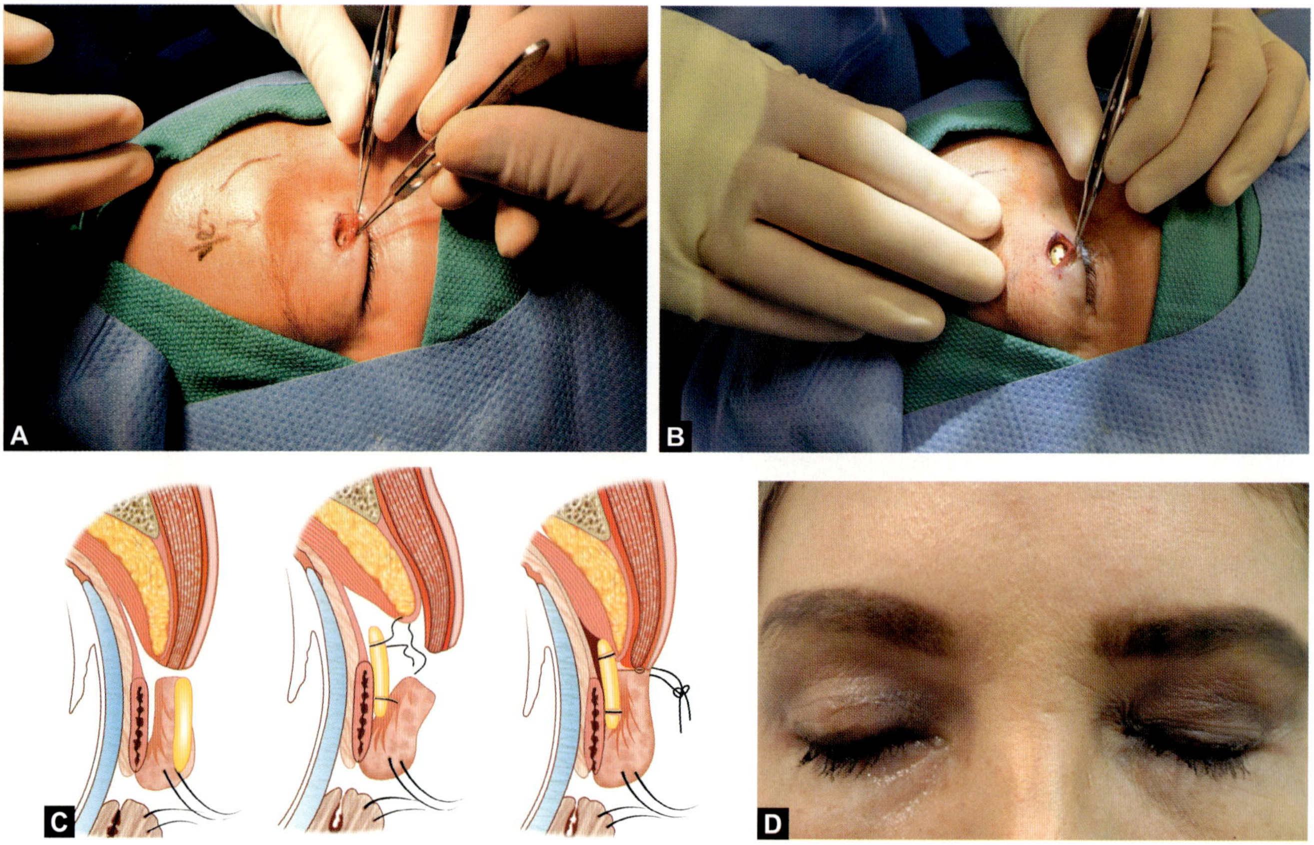

Figs 24.4A to D: (A) Creation of a pocket for gold weight implantation superficial to the tarsal plate; (B) Securing the gold weight implant. The two holes are superiorly placed; (C) Sagittal diagram of gold weight insertion; (D) Six-week follow-up with complete right eye closure with no effort and a good aesthetic result

whereby the eyelids are partially sewn together thus narrowing the palpebral fissure. Due to the inherent nature of the procedure, the degree of eyelid distortion is a deterrent for many surgeons. Additionally, if facial nerve function recovers, reversing the procedure may still leave the patient with a persistent eyelid deformity. For these reasons, the author does not use this technique and favors the lid-loading procedures instead.

Risks are minimal but include aesthetic deformity (inevitable), unsatisfactory results with reversing the procedure and rare infection.

Benefits

- Avoids potential ptosis with lid loading.
- Reversible.

Lifts

Lifting procedures such as a brow lift or a rhytidectomy can be useful adjuncts in the management of facial paralysis. These static procedures place minimal risk to injuring individual facial nerve branches while yielding an immediate benefit in appearance. They can be performed even while awaiting an expected return of facial nerve function.

Nasal Obstruction

Patients with facial paralysis often suffer from ipsilateral nasal obstruction. This results from a loss of the nasal elevator muscles which lead to slight nostril dilation and a lift of the upper lateral cartilage. When this is lost, the patient suffers from partial collapse of the internal nasal valve. In short, the patient with nasal obstruction from facial paralysis should be thoroughly questioned regarding his or her nasal history, and the work-up and approach for functional rhinoplasty is undertaken in a similar fashion as a patient without facial paralysis.

Temporalis Sling

The temporalis sling is a method by which a segment of the temporalis muscle with its fascial attachments

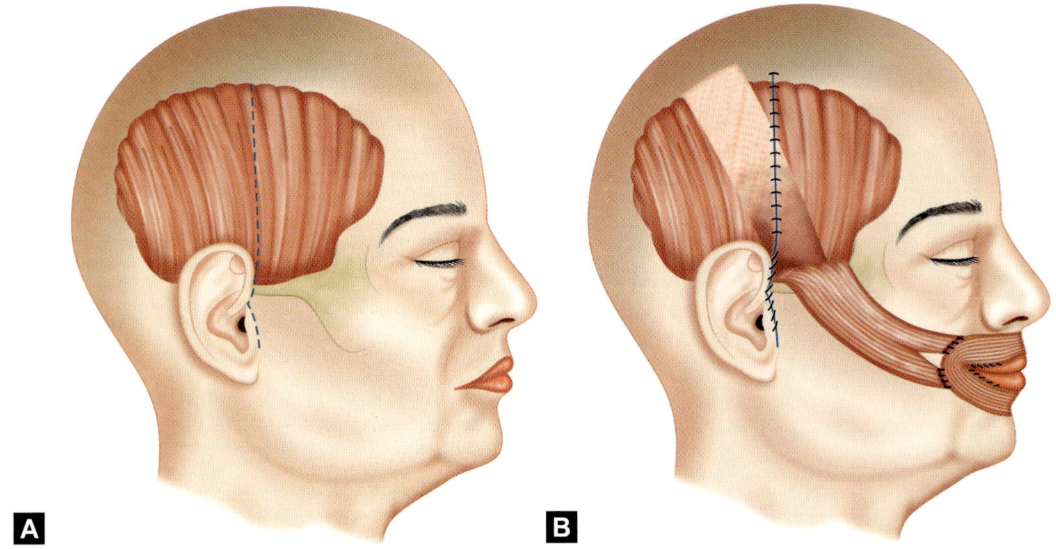

Figs 24.5A and B: The use of the temporalis muscle to lift the lower face

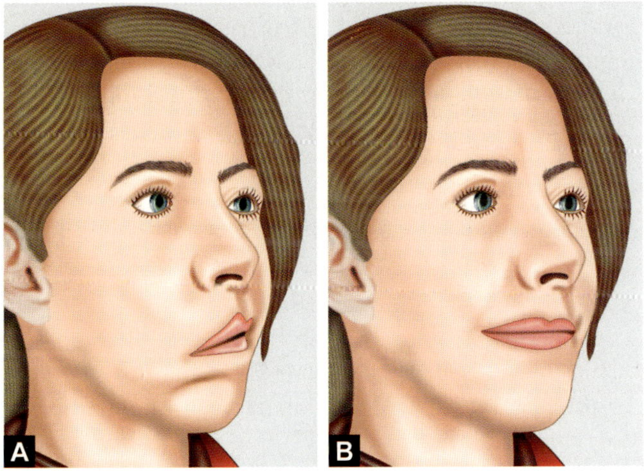

Figs 24.6A and B: Overcorrection of the lower one-third of the face is necessary with the temporalis muscle sling

is rotated and sewn to the obicuarlis oris muscle, and along the lips, to improve the lower one-third of the face. The superolateral vector of pull yields a favorable result for this region. However, results in the upper portion of the face have been less successful, and therefore it is generally reserved for the lower one-third of the face while reserving other procedures, such as lid-loading, for the upper face.

Risks include aesthetic deformity, hematoma, infection, loss of lift with time, dehiscence, scarring and alopecia.

Benefits

- Immediate benefit to the patient.
- Reliability.
- Can be used with nerve repair techniques.

Figures 24.5A and B demonstrate the concept behind the temporalis sling, Figures 24.6A and B show the results of a successful transfer.

Steps in temporalis muscle transfer are as follows:

1. Demarcate a preauricular incision and take it into temporal region as is done in a cheek and lateral brow lift.
2. Part the hair on each side of the incision and place in rubber bands. Shaving the hair is not necessary.
3. Mark the nasolabial fold and along the superior and inferior lateral vermillion borders of the ispsilateral side by having the patient smile to gauge symmetrical recreation of the nasolabial fold.
4. Administer preoperative antibiotics while the patient is undergoing general anesthesia.
5. Infiltrate these areas with local anesthesia containing epinephrine and while allowing time for the vasoconstrictive effect; prepare the face with an antiseptic solution such as an iodine- or chlorhexidine-based agent.
6. Make the temporal incision and take care not to injure the temporal artery or vein. Do not perform excessive cauterization as this may lead to alopecia. If bleeding occurs, try injecting more local anesthetic first or consider the use of Raney clips or suture.
7. Dissect to the loose aerolar tissue and locate the superficial layer of the temporalis fascia.
8. Create a tunnel between the superficial musculoaponeurotic system (SMAS) and the subcutaneous tissue to the nasolabial fold.
9. Incise at the nasolabial fold, dissect superolaterally and connect the tunnels.

10. Create a plane over the temporalis muscle and delineate the middle one-third of the muscle (~ 4 cm).
11. Sharply incise these borders and continue to dissect past the end of the muscle as some of the periosteum can be used for additional length.
12. Divide the muscle belly in two equal segments.
13. Use a 2-0 or 3-0 nonabsorbable suture through each end of the muscle bellies to pass through the tunnels.
14. The temporalis can be sewn with nonabsorbable sutures to the orbicularis at the melolabial fold with intentional overcorrection. A deliberate sneering appearance should be created as it will relax with time.
15. Additionally, the muscle (or periosteum) can be sewn more medially for additional support.
16. The vermillion incisions can be made and pockets created to the melolabial folds allowing for the muscle to be brought more medially and sewn to the lip in patients without a well-defined nasolabial fold.
17. Once overcorrection is achieved, the wounds can be closed in a standard fashion.
18. The remaining temporalis muscle can be sutured together to reduce the chance of a concavity as described by Cheney.[1]

The patient should expect a palpable bulge of the temporalis muscle over the zygomatic arch which will improve with time. Some patients are able to learn to bite down at the time during which they wish to smile which can allow for some dynamic rehabilitation with this technique.

DYNAMIC RECONSTRUCTION

The following are examples of procedures that are intended to help reanimate the face. They are useful procedures when the patient's distal nerve status is known to be intact, but the proximal segment is jeopardized (e.g. brainstem surgery). These procedures should not be used if there is a chance for spontaneous neural regeneration as these procedures inherently sacrifice the status of the nerve distally.

When dealing with facial nerve reinnervation, either spontaneous or through one of the reanimation procedures, an inherent risk of synkinesis is present. Simply put, synkinesis is the condition which results when the neural impulse is transmitted to several facial regions rather than just one. This mass movement of the face is aesthetically displeasing and functionally inefficient.

At their best, these procedures allow for volitional facial movement which is the goal of every patient with complete facial nerve paralysis. At their worst, the procedures fail to achieve successful reanimation, and in between, there may be enough innervations to help prevent muscle atrophy. Therefore, expectations must be managed, and the patient must understand that achieving complete reanimation is not yet possible.

XII-VII Graft

In a situation in which the contralateral hypoglossal nerve is at risk for future injury (e.g. surgical sacrifice) or involvement secondary to a neurologic process or disease (neural tumors, invasive malignancy), this procedure should not be performed. Bilateral hypoglossal nerve injury is devastating for a patient and will leave the patient with a severe oral disability. The patient must clearly understand that the XII-VII graft does not yield an immediate improvement. It may take up for a year for improvement to be observed.

Risks include dysarthria, dysphagia, failure to obtain reinnervation, synkinesis, scar, hematoma and infection.

Benefits include potential for reinnervation and low morbidity in healthy individuals.

The steps below are for a complete transection and sacrifice of cranial nerve (CN) XII. The use of jump grafts and splitting CN XII could be considered but are generally not the favored choice in this situation.

Steps in XII-VII grafting are as follows:

1. A standard parotidectomy incision is marked and infiltrated with local anesthesia. While taking effect, the face is prepared with an antiseptic solution.
2. Take a superficial parotidectomy approach and locate the pes anserinus.
3. Dissect proximally and distally for a short distance to ensure that closure will be tension free.
4. Follow the posterior belly of the digastric muscle anteriorly toward the digastric tendon. Retract this superiorly, and the CN XII should be just deep to this travelling toward the intrinsic tongue musculature. If unsure, and the patient is not paralyzed, stimulation with around 0.5 mA will result in obvious tongue movement.
5. Sever the nerves. Do not crush them while doing this. Use a cutting block and a new knife blade or fine serrated scissors.
6. Prepare the ends of the nerves for suturing as shown in Figures 24.2A and B.
7. Fine monofilament suture such as 8-0 nylon can be used. Ensure tension-free repair.

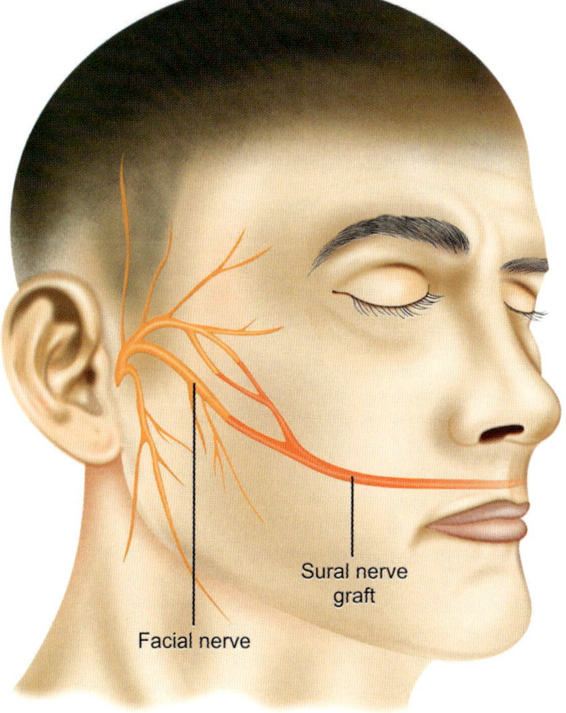

Fig. 24.7: Concept of cross-facial nerve grafting

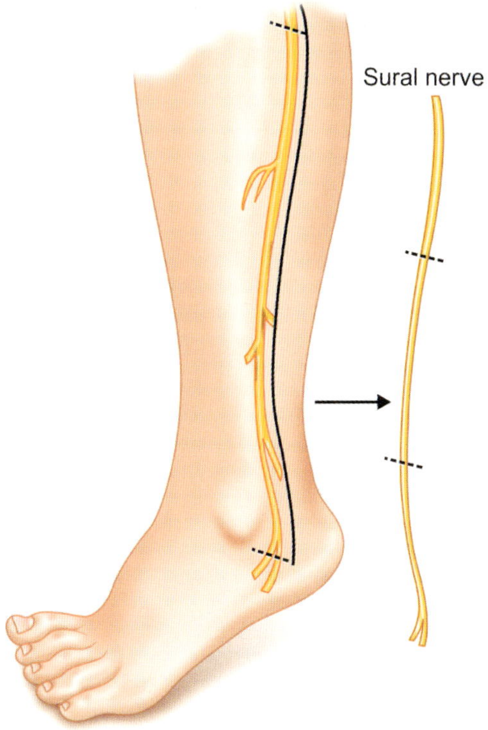

Fig. 24.8: Sural nerve harvest. Stair-step incisions can be made to harvest the nerve as well as the use of a nerve stripper to decrease the risk to adjacent structures

8. A Penrose drain can be brought out of the wound and the wound is closed in a layered fashion.

Cross-Facial Graft

As with the XII-VII graft, the patient must be willing to allow time for reinnervation to occur. As demonstrated in Figure 24.7, this surgery relies on an intact contralateral facial nerve, and through the use of an interposition nerve graft, the contralateral VII supplies the neural input for the paralyzed side. If successful, the cross-facial graft allows both sides of the face to move in sync with each other during volitional movement, thereby creating a desirable aesthetic. However, this invariably requires sacrifice of some of the contralateral (intact) CN VII. Logically, the more proximal the sacrifice, the larger the nerve with better potential for reinnervation, but this comes with the cost of increasing donor side morbidity. Additionally, the length of the interposition graft mandates a great deal of time for neural regeneration and innervations.

Risks include failure to obtain reinnervation, time for reinnervation, synkinesis, jeopardizing the contralateral CN VII, hematoma, synkinesis, infection and scar.

Benefits include potential for reinnervation and low morbidity in healthy individuals.

Steps in sural nerve graft harvest (Fig. 24.8) are as follows:

1. Consent the patient and explain the loss of sensation over the lateral aspect of the dorsum of the foot.
2. Mark the proposed incisions and infiltrate small amounts of local anesthetic with epinephrine.
3. Incise behind the lateral malleolus and locate the sural nerve.
4. Sharply transect the nerve and place a nerve stripper over the free end.
5. Use the nerve stripper to dissect off surrounding tissues while avoiding injury to adjacent structures.
6. Make the proposed incision on the calf for the necessary length of harvested nerve. Take more nerve than is deemed absolutely necessary to allow for a tension-free repair and some loss of length with preparing the ends of the nerve.
7. Use a suture to tag the distal end of the nerve for orientation purposes as this will be the end which is sutured to the paralyzed side.
8. Close the incisions in the leg and place a gentle compressive dressing.

Steps in cross-facial nerve grafting are as follows:

1. Determine the branches of the paralyzed side to be reinnervated and determine which branch(es) will be sacrificed on the donor side.
2. Expose the paralyzed side through a standard parotidectomy approach and dissect the branches to be repaired.
3. The sural nerve can be harvested simultaneously if the appropriate assistants are available.
4. Expose the donor side in a similar fashion.
5. Create a subcutaneous tunnel between the sites to undergo anastamosis. Typically this is around the lips so as to innervate the buccal region.
6. Maintain the known direction of the sural nerve.
7. Tunnel the sural nerve as atraumatically as possible (avoid stretching) through the plane. Ensure that the distal end of the sural nerve is going to the affected side of the face. This is the tagged end of the sural nerve from the harvest.
8. Through the neurrorhaphy techniques described earlier, prepare each of the facial nerves and each end of the sural nerve for suturing.
9. Anastamose the proximal end of the sural nerve to the donor side and the distal end to the paralyzed side.
10. Standard wound closure and drains as appropriate can be used.

REFERENCE

1. Cheney ML, McKenna MJ, Megerian CA, et al. Early temporalis muscle transposition for the management of facial paralysis. Laryngoscope. 1995;105(9):993-1000.

BIBLIOGRAPHY

1. May M, Schaitkin BM. Facial Paralysis: Rehabilitation Techniques. New York: Thieme; 2003.

CHAPTER 25

Microtia Reconstruction

Anthony P Sclafani

OVERVIEW

Congenital auricular deformities describe a wide range of anomalous auricular forms, from prominent to completely absent ears. These deformities may be associated with other congenital syndromes, but most often are found in isolation. Microtia is the presence of a malformed or underformed auricle, ranging from mild to severe forms. Microtia has a reported incidence in the United States of 1 in every 7000–8000 live births. Ethnic and national differences in incidence have also been described, with Hispanics, Asians and Navajo Indians more commonly affected in the U.S.; there and there is a high incidence of microtia in both Finland and Equador. Microtia is more common in boys (60–70%) than in girls; more microtias are noted on the right side (60%) than the left (30%), while approximately 10% are bilateral. Microtia can range in severity from grade I (small but relatively normally shaped ear), through grade II (abnormally sized and formed auricle with some recognizable components of the auricle) to grade III microtia (malformed remnants of skin and cartilage). Grade III microtia (Figs 25.1A to F) can be subdivided into lobule remnant (skin or skin and malformed cartilage is present which approximates a malpositioned earlobe) and conchal remnant (approximates a portion of the conchal bowl and earlobe). Anotia refers to the complete absence of and auricular structures.

SPECIAL CONSIDERATIONS

Microtia is very frequently associated with aural atresia and its associated maximal conductive (60 dB) hearing loss, although the affected individuals rarely suffer from auditory deprivation as hearing in the contralateral ear is usually normal. In school, the child should receive preferential classroom seating. In cases of bilateral microtia/atresia, auditory rehabilitation with bone anchored hearing aids is essential to allow for appropriate auditory cortical development and to facilitate normal speech development. Standard surgical management of microtia typically uses autologous costal cartilage, so the time of surgery must balance the desire of the patient and parents for early correction and the requirement for significant amounts of cartilage. Surgery is generally performed not earlier than 6–7 years of age, with some surgeons arguing that thicker and broader cartilage can be harvested if surgery is delayed until adolescence.

ALTERNATIVES TO PROCEDURE

Rather than surgically constructing an ear, a prosthesis can be created which in skilled hands can mirror the normal ear quite closely. This can be affixed to the scalp with adhesive or with osseointegrated pins. Some surgeons have described the use of alloplastic implants as an auricular framework, covered by a temporoparietal fascia flap and a split thickness skin graft. While some results have been stunning, reports of early and late implant exposure have limited the adoption of this technique.

TECHNIQUES

Most surgeons performing surgical treatment of microtia generally follow the techniques described by Tenzer and Brent, in which autologous costal cartilage is used to create a framework, which is later elevated from the temple to project laterally after it has been joined with the transposed lobule remnant. There are three basic stages to this procedure, although some stages may be combined while other ancillary procedures may be performed to maximally improve the appearance of the auricle.

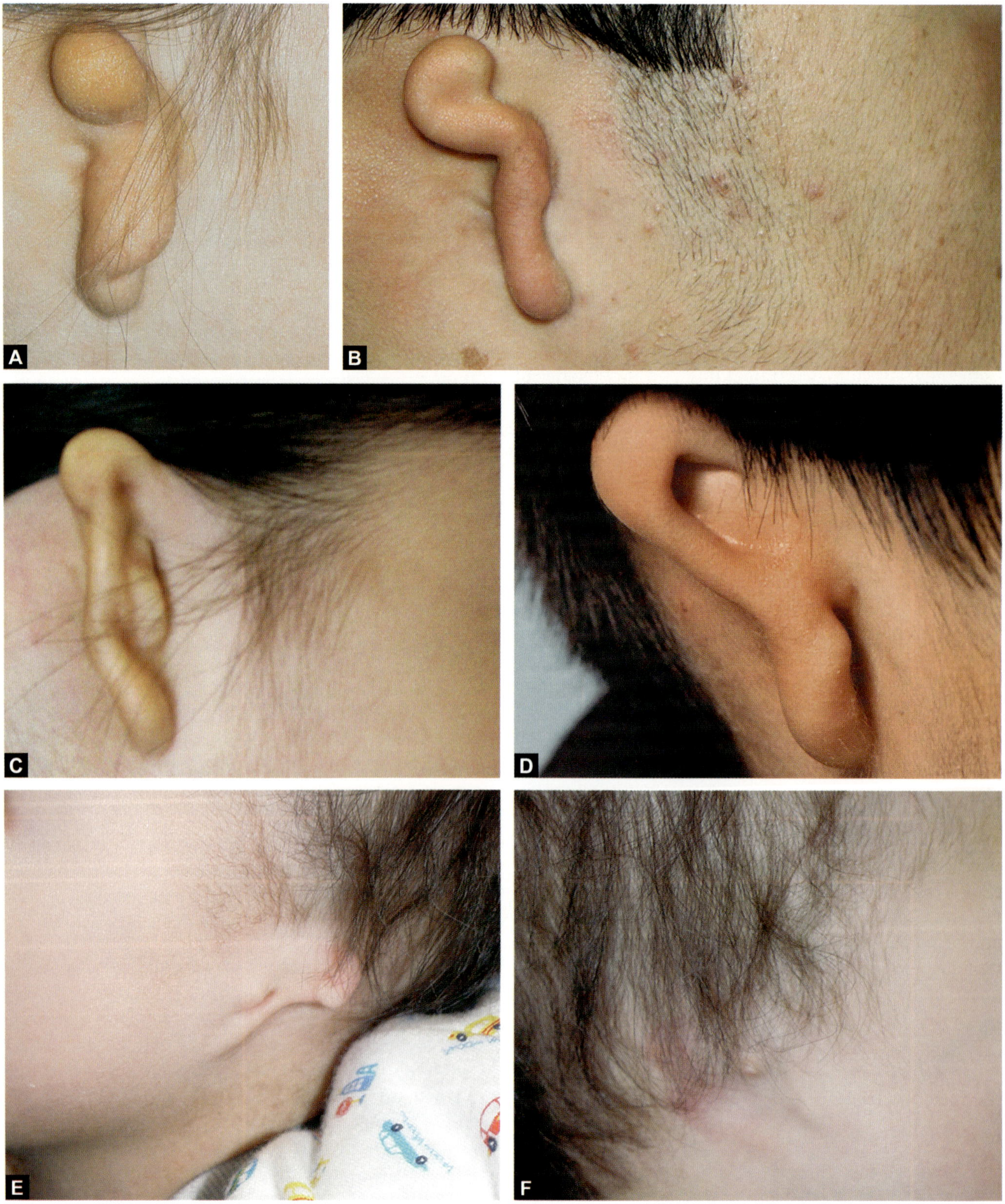

Figs 25.1A to F: Various forms of grade 3 microtia. (A) Classic grade 3 microtia with fleshy vertical lobule inferiorly and small nodular cartilaginous mass superiorly; (B) More formed cartilaginous portion superiorly; (C and D) Conchal remnant microtia shows varying degrees of a blind pouch in place of the conchal bowl; (E and F) Anotia has minimal to no markings or ear development

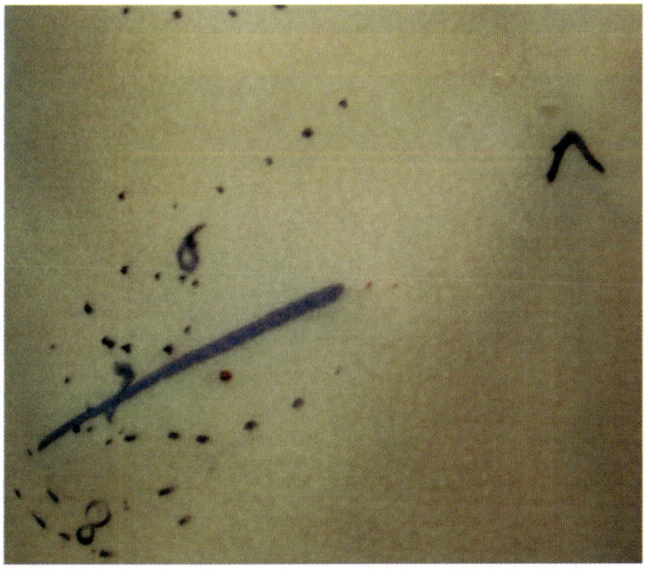

Fig. 25.2: Autologous rib cartilage may be harvested through an oblique incision two fingerbreadths above the costal margin

Stage 1

Reconstruction with autologous rib requires a staged approach. Surgery is generally begun after the patient is 6–7 years of age, so that adequate costal cartilage is available. A piece of clear X-ray film is placed over the normal ear and the outline of the auricular structure is traced. The position and orientation of the normal ear relative to the temporomandibular joint, lateral canthus and superior orbital rim are also drawn. Small perforations are made in the X-ray film with a needle along each of these marks, preserving these markings even after the template has been sterilized.

Incision Placement

A 7–8 cm incision is made across the lower ribs approximately two fingerbreadths above the contralateral costal margin (Fig. 25.2).

Extent of Undermining/Dissection

The inferior oblique and rectus abdominis muscles are transected. The perichondrium over the seventh rib is incised and elevated, and this plane is followed medially until the synchondrosis of the sixth and seventh ribs is exposed; this will form the core of the auricular framework. The eighth rib is identified and similarly exposed, and will be used to create the helix (Fig. 25.3).

Using the template made from the normal ear, an appropriate section of the seventh rib and its synchondrosis with the sixth rib is selected for en bloc

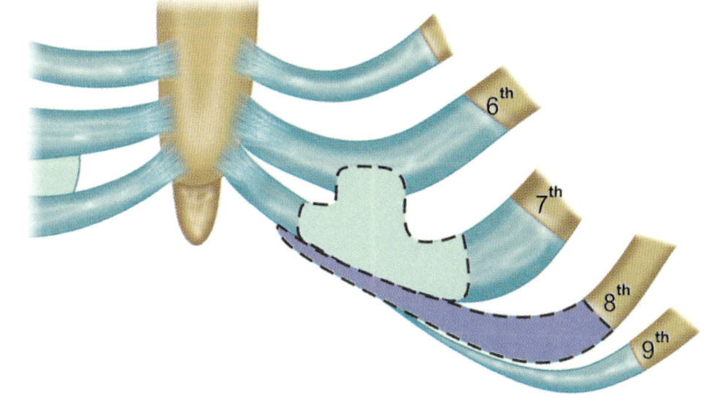

Fig. 25.3: Portions of the sixth and seventh rib are harvested and used to create the central portion of the framework; a segment of the eighth rib at least 8 cm in length is necessary to create an adequate helix

harvest. The superficial perichondrium is incised and then elevated to the upper and lower borders of the rib with a Freer elevator. The dissection is carefully continued around the rib to elevate the deep perichondrium for protection. Once the deep perichondrium has been fully elevated, the cartilage block is harvested by cutting through the cartilage with a #57 blade while the Freer elevator is positioned between the cartilage and deep perichondrium for protection. An 8–9 cm segment of cartilage from the eighth rib is similarly harvested; it is often easier to proceed medially to laterally, as the tip of the eighth rib is easily accessible after the seventh rib has been removed. Occasionally, the osseocartilaginous junction is fairly medial and limits the amount of available cartilage.

Elevation of the perichondrium is fairly simple on the anterior surface, but particular care should be taken to remain in between the cartilage and perichondrium when working on the posterior surface. Once the cartilage has been removed, the integrity of the posterior perichondrium and parietal pleura should be confirmed by filling the wound with warm saline and having the anesthesiologist perform a Valsalva maneuver. The presence of air bubbles indicates a pleural air leak; if present, the pleural violation should be identified and suction is applied via a soft red rubber catheter inserted into the pleural space. A chromic suture is placed as a purse-string around the tear; as the suture is tied, the catheter should be withdrawn.

Tissue Modifications

Excision

A pocket must be created to accommodate the cartilage framework to be created from the costal cartilage. The appropriate area of skin is outlined, mirroring the size,

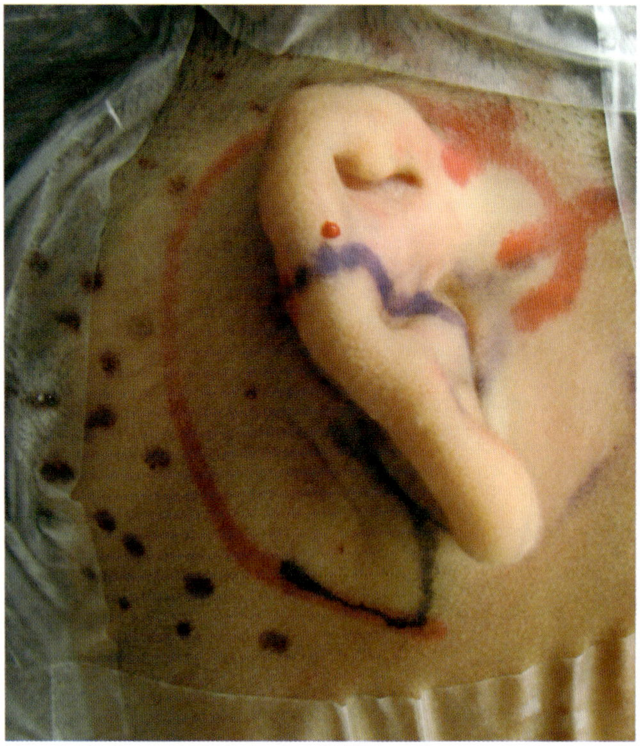

Fig. 25.4: Markings for stage 1 of the microtia repair. Red outlines the desired location of the helical edge of the framework, while the red cross-hatches indicated the orientation of the inferior and superior crura. Brown stippling indicates the area of subcutaneous dissection. The blue markings indicate the incisions necessary to transpose the lobule posteriorly

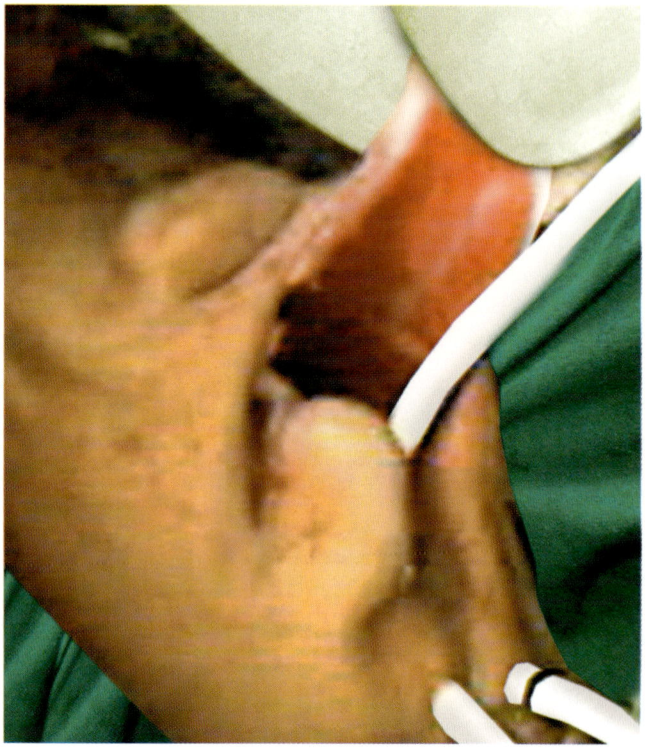

Fig. 25.5: To maximize postoperative auricular definition, it is essential to elevate skin flaps in the immediate subdermal plane

height, distance from the lateral canthus and angulation of the normal ear. Additional undermining should be performed to allow the skin to drape over the framework without tension (Fig. 25.4). The microtia remnant present typically includes a mostly fibrofatty skin appendage inferiorly, and a skin covered malformed cartilage portion superiorly. This cartilage generally cannot be incorporated into the constructed auricle and is generally removed through an anterior incision. Through this incision, a thin skin flap is raised just below the dermis to create a recipient pocket (Fig. 25.5).

Suturing

The harvested cartilage pieces are carved and sutured with 5-0 clear nylon sutures to form the auricular framework. Ideally, the synchondrosis between the sixth and seventh ribs forms the superior and inferior crura, fossa triangularis and superior part of the scaphoid fossa; the remainder of the scaphoid fossa, common antihelical crus, conchal bowl, antitragus and inferior auricle are formed with the bulk of the seventh rib. This piece is also left a bit long, with the extension ultimately being tucked into the midportion of the transposed earlobe (Fig. 25.6). Using the template, the cartilage block is carefully shaved to exaggerate the natural folds of the ear. The eighth rib is split longitudinally to produce a thin segment to form the helical rim. This portion is bent and sutured to this inner base framework to form the helix, resting atop the "shelf" created beyond the antihelix (Fig. 25.7). The remaining pieces are carved and used to increase the relief of the antihelix by splitting one end and suturing it over the common, inferior and superior crura. Another piece is sutured inferior to the lobule segment and curled anteriorly to be sutured at the helical root to provide bulk for the tragus. An additional piece should be sutured on the undersurface of the conchal bowl to add additional framework height to this area (Fig. 25.8). Remaining cartilage is then "banked" subcutaneously in the temporal region at least 2–3 cm superior to the helical position and retrieved for use to provide additional auricular lateralization in the stage 3 (elevation) procedure; if only small pieces remain, they can be included with the

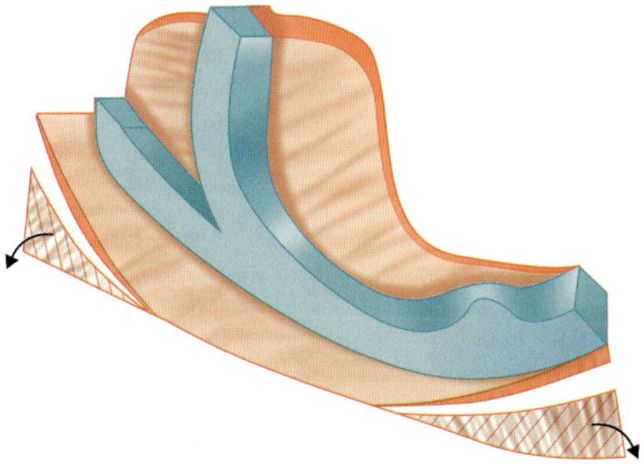

Fig. 25.6: The block of cartilage harvested from the sixth and seventh ribs is carved to form the scaphoid fossa, antihelic, fossa triangularis, antitragus and conchal bowl floor

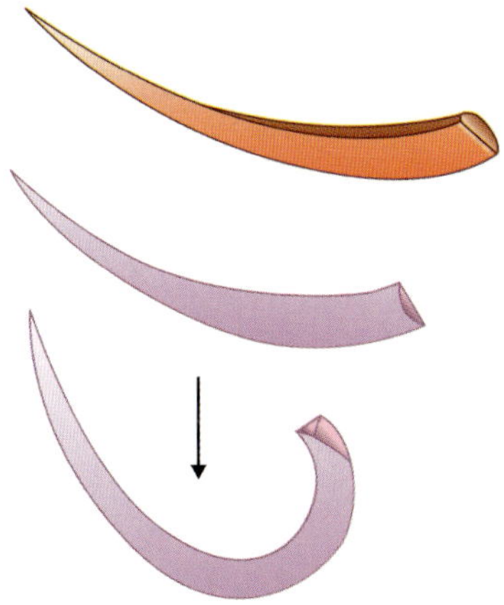

Fig. 25.7: The eighth rib is split longitudinally to allow greater flexibility to wrap around the base

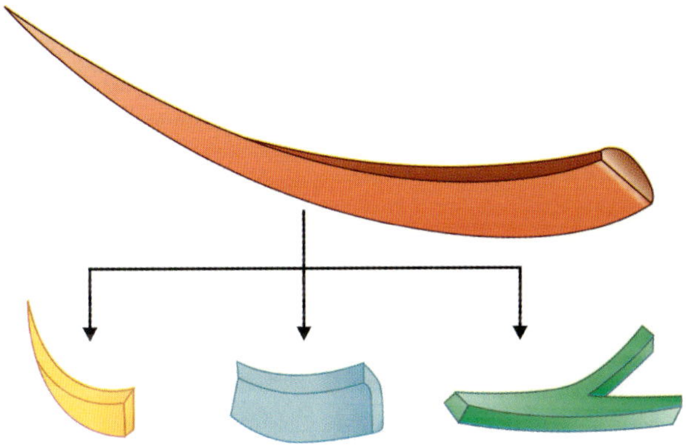

Fig. 25.8: Remaining portions of the eighth rib are carved to enhance the relief of the antihelix, form the tragus and to increase the height of the conchal bowl

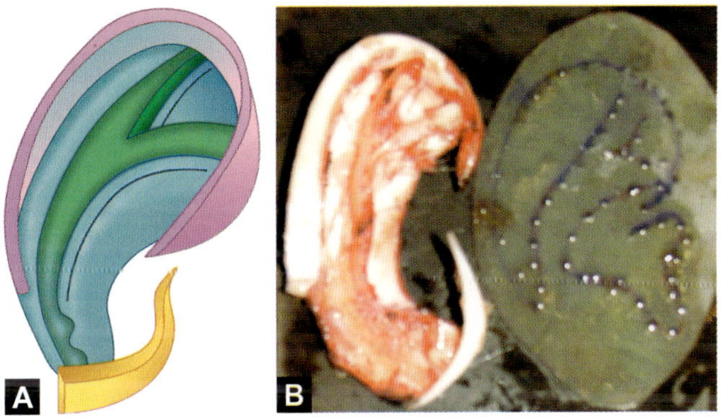

Figs 25.9A and B: The final framework is a high relief outline of the desired auricular features

deformed native ear cartilage and wrapped in Surgicel (Ethicon, Inc., Cincinnati, OH) before banking in temple. The completed framework is kept in saline until it can be placed in the temporal pocket (Figs 25.9A and B).

Closure

Chest Closure

- *Layers/sutures*: Transected rectus abdominis and oblique muscles are then reapproximated with 3-0 Vicryl sutures, and the skin is closed with 3-0 Monocryl sutures for dermal closure and running 5-0 Monocryl sutures subcuticularly.
- *Drains*: A 7mm Jackson-Pratt (JP) drains the supra-muscular space and is brought out of the skin through a separate stab incision.
- *Dressings*: A simple dressing of adhesive skin strips and an acrylic dressing (Steri-Strips and Tegaderm, respectively, 3M Corp., St. Paul, MN).

Auricular Closure

- *Layers/sutures*: Next, the template is again used to confirm the correct positioning of the framework. Skin incisions are closed with 3-0 Monocryl sutures at a dermal level to set the skin closure and to establish an airtight closure, and completed with a running 5-0 Monocryl suture for cutaneous closure.
- *Excision*: The cartilage from the superior portion of the auricular remnant having been removed, excess skin exists and typically covers a portion of the fossa triangularis. With drains placed on suction, some of this redundant skin fills in some of the desired concavities, but if excess skin is apparent, it is resected and closed as above.
- *Drains*: Prior to wound closure, two 4 mm drains (TLS Evacuated tube drainage system, Stryker Corp., Kalamazoo, Michigan, US) are placed to drain the conchal bowl and the scaphoid fossa, respectively.

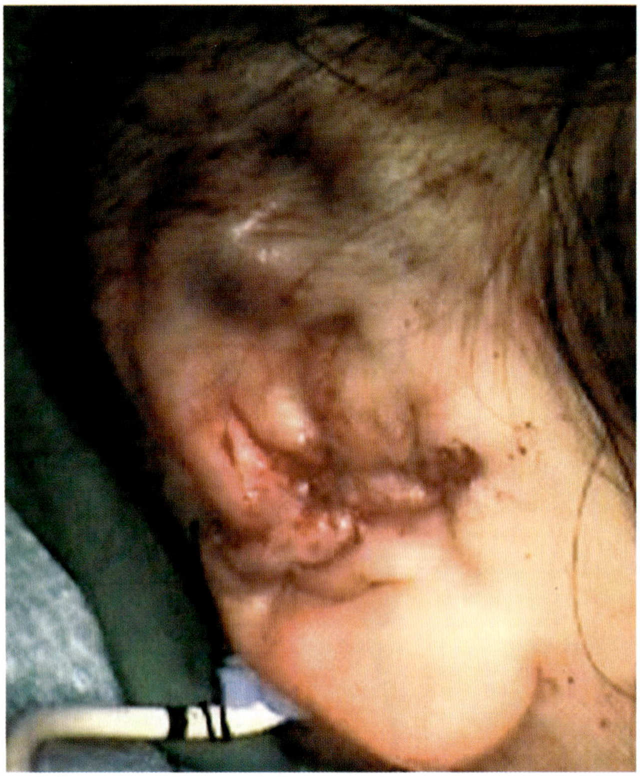

Fig. 25.10: After the framework is placed, skin closed and drains placed on suction, the shape of the auricle becomes apparent

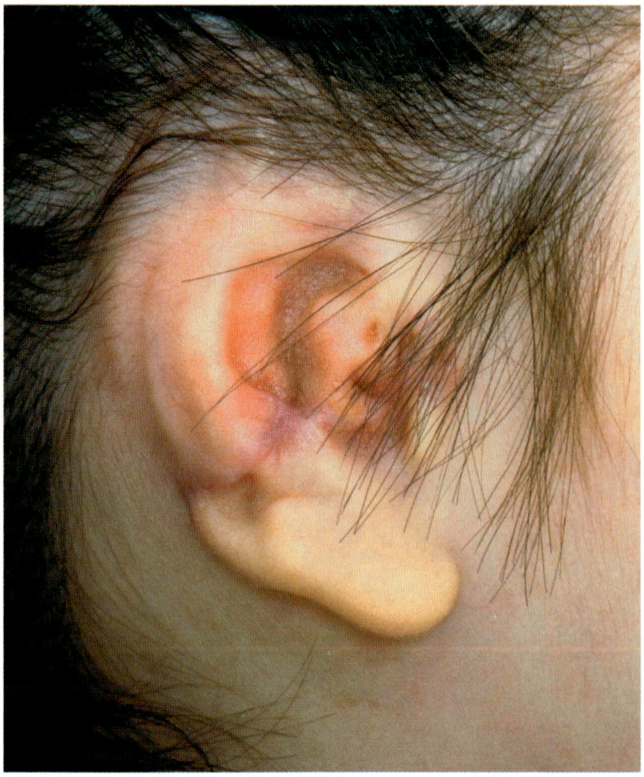

Fig. 25.11: Reconstructed ear 10 weeks after framework construction and placement with lobule transposition

Once placed on suction, the outline of the framework can be seen (Fig. 25.10), checked for proper placement and the framework adjusted as needed.

- *Dressing*: Sterile cotton soaked in mineral oil is then layered and compressed into the desired concavities of the constructed auricle. This is then covered with dry gauze and a mildly compressive preformed dressing (Glasscock dressing, OTOMED, Lake Havasu City, Arizona, US) is applied.

Stage 2

At least 6–12 weeks after the first stage (Fig. 25.11), the earlobe is created by transposing the lobular remnant. Alternatively, this stage can be performed at the same time as the framework construction and placement by extending the incisions from stage 1 into those described below.

Incision Placement

Remnant skin and cartilage is generally located at or just anterior to the temporomandibular joint, running vertically and crossing the desired conchal bowl position. An inferiorly based, V-shaped incision is made around the microtia remnant, and then continued posteriorly to extend up to the lower part of the auricular framework (Figs 25.12A and B).

Extent of Undermining/Dissection

The lobule portion of the flap is elevated at the subcutaneous level, as is the skin triangle posterior to the lobule.

Tissue Modifications

Incision

The lobule remnant is then bivalved, creating a pocket within the substance of the lobule. The inferiormost portion of the auricular framework is also exposed.

Tissue Advancement

The lobule is transposed posteriorly, while the other skin triangle is turned anteriorly as in a standard Z-plasty. The inferior end of the cartilage framework is tucked into the pocket created in the lobule remnant.

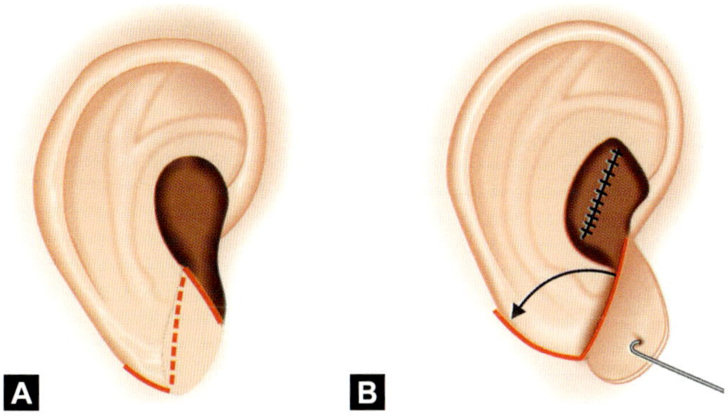

Figs 25.12A and B: Incisions for lobular transposition can be incorporated into the placement of the framework or be performed as a separate procedure. (A) Lateral view and (B) with lobule retracted. The cartilaginous portion of the microtia remnant (above) is excised

Suturing

The inferior framework is sutured to the deep tissues of the lobular pocket with 4-0 Monocryl. It is important to suture the dermis of the medial side of the lobule to the deep surface of the framework to avoid lateral protrusion of the lobule.

Closure

Layers/Sutures

Generally, the original site of the lobular remnant can be closed primarily, especially superiorly. Inferiorly, it is useful to utilize the transposed skin triangle to allow the lobule to fully rotate inferiorly and posteriorly. The skin is closed in layers, using 4-0 Monocryl sutures for dermal closure and a running 5-0 Monocryl suture for cutaneous closure.

Dressings

Triple antibiotic ointment is placed on all sutures.

Stage 3

Six to eight weeks after stage 2 (12–16 weeks after stage 1), the auricular framework and skin can be lateralized if desired, depending upon the amount of lateral projection that was obtained from the first stage.

Incision Placement

The skin approximately 5 mm beyond the helical rim framework is incised from just in front of the helical root to the postauricular sulcus medial to the lobule (Figs 25.13A and B).

Extent of Undermining/Dissection

The incision is carried down to temporalis fascia and the auricular framework is progressively elevated, leaving a generous cuff of soft tissue covering the medial aspect of the cartilage. The framework is elevated far enough anteriorly to allow the framework to be easily lateralized. Dissection is performed superiorly and the banked cartilage is retrieved. Posterior undermining is performed above the mastoid periosteum. Superior and posterior undermining is performed at least 4–6 cm from the skin incision. Inferiorly, fibers of the superior sternocleidomastoid muscle are encountered; cautery should be used to ensure appropriate hemostasis.

Tissue Modifications

Incision

The capsule which surrounded the banked cartilage restricts movement of the superior skin flap. Relaxing incisions parallel to the skin incision should be made to release this restriction and allow for the necessary skin mobilization. Similarly, the scar tissue from the stage 1 procedure posteriorly limits anterior mobilization of the skin, and relaxing incisions should be used here as well.

Tissue Advancement

The skin flaps are mobilized, advanced inward toward the postauricular sulcus and stabilized with multiple 3-0 polydiaxonone sutures from dermis to the mastoid periosteum and deep temporal fascia, so that the skin edges rest at the apex of the postauricular crease.

Excision

A full thickness skin graft the dimensions of the uncovered portion of the postauricular crease is harvested from the inguinal region centered over a line drawn from the anterior superior iliac crest and pubis (Fig. 25.14). With the skin flaps covering the medial aspect of the postauricular crease, the skin graft is used to cover only the medial surface of the elevated auricle.

Suturing

A small incision is made superiorly in the soft tissue covering the deep surface of the central portion of the framework, and a pocket is created. The banked cartilage is carved into a semilunate shape and placed into this precise pocket (Fig. 25.15). Placing this cartilage below the carved antihelix on the lateral side of the framework

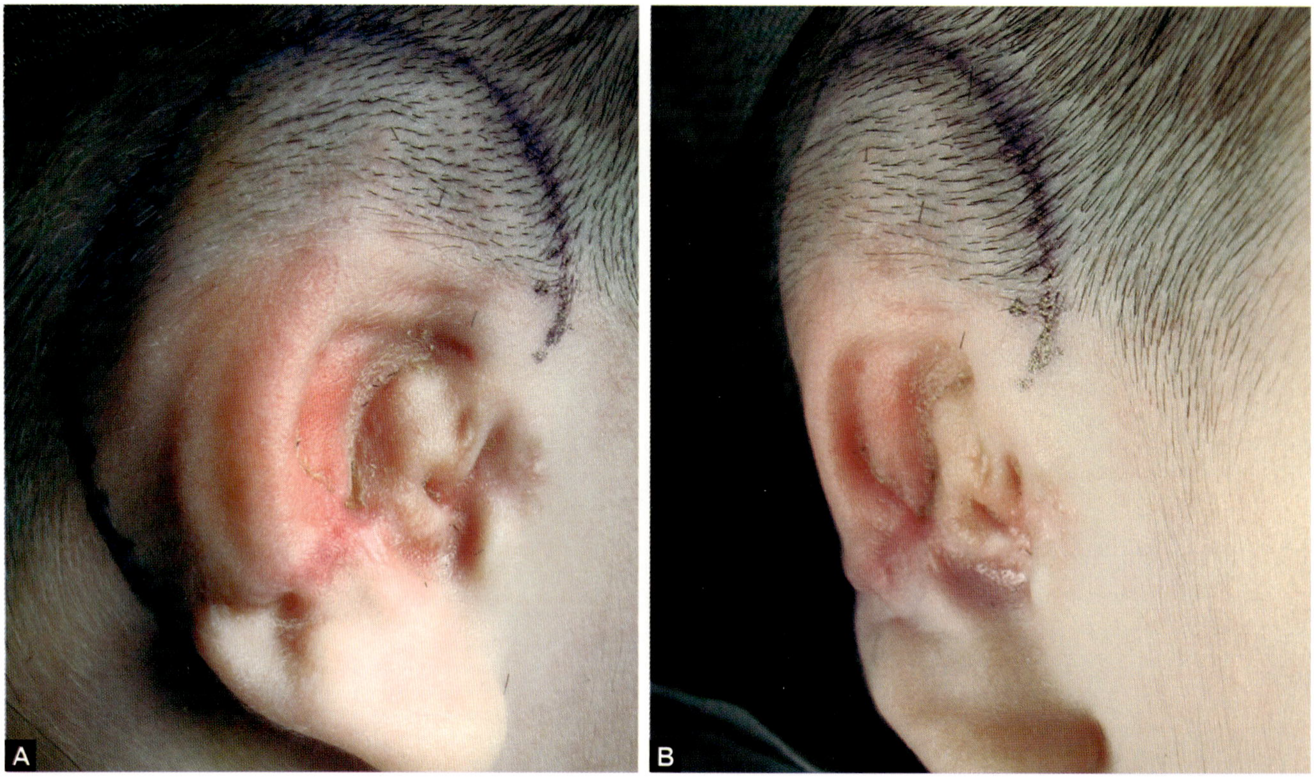

Figs 25.13A and B: Markings for framework elevation

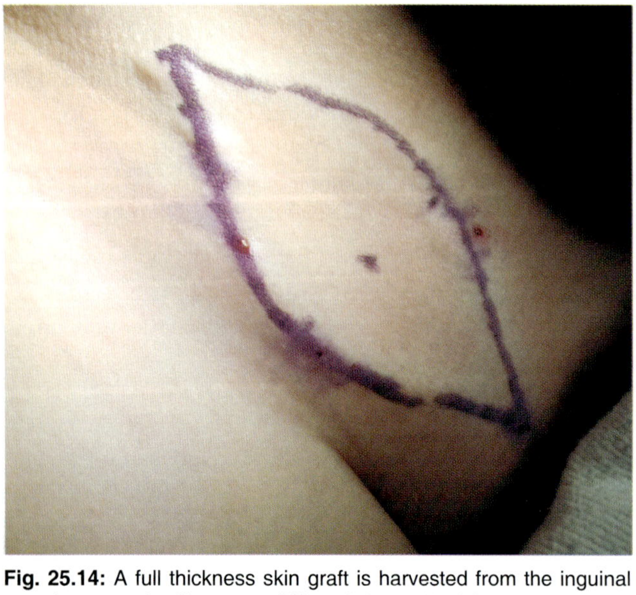

Fig. 25.14: A full thickness skin graft is harvested from the inguinal area between the iliac crest (IC) and the pubis (P)

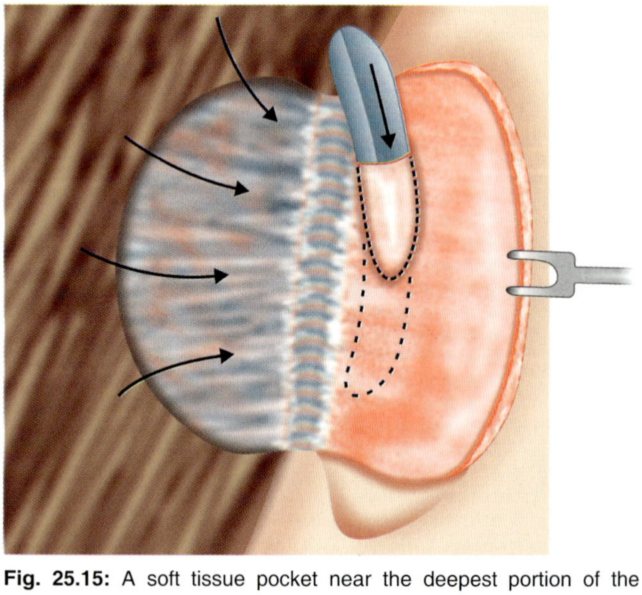

Fig. 25.15: A soft tissue pocket near the deepest portion of the postauricular crease is dissected from the framework and the banked cartilage is pocketed to increase the lateralization of the auricle

maintains the lateralized position of the auricle. The full thickness skin graft is then sutured to the skin at key points along the helical rim and at the corresponding portions of temporal skin across the postauricular sulcus with 3-0 Monocryl sutures.

Closure

Layers/Sutures

The skin graft on the medial surface of the auricle is sutured around its periphery with a running 5-0 Monocryl

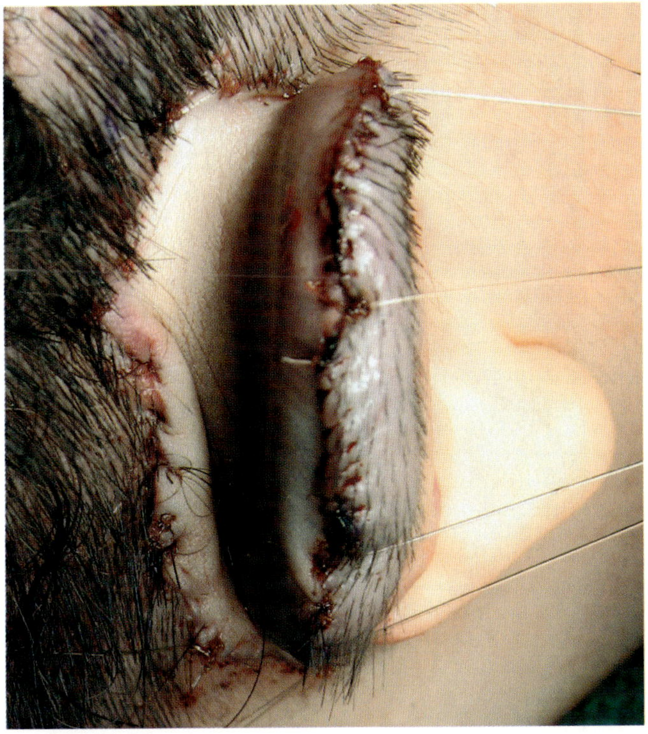

Fig. 25.16: Full thickness skin graft sutured to the back of the framework

suture in a single layer (Fig. 25.16). The inguinal donor site is closed primarily after peripheral undermining with interrupted 3-0 and running subcuticular 5-0 Monocryl sutures for dermal and cutaneous closures, respectively.

Dressings

An antibiotic/petroleum gauze bolster packed into the postauricular sulcus and is tied in place over the skin graft using the 3-0 Monocryl sutures previously placed (Figs 25.17A and B).

POTENTIAL COMPLICATIONS

The most significant potential complication from this surgery is a pneumothorax. Careful inspection as described above is essential in making this diagnosis. Should a pneumothorax be diagnosed after surgery, it can be followed radiographically for progression, and early intervention with a chest tube should be strongly considered. Postoperative pain can lead to atelectasis and pneumonia and should be appropriately managed. Excessive resection of cartilage has been associated with the development of scoliosis; maintenance of the structural integrity of the sixth rib is important. While the pocket created for the auricular framework should not be excessively large, a tight pocket or quilting sutures may lead to necrosis of the overlying skin and cartilage exposure. If the area is small, local tissue flaps should be advanced or transposed to cover the cartilage as soon as is feasible; larger areas may require salvage with a temporoparietal flap. Frank infection and chondritis will lead to rapid loss of the cartilage framework. Drains should be maintained until there is little chance of a hematoma developing. Hypertrophic or keloid scars can develop but are relatively uncommon and should be treated as in any other area.

AFTERCARE

Stage 1

A mildly compressive dressing can be changed but maintained for 3–4 days, while the drains around the framework are kept on low suction and removed when the drainage decreases to less than 5 cc per day. The JP drain in the chest is removed 1–2 days, once drainage decreases sufficiently. Chest X-rays should be performed in the recovery room as well as on the morning after surgery to evaluate not only for a pneumothorax but atelectasis and pneumonia as well. Early ambulation, with analgesics as required, will reduce the risk of postoperative pneumonia.

Stage 2

Sutures can be removed 7 days after surgery.

Stage 3

The postauricular bolster dressing is left in place for at least 7–10 days, at which time all sutures can be removed.

ANCILLARY PROCEDURES

After the first three stages, patients seeking hearing restoration can undergo aural atresia repair. At that time or at a subsequent surgery, an anteriorly based skin flap can be raised from the conchal bowl (which can then be deepened) and used to wrap around previously placed cartilage for tragus reconstruction, or simply used as the lateral tragal surface while a composite graft from the contralateral conchal bowl is used for tragal structure and medial surface coverage. Also, patients whose remnant

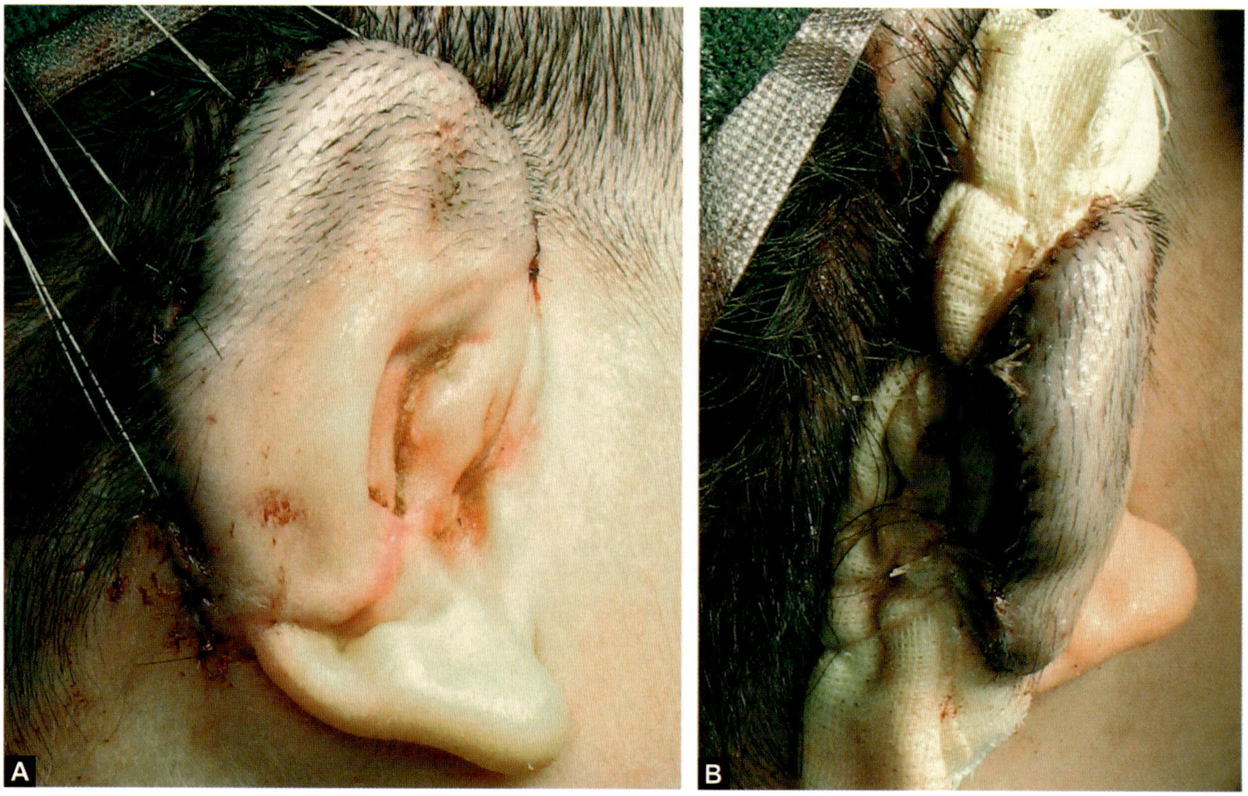

Figs 25.17A and B: A Xeroform dressing bolster is sutured in place over the skin graft

skin was based too superiorly will have an elevated earlobe after stage 2; this can be transposed to a more symmetric, lower position if needed.

BIBLIOGRAPHY

1. Brent B. Auricular repair with autogenous rib cartilage grafts: two decades of experience with 600 cases. Plast Reconstr Surg. 1992;90(3):355-74.
2. Brent B. Technical advances in ear reconstruction with autogenous rib cartilage grafts: personal experience with 1200 cases. Plast Reconstr Surg. 1999;104(2):319-34.
3. Porter CJ, Tan ST. Congenital auricular anomalies: topographic anatomy, embryology, classification, and treatment strategies. Plast Reconstr Surg. 2005;115(6): 1701-12.
4. Tanzer RC. Microtia—a long-term follow-up of 44 reconstructed auricles. Plast Reconstr Surg. 1978;61(2): 161-6.

Index

Page numbers followed by *f* refer to figure.

T

U

V

W

Z